CW00642413

A HISTORY OF IRELAND
IN TEN BODY PARTS

A
HISTORY
OF IRELAND
IN TEN BODY
PARTS

DR IAN MILLER

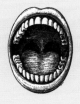

GILL BOOKS

Gill Books
Hume Avenue
Park West
Dublin 12
www.gillbooks.ie
Gill Books is an imprint of M.H. Gill and Co.
© Ian Miller 2024
978 18045 8041 7

Designed by www.grahamthew.com
Edited by Bríd Nowlan
Proofread by Ruairí Ó Brógáin
Printed and bound by FINIDR, s.r.o., Czech Republic
This book is typeset in Elena basic 10.5.

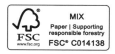

For permission to reproduce photographs, the author and publisher gratefully acknowledge the following: © Adobe Stock: 49, 75, 78, 140, 179, 222, 240; © AlamyPuripat Lertpunyaroj / Alamy Stock Photo: 51; © Album / British Library / Alamy Stock Photo: 85; © Alpha Stock / Alamy Stock Photo: 106; © Anterovium / Shutterstock: 9; © Antiqua Print Gallery / Alamy Stock Photo: 258Aren8906754 / Wikimedia: 289; © Associated Press / Alamy Stock Photo: 110, 115; © Battle of Clontarf, oil on canvas painting by Hugh Frazer, 1826 (Isaacs Art Center): 66; © Beaumain / Wikimedia Commons (CC BY-SA 2.0): 137; © Ben Arch / Alamy Stock Photo: 119; By permission of the Royal Irish Academy © RIA: 89; 'The Giant Magrath' by Pietro Longhi (Ca' Rezzonico Collection): 56; © Causeway Coast and Glens Museum: 71; © Ciaran Walsh: 30; © colaimages / Alamy Stock Photo: 144; Colin Waters / Alamy Stock Photo: 166; Courtesy of Liam Campbell: 220; © CPA Media Pte Ltd / Alamy Stock Photo: 88; CSA Images / Getty Images: 80, 81, 116, 184, 231, 270; © CSA-Archive / Getty Images: 271, 293; CSA-Printstock / Getty Images: 230, 292; © Daniel / Adobe Stock: 207; © Danvis Collection / Alamy Stock Photo: 197; © Darren / Adobe Stock: 226; David Matthew Lyons / Adobe Stock: 52; © David Matthew Lyons / Adobe Stock: 95; © Dawid / Adobe Stock: 85; © De Luan / Alamy Stock Photo: 242, 296; Dromoland Castle: 18; © duncan1890 / Getty Images: 44, 143, 209; © Eddie Kelly/ The Irish Times: 178; © Emilio Ereza / Adobe Stock: 160; © EMU history / Alamy Stock Photo: 8;[FED 90] Courtesy of Dublin City Library & Archive: 129; © fhwrdh / Flickr (CC BY 2.0): 155; © Flickr / Bord Fáilte- Irish Tourist Board: 188;Frank Murphy Collection. Picture by kind permission of the Old Dublin Society: 150; © Gainew Gallery / Alamy Stock Photo: 149; © Galway City Museum: 102; © George Andrew Lutenor / Wikimedia: 308; © Getty Images: 61, 93, 142, 282; © Gwengoat / Getty Images: 208; © Hemis / Alamy Stock Photo: 69; © Historic Collection / Alamy Stock Photo: 214; © Historic Images / Alamy Stock Photo: 22, 181, 257; © History and Art Collection / Alamy Stock Photo: 65; © Homer Sykes / Alamy Stock Photo: 28, 317; © IanDagnall Computing / Alamy Stock Photo: 200; © ilbusca / Getty Images: 117, 123, 304; © iStock / mammoth: 47; © iStock / John Duncan / Wikimedia: 72; © Jon Bower / Alamy Stock Photo: 132;© Lakeview Images / Alamy Stock Photo: 253;Library of Congress Prints and Photographs Division. Brady-Handy Photograph Collection: 157; © Library of Congress. National Photo Company Collection: 171; © The Library of Trinity College Dublin: 32; © Magite Historic / Alamy Stock Photo: 266; © Marcus Harrison - adverts / Alamy Stock Photo: 250;Medical Historical Library, Harvey Cushing/John Hay Whitney Medical; Library, Yale University: 169; © Michael Siluk / Alamy Stock Photo: 228; © MNStudio / iStock: 14, 187; © Nastasic / Getty Images: 185; © National Folklore Collection, University College Dublin: 37, 41, 311; National Museums NI: 223, 261; reserved; collection National Portrait Gallery, London: 195; © Nheyob / Wikimedia Commons (CC BY-SA 4.0): 97; © Nickstonberg / Wikimedia (CC BY-SA 4.0): 114; © Niday Picture Library / Alamy Stock Photo: 25; © North Wind Picture Archives / Alamy Stock Photo: 77; © NSA Digital Archive / Getty Images: iii; © PA Images / Alamy Stock Photo: 138, 182; © Penta Springs Limited / Alamy Stock Photo: 98; © Pictorial Press Ltd / Alamy Stock Photo: 234, 237; © piemags/NSC / Alamy Stock Photo: 131; © Poligrafistka / Getty Images: 111; © powerofforever / Getty Images: 157, 281; © Pryderi / Wikimedia (CC BY-SA 3.0): 152; © Public Record Office of Northern Ireland (PRONI): 198; © Rama / Wikimedia: 211; Reproduced by kind permission of the Honorable Society of King's Inns: 82; © Rik Hamilton / Alamy Stock Photo: 2; Ripley's Believe It or Not (1953): 113; © RTÉ Archives: 146; © Science History Images / Alamy Stock Photo: 175; © Smith Archive / Alamy Stock Photo: 173, 244; © stevie / Adobe Stock: 104; © Stocktrek Images, Inc. / Alamy Stock Photo: 45;Stromeyer & Wyman, published by Underwood & Underwood, Washington D.C.: 298; © Stuart Borthwick / Alamy Stock Photo: 190; © The Historical Picture Archive: 303; © The National Library of Ireland: 100, 120, 128, 192, 204, 248, 274, 278; © The National Museum of Ireland: 12, 124, 126, 203; © The Picture Art Collection / Alamy Stock Photo: 215; © Tim Graham / Alamy Stock Photo: 4; © Tony Baggett / Adobe Stock: 10; © TV Times / Getty Images: 263; © Von Silvio / Adobe Stock: 161; © Warren Rosenberg / Adobe Stock: 90; © Wayne Whitty: 301; © Wellcome Collection: 60, 216, 287; © WHPics / Alamy Stock Photo: 11; © Wikimedia: 194; © Wirestock, Inc. / Alamy Stock Photo: 213; © World History Archive / Alamy Stock Photo: 256, 306.

For Laura Garland

CONTENTS

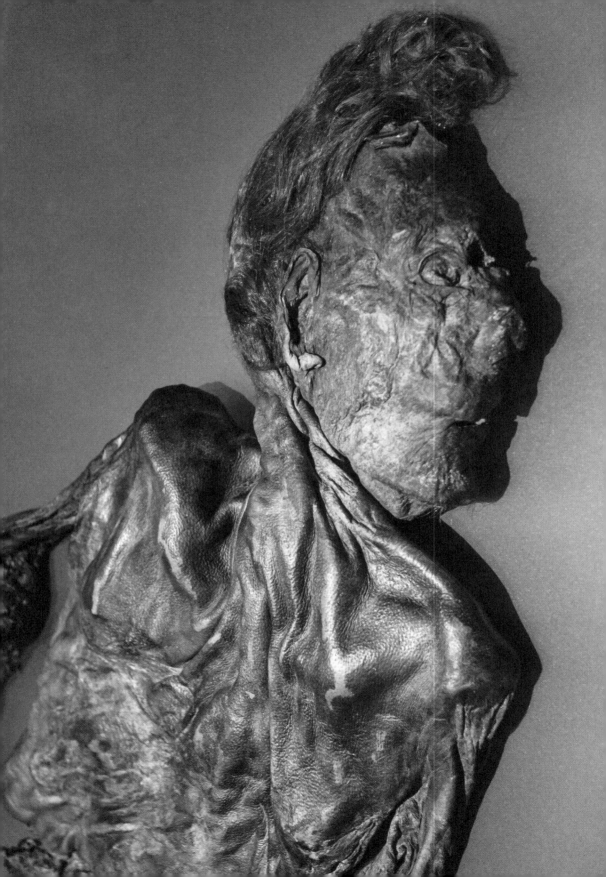

INTRODUCTION

Sometime between 392 and 201 BC, in a part of Co. Meath now known as Clonycavan, a 25-year-old man stooped down on his knees before an executioner and awaited his death. With a blunt axe, the executioner delivered an initial blow that split open the top of the man's skull. A second blow lacerated the top of the man's head, leaving a deep, gaping wound. A third and final laceration was struck across the bridge of the man's nose, cutting deep under his right eye. This blow killed him. The young man's nipples were pinched and sliced, his insides disembowelled and his mutilated bodily remains thrown into a bog.[1]

Usually, bodies start to decay immediately from the moment of death, but not this time. As the body sank rapidly, the properties of the bog shut off the oxygen supplies that normally cause decay. Anaerobic conditions, high acidity and the bog's cold temperature prevented bacteria from growing. Sphagnum moss further shielded the corpse from decay-causing microbes. Over time, the bones disintegrated due to the corrosive effects of acids, but the soft organs – the skin, stomach, hair, nails – were preserved in a chemical process not too dissimilar from the way soft fruit and vegetables are pickled. As the bones wore away, the corpse adopted an eerily contorted position, and the skin became darkly discoloured. There the man remained for thousands of years, undisturbed and unknown to those passing by on the surface above. Until March 2003.

Bogs are scattered across the Irish landscape. These waterlogged patches of land provide fuel for humans in the form of turf and nutrients for wildlife. They also remind visitors of the sprawling wilderness that once existed before modern humans forever changed Ireland's physical environment. Things easily go missing in bogs, and numerous artefacts from the past have been found submerged in them, perfectly preserved by the bogs' chemical qualities. Human bodies are among them, eerily intact, with flesh and sometimes even hair. Most were victims of violence. Ireland's bogs are perfect places to ditch a body should someone find themselves inclined to commit murder. The physical evidence is unlikely to be found any

Clonycavan Man, an Iron Age bog body, discovered near Ballivor, Co. Meath, in 2003.

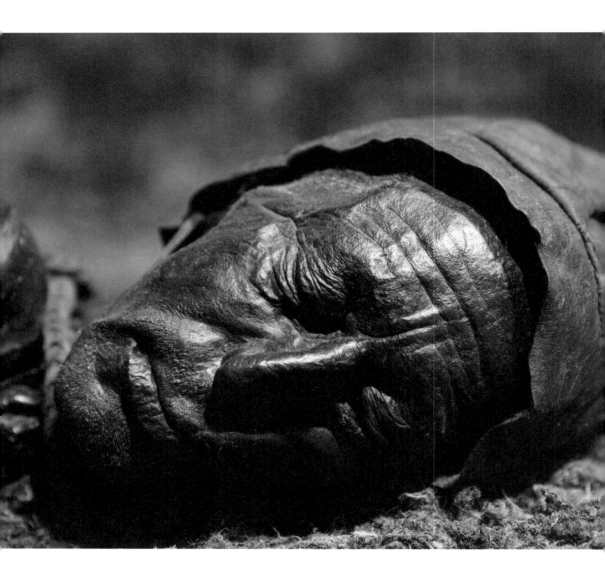

A well-preserved bog
body from Denmark.

time soon. The oldest bog bodies, including the so-called Clonycavan Man, are thought to have been human sacrifices.

To date, 17 bog bodies have been found in Ireland, although some deteriorated soon after their discovery. Cashel Man is perhaps the best known, dating from around 2000 BC and discovered in Co. Laois in 2011. Buried in a crouched position with knees against his chest, his arm wrapped around his body, Cashel Man came to his end with a broken arm, a wound on his back and his spine broken in two places. He was ditched in the bogs nearby to a hill believed by archaeologists to have once been used for kingship initiations, alongside wooden stakes, a common feature in ritualistic sacrifices.

In many ways, Clonycavan Man is far more intriguing. The body was found in a peat harvesting machine and the lower torso was never discovered; it remains unclear whether this was removed as part of the sacrificial ritual or accidentally severed in modern times by the machine. Most striking about the preserved remains is Clonycavan Man's dashing red hair, which remains intact and visible. Admittedly, Cashel Man also has a well-preserved face but, unlike Clonycavan Man, his eyes give the appearance of being closed, and his hair is less visible.

Approaching Clonycavan Man in his current home, the National Museum of Ireland (also home to Cashel Man), is a disconcerting experience. When we look at the body, Clonycavan Man's eyes appear to stare directly back at us, a time traveller staring with reciprocal wonder and fascination into a strange, futuristic world. Gazing upon the preserved face provides us with a glimpse into how people – not too dissimilar from ourselves – looked in distant, ancient times. Far from alien, the face seems ominously familiar. It's an experience drastically different from looking upon a fleshless skull or skeleton. Clonycavan Man's preserved facial features offer a more intimate portal into Ireland's ancient past. His hair, eyes and skin remind us that this head once belonged to a real person, with feelings, thoughts and behaviours much like our own.[2]

In reality, our bodies are constantly changing. Even since Clonycavan Man's time, humans have grown taller. Female hip size has increased. We start puberty at a younger age and menopause at a later one. Changes have occurred in our hair colour, birth weight and body mass index.[3] Of course, evolution hasn't magically ironed out all our problems. We may live for longer, but our bones and organs fail us as we age. Throughout our extended lives, we require glasses, teeth braces, pacemakers and even artificial limbs. We rely increasingly upon technology to replace body parts and functions gone awry, leading some philosophers to argue that we are living in a 'post-human' era, having begun to transcend the limitations of our natural bodies.[4]

Approaching history from the perspective of the body offers a novel way of understanding how people experienced life in the past, whether living through momentous periods of historical change or simply getting on with their daily lives. Those experiences were lived largely through their bodies. Today, in Western countries including Ireland, our bodies are fortunate enough to be relatively shielded from infectious diseases that in the past might have prematurely ended our lives. This was made possible by curative developments in medicine over the past century (termed by scientists the 'epidemiological transition' or 'golden age of medicine').[5] However, the COVID-19 pandemic that struck in 2020 reminded us of our vulnerability to germs and microbes and the enormous social effort required to protect us.[6] Now though, rather than die at a young age from an infection, we live longer but suffer from chronic illnesses often stemming from our lifestyle choices. Our bodily experiences (including mental and psychological) have changed considerably, even in living memory.

This book examines Irish history through a unique lens: 10 different body parts. (Admittedly, I cheat a little. 'Blood', 'height' and 'corpses' are technically not 'body parts'.) It provides a fruitful and entertaining way of introducing readers to the complexities of Irish history by revealing how physical (and mental) experiences shaped that history. The book aims not to be comprehensive but to be informative, engaging and insightful.

In the pages that follow, we will consider ancient skulls stolen from islands off Ireland's scenic west coast; the giants believed to have once roamed Irish lands; and fairies, leprechauns and banshees. We will meet the famous scribes, including St Patrick, who, all by hand, preserved our knowledge of ancient Ireland. We will look at not only old traditions such as Irish dancing, Sheela-na-gigs and Irish sports but also the empty Irish stomachs that accompanied the Great Famine and the mental health crisis that soon followed, at the time blamed on excessive tea drinking and ether drinking. Great orators such as Daniel O'Connell, whose speeches changed the course of Irish history, and controversial romantics including Charles Stewart Parnell, Maud Gonne, W.B. Yeats and Oscar Wilde make their appearance, as do the doctors who revolutionised Irish medicine in the nineteenth century (and the bodysnatchers who helped them), as well as the scientists, anthropologists and literary figures who, from the late nineteenth century, sought to uncover and better understand the ways of the ancient Irish. And much more too.

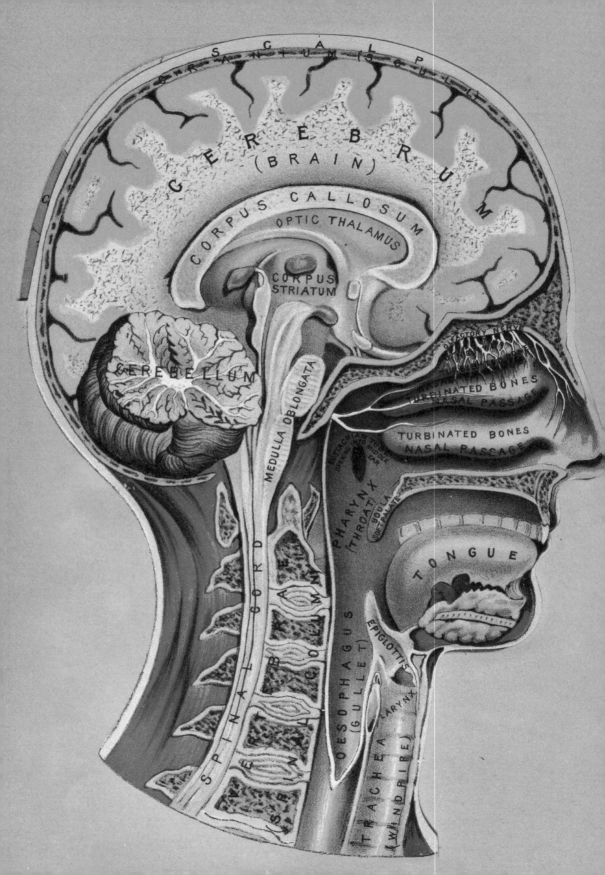

CHAPTER 1

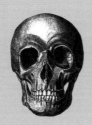

SKULLS
AND HEADS

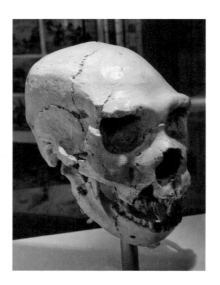

A typical Neanderthal skull.

The human skull has changed significantly over time. Think of the Neanderthal skull, with its large middle face, angled cheekbones, hefty brow ridges and huge nose. Neanderthal skeletons look recognisably human but contain not-too-subtle differences that remind us of how fundamentally different earlier types of human beings once appeared. Over the past 10,000 years, as the Ice Ages receded, the bodies and faces of most large animals grew smaller, including humans. Our brains shrank slightly too. Humans no longer depended as much on large jaws because we began to chew softer, more processed foods than our predecessors. Some scientists even believe that our faces are generally smaller than those of humans living only 300 years ago.[1]

Skulls are useful for protecting our brains and housing our facial muscles. Faces have a crucial psychological function for humans. They are central to perception, cognition and behaviour. The uniqueness of each and every one of our faces makes us singularly identifiable to others. We rely heavily upon facial recognition to remember the myriad of individuals we encounter throughout our lives. As our brains perceive, process and remember faces, they also guide the presumptions we make about other people's behaviours and personalities. It's for such reasons that skulls, heads and faces have acquired such symbolic importance in human culture. This symbolism also helps explain why many figures of historical importance ended up having their heads brutally removed.

CLONYCAVAN MAN'S HEAD

While gazing upon the remains of Clonycavan Man, our neural pathways recognise a human face. The remnants of his facial features automatically prompt our brain to process the neural mechanisms of face perception. So, when looking at him, we start to pose fundamental questions. What type of person was Clonycavan Man? What was his personality like? How did he behave? How did he live his life? Faces are very communicative, explaining why Clonycavan Man's contorted expressions, the apparent eye-to-eye contact and the preserved mouth and ears all unnerve the observer. His ancient facial expression looks far from happy, encouraging us to empathise with the pathos and sadness of a man being brutally murdered.[2]

Clonycavan Man is one of Ireland's oldest faces. His head is contorted and flattened due to the weight of the peat and his skull having dissolved in the bog. Nonetheless, in the 2000s a team of forensic anthropologists and artists used a state-of-the-art computer system to recreate his facial appearance. He looks surprisingly modern. His hair sweeps backwards from the front to form a bun on top of the head, in a tall arrangement. He also had short stubble above and below his lip and under his chin, resembling a moustache and goatee beard. Remnants of a hair tie were found too.[3]

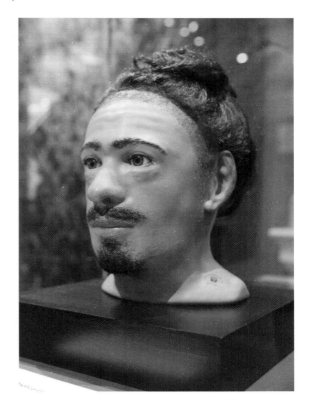

The reconstructed face of Clonycavan Man.

Visitors find themselves curiously drawn to the hair still appended to Clonycavan Man's skull. Human hair is simply not meant to survive through the millennia. It is an extremely rare occurrence when ancient hair becomes miraculously visible to us. In 1780, the Drumkeeragh body was discovered in Co. Down, the remains of an ancient woman found by surveyors near Drumkeeragh Mountain, close to Ballynahinch. A braided lock of hair from

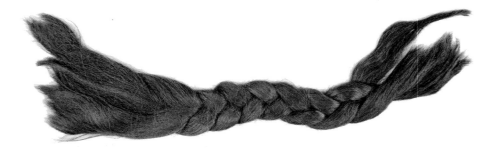

16.5-inch hair plait saved by Lady Moira in the 1780s. Still undated, it might be medieval.

the body was given to Elizabeth Rawdon (also known as Lady Moira) in 1781, whose interest in the body encouraged her to publish an article in the *Journal of Archaeologia*. In this, she recalled how Lord Moira had ordered a survey to be undertaken of a farm on his estate. It was the surveyor who brought the plait of hair to Lady Moira, informing her that he had taken it from a human skull recently dug up by a tenant.

In a small turbary situated at the foot of the Drumkeeragh Mountain, not far from Slieve Croob, the heart of the mountainous region known as the Dromara Hills, the tenant had been cutting turf for his winter's fuel at a depth of four-and-a-half feet when he came across some hard gravel. Digging further, he discovered the skeleton of a young woman. Around the bones lay many preserved garments. Further investigation revealed that the tenant's father had been digging in the very same area some fifty years earlier to a depth of eleven feet and had been the first to discover, and then rebury, the corpse. After being bribed with a handsome payment, the tenant handed over the plait of hair.[4]

This was the first documented scientific investigation of the remains of a bog body, and the lock of hair and some cloth fragments still survive today. A nineteenth-century description by prominent doctor William Wilde (father of Oscar) read:

> The hair of the individual was long, silky and of a deep chestnut colour, but how far this brownish-auburn tint is the original shade of the hair, or the result of the bog colouring, is questionable. Its present hue would be much coveted in our own day. The plait was formed of three strands, interwoven after the manner depicted in the adjoining woodcut, and closely resembles the mode of wearing the hair in vogue among children and young girls a few years ago. The entire plait is now fourteen inches long.[5]

But Clonycavan Man was much older, making the survival of his hair all the more fortuitous. The hair is also of interest because of the insights which it reveals into ancient Ireland. It seems that Clonycavan Man lived at the height of the Celtic Iron Age. At the time, the Celts were divided into a bewildering 150 kingdoms across Ireland. To confuse matters further, each had its own ruler. Ireland's Ice Age ended around 15,000 BC, and Ireland and Britain separated from the European continent around 12,000 BC. The first evidence of permanent human residence in Ireland dates from around 10,500 BC. Ireland's prehistoric period ended around AD 400, somewhat later than the rest of Europe and Near East, and the island was probably fully populated by hunter-gatherer humans between 7000 and 6500 BC. Ireland's Bronze Age commenced around 2500 BC and merged into the Iron Age when the Celts arrived between 500 and 300 BC.[6] Clonycavan Man seems to have lived towards the end of that period. Further afield, the Romans were conquering much of Europe, but Ireland remained unconquered.

The Celts were composed of various groups who gradually developed a single culture based largely upon the use of bronze and iron. They arrived in Ireland with a working knowledge of iron and ordered their society into a

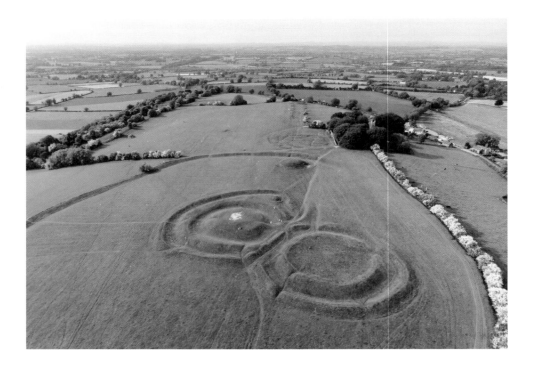

Aerial image of
the Hill of Tara.

hierarchy of warriors, with druids at the top of the social scale. Their kings were crowned at the Lia Fáil, a summit on the Hill of Tara, close to the bog into which Clonycavan Man was thrown. The three blows which felled him were not applied arbitrarily. For the Celts, three was a sacred number. The blows may have represented the three different forms of the goddess to whom the sacrifice was being made.[7]

The hair reveals much about the ancient grooming habits of Celtic men. People in the distant past, just like us, combed and styled their hair. Clonycavan Man's modest height, 5 feet 2 inches, set off speculation that he preferred to coif up his hair with gel to appear taller than he actually was. When archaeologists investigated the mysterious gel still contained in the bog body's hair, they established that it was made of vegetable plant oil mixed with resin from pine trees found only in Spain and south-west France, suggesting strong evidence of Iron Age trade across western Europe. This discovery of Iron Age hair gel caused considerable interest

Clonycavan Man also had well-manicured nails. The healthy state of his fingertips and hands, and absence of bodily scars, suggest that he was not a man accustomed to carrying out manual labour. Instead, he was most likely from the upper echelons of society, a wealthier individual who enjoyed interactions with continental neighbours. Someone important had to be sacrificed for the desired results to occur.[8] Perhaps Clonycavan Man was even a king.

After being subjected to all these examinations, Clonycavan Man's body was impregnated with a water-soluble wax solution and freeze-dried. The drying process took approximately six weeks.[9] He now forms part of a National Museum of Ireland exhibition, resting beside various materials connected with ancient rituals: weapons, jewellery, feasting utensils, wooden carvings, quern stones and butter deposits known as 'bog butter'. Archaeologists speculate that these objects may have been associated with the inauguration of a new king.[10] What is most striking, however, is the multitude of secrets which even half a preserved body, and specifically the head, can disclose about everyday life in ancient Ireland. A few strands of gelled-up hair reveal a wealth of information on ancient trading patterns and Ireland's ancient interconnectedness with nearby European countries, but they also prompt our brains to imagine an ancient Celtic world now long lost to us.

THE RED-HAIRED IRISH

Although Clonycavan Man's hair colour was probably dark, its preserved remnants give the impression that he had naturally red locks. This erroneous impression links to stereotypes of the Irish being a nation of redheads (or, more derogatorily, 'gingers'). Leprechauns, for instance, are always depicted with red hair flowing from under their tall, oversized green hats.

Debates on this matter have endured for centuries. In 1892, Catholic-oriented Boston periodical *Donahoe's Monthly Magazine* ran an article entitled 'Are the Irish a Red-Haired Race?' This question followed on from observations made in 1860 about the colourful hair of Irish members of the Papal Brigade. At the time, the Papal States were under threat from Italian nationalism, which sought the unification of the various regions in the Italian peninsula. Pope Pius IX dispatched a group of papal emissaries to Ireland to recruit an Irish battalion to fight in Northern Italy.[11] The author, who anonymously signed off as 'Irish Citizen, Chicago', noted that:

> As far as our observation has extended, only about two or three per cent of the Irish can be truthfully described as being red-haired. There is a beautiful shading of auburn in the dark locks of many Irish women – the most beautiful hair to be found among mortals; heavy, glinting and luxurious – but nobody, unless he was colour blind, could call them red or strawberry tresses.

The author added:

> There is a great deal of beauty in brilliant red hair – not the brick-coloured type – and a handsome woman, with a mass of red locks, is all the more beautiful in consequence, especially as snowy skin is a usual accompaniment of such hirsute adornment, particularly in Irish women.[12]

Similarly, in 1887, barrister Alexander George Richey wrote about a specific physical type of Irish person also characterised by red hair, in his influential *A Short History of the Irish People*, although he noted that this appearance was particularly common only among the 'Scottish colonists in Ulster'. Elsewhere across the island, 'the asperities and angularities of this type have been softened down, probably by a mixture of Iberian blood'.[13]

While obviously appreciating the pale-skinned, red-haired variety of Irish woman, these authors concluded that, despite the myth, red hair wasn't any more prevalent in Ireland than in Scotland or England. They were correct. Nowadays, around 10 per cent of Irish people (roughly 500,000) have red hair, but Scotland does indeed have a slightly higher proportion, with about 13 per cent of Scots having red hair. The Vikings are thought to have introduced red hair into the Irish gene pool from the ninth century AD. One Norse document describes Thor, son of one of the gods of Asgard, as having a head full of red hair, a bushy red beard and a quick temper. Scientists associate red hair with a recessive gene called MC1R. Rare, this gene is found only in around 2 per cent of the world's population. To produce a red-haired child, both parents must carry a copy of the gene, although the trait can skip generations, adding to the rarity of red hair. Redheads with blue eyes are especially scarce.[14]

Negative cultural stereotypes abound about red-haired Irish people. In *Gulliver's Travels*, Dublin-born Anglo-Irish author Jonathan Swift (1667–1745) wrote of the Yahoos (crude, dirty brutes who lived in the land of the Houyhnhnms) that 'the red haired of both sexes are more libidinous and mischievous than the rest, whom yet they much exceed in strength and activity'. Not all Yahoos had red hair, but those that did, particularly the females, were the most dangerous. A female Yahoo who attacked Gulliver sexually was a redhead. Evidently, Swift's portrayal of the Yahoos was not flattering and is believed to represent the Irish. An irrational people, they represented humanity's worst side, being 'the most filthy, noisome and deformed animals which nature ever produced'.[15]

Swift drew from millennia-old stereotypes, presumably recognisable to his contemporary readers. Satan himself was covered with red hair, according to the Bible. Jewish communities were traditionally associated with red hair (the so-called 'Red Jews') and for centuries faced persecution and discrimination. Early Christians associated red hair and beards with evil and sins.[16] In Irish mythology, Badb, the goddess of war and death, who commonly took the form of a crow, used to meet heroes in the guise of a red-haired woman.[17]

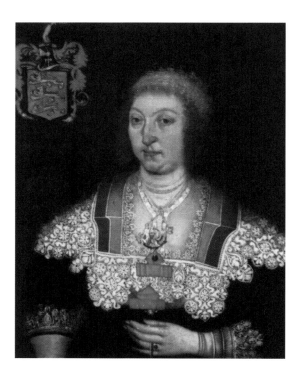

Máire Rua O'Brien (also known as Red Mary).

While today red hair is more commonly associated, sometimes erotically, with images of pale-skinned female Irish beauty, red-haired women were historically held in low repute. In folk culture well into the twentieth century, encountering a woman with red hair first thing in the morning was an omen that forebode bad luck and evil. As one proverb stated: 'Let not the eye of a red-haired woman rest on you.'[18] To counteract the negative effects of coming across a red-haired lady, the unfortunate victim had to return to his starting point. If he met a white horse along the way, any spells cast were averted.[19] However, red-haired men enjoyed a far better reputation. The Red Captain was a spirit thought to appear in the form of a red-haired young man whose presence, unlike that of his female counterparts, brought good fortune.[20]

The most notorious female redhead was Máire Rua O'Brien (1615–1686), an Irish aristocrat who married three times to retain family lands. Her nickname, Red Mary, derives from her rouge hair. She is a notorious figure in Irish folklore, and numerous (exaggerated) stories and legends are associated with her. She lived during the Irish Confederate Wars (or Eleven Years' War), which took place between 1641 and 1653. As with many Irish conflicts, the main issues revolved around whether Catholics or Protestants should hold political power and whether Ireland should be self-governing or subordinate to the parliament in England. In 1649, a large English Parliamentarian army, led by

Oliver Cromwell, invaded Ireland, massacring many soldiers and civilians. The conflict ultimately led to the repression of Catholicism from the 1650s after the end of the Cromwellian War (1649–53). The death toll was huge. An estimated 400,000 to 600,000 people died on Irish soil.[21]

During this conflict, Máire backed the Royalist cause against Cromwell's forces. With her first husband, Conor O'Brien, she built one of the finest houses erected in seventeenth-century Ireland. However, he died at the hands of the Cromwellians, and the property was forfeit. Máire became determined to marry a Cromwellian to regain her property. John Cooper was her chosen candidate, although he soon died after Máire reportedly kicked him in the stomach when he insulted O'Brien. According to some rumours, she threw her third husband out of the window before marrying another 22 men, most of whom met a grisly end. She was also rumoured to enjoy hanging her maids from the tower by their hair. Eventually, she suffered a witch's curse and was fastened in the hollow of a tree, her red hair entangled with its roots. However, her ghost escaped to forever haunt Leamaneh Castle. Another legend states that she was hanged by her hair from a tree. Either way, Máire's red hair figures prominently in her mythology.[22]

DECAPITATION

Red Mary would probably have approved of Cromwell's ultimate fate. In 1659, Charles II of England was restored as King of England following a brutal Civil War. Upon his restoration, Charles announced that Cromwell must be executed for regicide. (His father, Charles I, had been beheaded.) Cromwell had died in September 1658, but Charles didn't let this deter him. In 1660, Cromwell's corpse was taken from Westminster Abbey, dragged through London's busy streets and hanged in chains at Tyburn, an area of London synonymous with the gallows. Cromwell was then posthumously beheaded in front of a rapturous, although somewhat bemused, audience. His head was placed on a 20-foot spike on the roof of Westminster Hall, where it rested until 1685, when a storm blew it down.[23]

The word decapitation comes from the Latin *capitis*, which translates as 'of the head'. Severing the head swiftly deprives the brain of oxygen and causes the body's organs to fail. Human heads are notoriously tricky to dislodge from a living body, and executioners commonly botched beheadings, requiring multiple attempts and causing excruciating pain to the soon-to-be headless person. When Cromwell's corpse was decapitated at Tyburn, it took the executioner eight blows to cut through the layers of cerecloth that wrapped his body. A successful decapitation requires powerful, accurate action, and a sharp, heavy blade. Even the most experienced executioners usually had to inflict a few blows before a person's head was fully cut off.[24]

Interestingly, the severed heads of some sea slugs can grow a new body. In the 1940s a chicken named Miracle Mike attracted international fame for living 18 months without his head.[25] Humans are not so fortunate. How long we can remain conscious after decapitation is unclear, although numerous macabre experiments have taken place. The guillotine is often remembered as a grotesque, barbaric invention of the French Revolution, but it was actually intended as a humane execution contraption which got around the problem of botched beheadings and the cruelty of inflicting several blows on the neck of a living person. Death under the guillotine was meant to be instantaneous but was still a bloody business.[26] Promises of a speedy, relatively painless death led to the replacement in France of the executioner's axe with the guillotine, but onlookers insisted that many of these heads continued to blink, breathe, blush, grind their teeth and even communicate for some time after being severed.[27]

One French physician who attended an execution approached as soon as the severed head, dislocated from its body, had fallen into the blood-stained basket below. He called out the name of the executed man and was convinced that the head made eye contact with him before lowering its gaze. Once again, the physician called out the man's name and noticed similar signs of consciousness. Based on this apparent communication, the physician concluded that human heads could retain consciousness for 25–30 seconds.[28] Subsequent experiments involving slicing off the heads of laboratory rats appear to confirm this.[29]

There is another interesting, and little-known, fact about the guillotine. The Irish might well have invented it. In 1307, Murcod Ballagh was the first person in the world recorded as having been executed by guillotine. The death took place in Merton, Co. Galway, according to *Holinshed's Chronicles*, published some centuries later in 1577, and the executioner was named David de Caunteton. Both names appear in the justiciary rolls for January 1308, which hints at the veracity of this story. Ballagh was an outlaw, which meant that his captors had the right to execute him upon apprehension without going through any legal process. Ironically, two years after Murcod's death, his executioner, David de Caunteton, suffered the same fate.[30]

In some ways, this is reminiscent of the beheading game, a literary trope found in Irish mythology, which tells of a mysterious stranger arriving at a royal court to challenge a hero to an exchange of blows. In this game, the hero might decapitate the stranger, but the stranger then inflicts the same wound in return upon the hero. The stranger is a supernatural figure, which explains how this unlikely event is possible, although this fact only becomes evident to the hero when the stranger unexpectedly retrieves his own decapitated head. If the hero submitted to the return blow, he was rewarded for his valour and suffered only a minor wound. Metaphorically, the tale is thought to represent the hero coming of age through a symbolic death and rebirth.

The story originates in the Fled Bricrenn legend, in which three heroes – Cú Chulainn, Conall Cernach and Lóegaire Búadach – are invited to a feast in which they are put through a series of trials, some involving supernatural figures, to establish who was superior. The beheading game subsequently featured in several Arthurian romances, most notably those featuring Sir Gawain and the Green Knight.[31]

Much to the distaste of modern sensibilities, decapitation was a historically common form of human execution (although it was usually performed on living, not dead, victims). Across Ireland, archaeologists have discovered a total of 56 sites

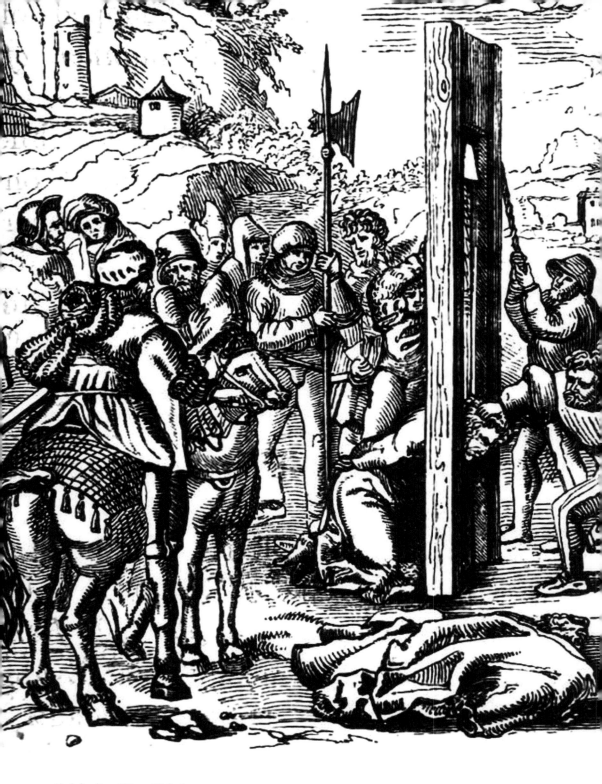

The beheading of Murcod Ballagh
in 1307 with a contraption similar
to a guillotine.

containing evidence of 68 beheadings dating from ancient times.[32] A beheading could signify a military victory, or it could be used to punish serious crimes.

From around the fifth century, Ireland became predominantly Christian, following on from a mysterious period between AD 100 and 300 which saw population levels and living standards plummet, for unknown reasons.[33] The years 800 to 1000 witnessed Viking raids and Norse settlements along the coast. Around this time, many of Ireland's ports sprang up: Dublin, Wexford, Waterford, Cork and Limerick. At the lake dwelling of Lagore, Co. Meath, 14 skulls have been found showing evidence of decapitation, probably dating from the period 500–1000. They might have been displayed around the edge of the site. Far more extensive evidence of decapitation has been found at a Viking enclave in Dublin, established in the 900s. The skulls discovered there are similar to written descriptions of trophy heads from that time. After 1171, when Henry II arrived, human remains continued to be used extensively as trophies, including heads.[34]

Ireland consisted of many different territories ruled over by many different factions before the Norman invasion of 1169–71. The Normans had invaded Britain the previous century, and King Henry II encouraged his Welsh barons to invade Ireland to strengthen his western border – and keep his barons busy. When he landed in Waterford with a large fleet in 1171, Henry was the first English king known to have set foot on Irish soil; he conferred the title Lord of Ireland on his son John. However, a Gaelic resurgence between 1350 and 1500 testified to two contrasting groups then existing on the island, each of which identified primarily with either English or Irish culture.[35] Decapitation was still common, either as punishment for crime or tactic of warfare. Most headless corpses discovered have been men, suggesting strong links between beheading and warfare. In earlier times, severed heads would be thrown into the grave along with the rest of the body, but the absence of buried heads in later periods suggests that they were used instead for trophy or display purposes.[36]

As punishment for treason and serious crimes, beheading formed one part of being hanged, drawn and quartered. One execution sentencing read:

That you be led to the place from whence you came, and from thence be drawn upon a hurdle to the place of execution, and then you shall be hanged by the neck and, being alive, shall be cut down, and your privy members to be cut off, and your entrails taken out of your body and, you living, the same to be burnt before your eyes, and your head cut off, your body to be divided into four quarters, and head and quarters to be disposed of at the pleasure of the King's majesty. And the Lord have mercy on your soul.

After this ordeal, the executioner held the head aloft shouting, 'Behold the head of a traitor. So die all traitors.' The heads and quarters were then mounted on the city walls and gates. Sometimes the heads would be parboiled in heavily salted water to impede decay and discourage birds from feeding on the remains. The process of quartering the body was also believed to risk eternal damnation for the executed person.[37]

From the mid-1530s, decapitation became even more common as the Tudor dynasty sought to cement its control of the country.[38] English expansion outside of 'the Pale' (that part of eastern Ireland controlled by the English government in the Late Middle Ages) was attempted, and sustained efforts were made to replace the Irish language with English.[39] At Dublin Castle, seat of the English government, the heads of rebels, outlaws and cattle thieves adorned the outlying forts. The government kept its cash reserves at Dublin Castle, so bounty hunters would travel to the capital to deliver their bloody, severed heads and obtain their 'head money' from the treasury. Archaeologists working around Dublin's city walls regularly discover portions of human heads, an indication that these were of executed men whose heads were displaced and displayed. Among these sites was Isolde's Tower, located at the north-east corner of the walled city. Overlooking the river that served as an entry point into the city for many travellers, it would have been one of the first sights visible to anyone approaching the city by boat.[40] This grotesque display of severed heads reminded onlookers of the Crown's authority and power. Severed heads differ from skulls. They serve vastly different

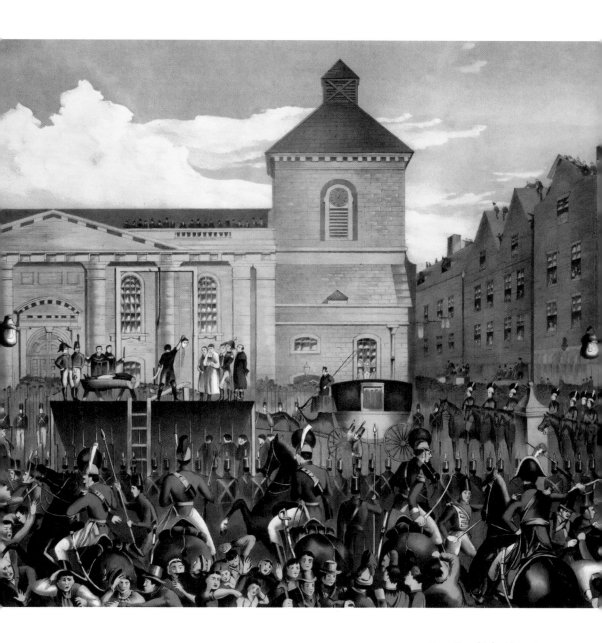

Execution of Robert Emmet
in Thomas Street, Dublin,
20 September 1803.

symbolic purposes. Still resembling the living, they were publicly displayed to remind onlookers of the consequences of disobedience, crime and rebellion.[41]

That said, the Irish also enjoyed head-taking.[42] The Greeks and Romans wrote regularly of the Celts' reputation as head-hunters and of an enthusiasm among Celtic warriors for cutting off the heads of their enemies slain in battle, hanging them from their horses' necks and finally nailing them up outside their homes.[43] Sometimes, they embalmed the heads of their enemies in cedar oil and put them on display.[44] Heads played an iconic role in Celtic religion, and some historians discuss a 'cult of the severed head'.[45]

By all accounts, in the Tudor period, the 'native' Irish still possessed a predilection for severing heads, and this motif appeared regularly in representations of the 'Wild Irish' on the Elizabethan and Jacobean stage. The English regarded this as barbaric and bloodthirsty, despite being similarly predisposed to removing the heads of enemies and traitors. A thin line existed between atrocity and justice, and much depended upon who was doing the head-chopping. From the Irish perspective, the practice, when performed by the English, offered firm evidence of English brutality. When performed by themselves, it was simply justice.[46]

Only after the eighteenth century did such practices fall out of fashion, partly because of a growing distaste for public executions, concern about the public revelry surrounding the gallows and the availability of alternative punishments such as transportation to Australia and long-term imprisonment.[47] By then, judges could only authorise decapitation after a criminal had been executed. Even this was only used in a handful of more serious cases of crime. Death by hanging became the most common execution method.[48] When Robert Emmet was sentenced to be hanged, drawn and quartered for high treason in 1803, following a failed attempt at overthrowing the British government after the Act of Union (1800–1), he was hanged until death before being beheaded. The executioner refrained from cutting the body into four pieces. By this time, the medical profession was actively seeking bodies for public dissection, which further discouraged the mutilation of bodies and corpses.[49]

Taking all of this into account, it should now be clearer why the Irish population greeted news of Cromwell's beheading with much glee. The removal of his head symbolically confirmed perceptions of Cromwell as a war criminal. The aforementioned Cromwellian War of 1649–53 saw Cromwell imposing harsh times on the Irish Catholic population, partly to punish them for the 1641 Rebellion, which had seen Protestants massacred in Ulster. Catholic landowners had land confiscated and Catholics were no longer allowed to live in towns. Catholicism was banned, and priests were hunted and executed. Even after the Restoration of 1660, Catholics were barred from public office.

The Drogheda Massacre of 1649 still looms large in Irish popular memory for its remarkable severity and brutality. Cromwell's troops killed priests and monks on sight and set light to Catholic churches with people inside. Civilians and soldiers were massacred, and few Royalist soldiers survived. These atrocities were then replicated in Wexford and Clonmel.[50] Most shockingly, around 50,000 Irish people were transported to Barbados between 1652 and 1656, where they were treated cruelly.[51] Few people in Ireland mourned when news reached them that Cromwell had lost his head.

This brings us to yet another famous head in this fraught period of Irish history. From its earliest times, Christianity had demonstrated an interest in fragmented human bodies and used pieces of heads as relics. In the Middle Ages and Early Modern period, some skulls were carefully severed after death to create a relic. Saintly heads tended to be passed around a lot. It was believed that some saints managed briefly to stay alive after execution, being able to pick up their detached head and take it in their arms while they walked to a place where they wished to rest forever. These were known as 'head carriers'.[52]

In St Peter's Church, Drogheda, rests the preserved head of St Oliver Plunkett, encased in an intricate golden shrine. It reminds onlookers of the religious persecution that accompanied the Cromwellian period, and beyond. Born in Co. Meath in 1625, Plunkett became a Catholic priest in 1654, and the Irish bishops appointed him as their representative in Rome. However, this coincided with the aftermath of Cromwell's conquest of Ireland and the subsequent banning

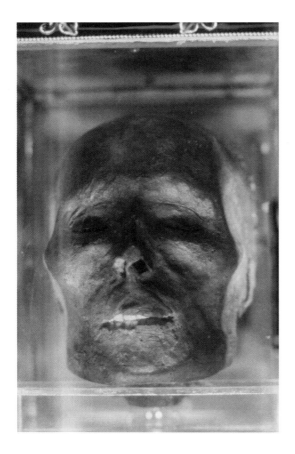

St Oliver Plunkett's
preserved head at St Peter's
Church, Drogheda.

of Catholic practice. Quite sensibly, Plunkett decided against returning to Ireland for many years. In 1669, he was appointed as the Catholic archbishop of Armagh and Primate of All Ireland and eventually set foot again in Ireland only in 1670.

Plunkett was the last victim of the Popish Plot, a fabricated conspiracy that stoked anti-Catholic hysteria between 1678 and 1681. Fictitious fears that Catholics were conspiring to assassinate Charles II heightened social tensions. Plunkett was arrested in Dublin on 6 December 1679, imprisoned in Dublin Castle, found guilty of high treason by an all-Protestant (and hardly impartial) jury and sentenced to death. He was hanged, drawn and quartered on 1 July 1681 at Tyburn, England. His body parts were buried in the courtyard at St Giles-in-the-Fields, although they were later exhumed. Then, Plunkett's dismembered head began its travels. Over the centuries, it enjoyed time in Germany, Rome and Armagh before arriving in Drogheda in 1929, where it remains. The majority of the body can be found in Downside Abbey, England, although a few parts remain in Germany.

Plunkett was beatified in 1920 and canonised in 1975. This was big news. Plunkett was the first new Irish saint for almost 700 years (although 17 other Irish martyrs have since been beatified). In 1997, Plunkett was promoted to a new position: Ireland's patron saint for peace and reconciliation. Pilgrims still travel to Drogheda to view the shrine, with its encased head. The head is more than just a skull. It survives in relatively good condition. Scorch marks are still visible from when it was thrown into a fire shortly after its removal, before being quickly saved. Although the eyes appear closed, the nose, teeth and basic outline of a human face are discernible, and even a few hairs rest peacefully on the brown-coloured head. To some, this remarkable facial preservation itself offers evidence of the miraculous nature of Plunkett's head.[53] In contrast, Cromwell's head is still associated with shameful behaviour, so much so that it remains buried in an unmarked location in Cambridge. No one would think to display Cromwell's head, perhaps for fear that it would swiftly be vandalised, probably by an Irish person if they got the opportunity.

THE STOLEN SKULLS OF INISHBOFIN

In 2023, Trinity College Dublin made international headlines for all the wrong reasons after finally agreeing, following years of public campaigning, to return a set of skulls taken in the 1890s from Inishbofin, an island off the coast of Galway. Trinity publicly apologised for having kept 13 skulls snatched by two 'academic head-hunters', although only after much public discussion and the signing of a petition by all of the island's 170 inhabitants demanding the skulls' return. The stolen skulls were returned in a broader international context of debate about colonial legacies in Western museums, heritage and commemoration, and the housing of human remains in anthropological collections that were tainted by nineteenth-century colonial violence and scientific racism. At the time, statues of former slave merchants were being regularly tossed into the sea in cities such as Liverpool and Bristol. But what had motivated the academics to abscond with the skulls in the first place?

In 1890, British ethnologist Alfred Cort Haddon, with his student Andrew Francis Dixon, sailed to Inishbofin under the pretence of carrying out a fishing

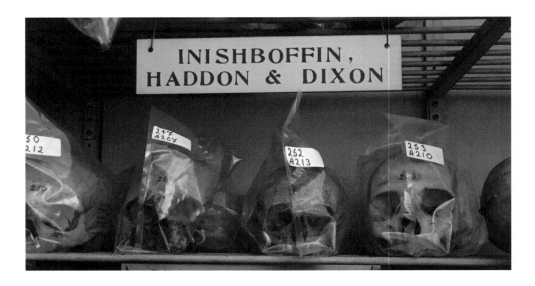

Inishbofin's stolen skulls, housed for over a century at Trinity College Dublin.

survey. While there, they secretly stole the 13 skulls from St Colman's Monastery, convinced that they had stumbled across specimens of Ireland's indigenous people. Even the boatman who ferried Haddon and Dixon away from the monastery was unaware of the pilfered goods being harboured on his vessel. In those stolen skulls, Haddon and Dixon thought, rested physical evidence of an original Irish people – a pure, uncontaminated prototype largely untouched by civilisation and modernity, perhaps even more ancient than Clonycavan Man. The academics deposited the skulls at Trinity, where they were stored in a collection for over a century alongside others taken from elsewhere on the Aran Islands and from St Finian's Bay in Co. Kerry. The university has not yet returned these other skulls.

A Cambridge-educated anthropologist and ethnologist, Haddon was appointed Professor of Zoology in 1880 at the College of Science, Dublin. His early papers researched embryology and marine biology, and his most famous fieldwork took place on the Torres Strait Islands, in the western Pacific Ocean, between north-east Australia and the island of New Guinea. The indigenous people of the islands interested Haddon as he believed them to be relatively unadulterated specimens of human beings, a living portal into how humans once looked and behaved before we became modern. It was usual at the time for anthropologists to collect ethnographical specimens and deposit them somewhere back home. The British Museum in London is full of them. In Australasia, Haddon justified his removal of 'native' body parts by claiming that their safety was under threat from missionaries determined to obliterate non-Christian traditions.

Haddon remained in Dublin until 1893, before moving to Cambridge, although he continued to publish his thoughts on Irish skulls for some decades. By the nineteenth century, Irish people's enthusiasm for cutting off heads had thankfully waned. Anthropologists such as Haddon now presented observations of the practice elsewhere in the world as a curious relic of a pre-'civilised' past which Westerners had transcended and left behind. In 1901, Haddon published his research on the Torres Straits Islands in the aptly titled *Head-Hunters: Black, White and Brown*.[54] Intended for a scholarly audience, *Head-Hunters* offered readers a captivating glimpse into how other people lived across the globe and how our ancient predecessors might have organised their societies and cultures. In the days before global interconnectedness, such books allowed Westerners opportunities to get to know people living in distant regions, with anthropologists presenting themselves as intrepid global explorers.

Haddon was fixated with 'native' traditions of chopping off human heads, and *Head-Hunters* listed an array of reasons for head removals in the Torres Strait Islands. Among some tribes, procuring a human skull was an indispensable necessity for young men looking to take a young maiden's hand in marriage, for it suggested that he was brave and strong enough to protect her, theorised Haddon. Women were known to actively propose to men known to have secured a skull. Some tribes believed that the person from whom the head had been separated would be their slaves in the next world. Other reasons included reprisal for injuries, a vendetta or blood feud and bringing home war trophies.[55]

Skulls were of particular interest to anthropologists due to the popularity of craniology, an investigative discipline which categorised the various ethnic

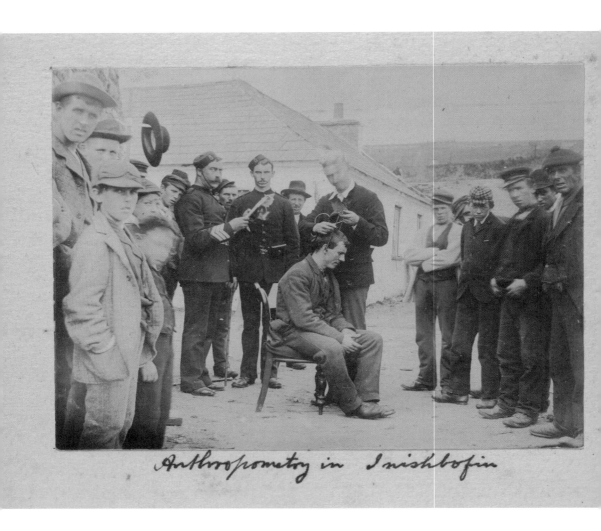

Anthropometry in Inishbofin

Inishbofin islanders
having their skulls
measured in 1892.

groups (or human races) using bodily measurements, including those of the skull. Many craniologists were influenced, knowingly or otherwise, by the racial prejudices of their day. Claims that Africans and Aborigines had smaller skulls than white Europeans supported racist ideas about the alleged inferiority of 'native' communities, their unsuitability for self-rule and the need for a paternalistic colonial presence. Most damaging to the reputation of non-Europeans was the (inaccurate) assumption that smaller skull size meant lower intelligence.[56]

Until the nineteenth century, the mind had been thought to exist in the lower organs, typically the stomach or heart, but phrenologists, most prominently Franz Joseph Gall, popularised the new idea that our minds are located in our brains.[57] Hence, the secrets to our personalities now rested inside the human head. However, brains were hard to investigate. Extremely messy organs, they disintegrate rapidly once removed from a human corpse and are difficult to keep in shape when detached from the skeletal frame. Skulls were the next best thing. Retaining their hard, durable shape, they proved much easier to measure.[58] Craniologists meticulously measured skulls, hoping to accurately decipher and categorise human 'types', 'races' and 'species'. With their human skulls, craniologists held in their hands a unique three-dimensional object replete with eye sockets, arches, protuberances and apertures available for quantifying. They devised a plethora of ways of measuring the various parts of a human skull.[59]

Haddon was not the first scientist who indulged in measuring Irish skulls (although he became the most notorious). Belfast-based naturalist and anthropologist John Grattan had undertaken considerable research into Irish skulls.[60] Grattan started off his career as a pharmaceutical chemist in 1825, and in subsequent decades he became enthralled by Gall's phrenological ideas. When one of his friends, Edmund Getty, undertook an archaeological survey of the round towers of Ulster, he chanced upon a large number of skulls buried in the floors of these towers, presumably the remains of the beheaded from some centuries previous, which he asked Grattan to examine. In 1857, Grattan presented his findings at a public talk in Dublin and took the opportunity to exhibit a craniometer, which he had invented for measuring skulls. Like Haddon, Grattan was intrigued by the 'origin stories' of the Irish people. He also saw the purpose of ethnology as being to 'investigate the progressional history of the various races of mankind'. The use of the term 'progressional' suggests that Grattan perceived the skulls as having once belonged to a race of people not yet civilised or modern. He wanted 'to decipher the faint and fading records of antiquity' and 'penetrate the mystery that enshrouds the earlier conditions of our race'.[61]

Grattan was fascinated by the idea of getting to know the human races who had once lived untouched by modernity and believed that remote communities still existed who were yet to fully progress into a civilised state. In the Society Islands of the South Pacific, Grattan observed, could be found stone hatchets, flint arrowheads and bone implements 'identical to those of the remote ages of our own country'. This somewhat simplistic model of human progression convinced Grattan that observing 'native' communities might offer a direct window into the lives and appearance of ancient people.

Undoubtedly, Grattan overestimated the lack of contact with modernity, and the extent of genetic change within those communities over the millennia, but his ideas were nonetheless influential. He was particularly intrigued by understanding what the Celts had looked like before their genetic intermingling with Vikings, Normans and the British.[62] Grattan died in 1871, leaving his ongoing research into Irish skulls unfinished. One of the most morbid publications of the time, which can still be read at the spectacular Linen Hall Library in Belfast, is a catalogue of 63 skulls from across Ireland collected by Grattan and bequeathed in the 1870s to the Belfast Natural History and Philosophical Society.[63]

Grattan's sisters later granted Haddon permission to consult Grattan's private notes. Haddon also had access to the notes of esteemed British ethnologist John Beddoe. In 1867, Beddoe published a prize-winning essay entitled 'The Origin of the English Nation', which he later expanded into an 1885 book, *The Races of Britain*. In his book's opening pages, Beddoe noted that 'it was the ancient controversy respecting the colour of the hair of the Celts, then burning briskly enough, and even now still smouldering, that led me to begin systematic numerical observations in physical anthropology'. Here, Beddoe referred to the ongoing fascination with the famed red hair of the Irish and wondered if this was a remnant of original Celtic features.

Impressed by Darwinian ideas of heredity, Beddoe thought that hair and eye colour retained more permanence over time than other physical characteristics, as 'whenever a distinct and tolerably homogeneous breed has been established, its colours may remain very much the same so long as the conditions of natural selection remain nearly identical'. However, Beddoe noted that samples of ancient hair were hard to find. 'As to whether red hair was more common then than now, we cannot have the same assurance,' he wrote, adding that 'such hair as has come down to us from individuals of ancient races is generally stained and altered, so as to be untrustworthy evidence'.[64]

Skulls provided more concrete physical evidence. Beddoe believed that the Gaelic Irish racial type derived from a large-jawed 'Africanoid' stock and visited Ireland several times to observe 'the physical characteristics of the natives'. He investigated 31 skulls in Dublin's museums, mostly from Co. Kerry and Connacht, while observing living heads in Munster. He concluded that 'the modern Irish skull is usually rather long, low and narrow, when compared with the average of English skulls, and these characters are still more marked when the comparison is extended to other European races. It seems probable that the Irish have narrower heads than the Welsh.' He recorded a strongly marked superciliary ridge extending across the nose, making a horizontal line below the eyebrows, as well as a low forehead, with a long, prominent nose featuring a large tip. Beddoe was convinced that people resembling the true 'native' Celt still lived in remote regions of Ireland that Norsemen, Englishmen and Scotsmen had never fully reached – romantic regions protected by mountains or the sea. He blamed Cromwell and his troops for diluting the original Celtic gene pool.[65]

This fascination with the secrets contained within Ireland's ancient bodily remains ultimately motivated Haddon and Dixon to steal Inishbofin's skulls. Unlike many of his contemporaries, Haddon's interest in Irish peasant life rested not in finding solutions to the country's relative lack of industrialisation or offering suggestions for social improvement, but instead, as a naturalist, in documenting how 'ordinary' people, or peasants, lived. Nor does he come across as overly prejudiced against the Irish, unlike many of his contemporaries. Haddon described the men whom he encountered in the Aran Islands as 'extremely pleasing people', slightly below the average height, with 'pleasant open countenances' and 'fairness of the complexion'. As he elaborated, 'these people are very kindly and friendly, fearless, independent, and manly, and they used to be extremely honest, so much so, that if you lost a purse, you would always find it the next Sunday or saint's day on the altar of the chapel'. Nonetheless, Haddon noted, this honest character had faded in the last half century due to (unspecified) negative external influences.

That said, the people of Inishbofin were a different kettle of fish. Haddon encountered there 'a darker and more burly people, who are also of a more truculent disposition. They are suspicious of strangers, and there is not much good feeling between them and the people on the mainland, each giving the other rather a bad character.' Haddon seemed oblivious to the fact that the 'natives' might well have good reasons to be suspicious of him and the unwelcome enthusiasm of Dublin-based researchers for arriving on their island, poking into their lives and, as it turned out, stealing the skulls of their ancestors.[66]

In a lecture delivered to the Royal Irish Academy in 1892, Haddon announced that 'it is a remarkable fact that there is scarcely an obscure people on the face of the globe about whom we have less anthropographical information than we have of the Irish'.[67] Perhaps the Irish had been too close to home to interest many ethnologists, or too white to appeal to the anthropologist's pressing concern with demarcating difference between white and non-white people. Other contemporary researchers had to rely upon chance finds such as 50 skulls dating back to the eighth century AD found in Donnybrook, the best preserved of over 600 humans massacred there.[68]

However, the skulls discovered by Haddon, having been snatched from a remote, isolated island, seemed potentially more revealing about Ireland's

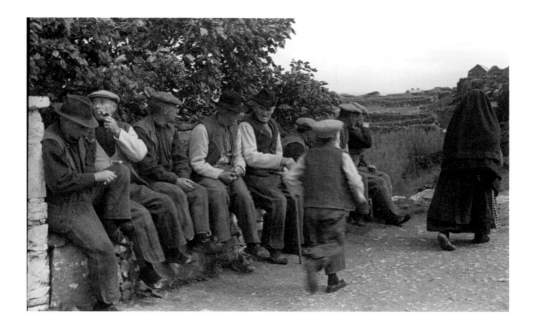

ancient past. Haddon explained to his captive audience that he had given the 13 skulls to Trinity's Anthropological Museum (which operated between 1891 and 1903, with its collections subsequently held in storage), but quietly overlooked his dubious pilfering of the skulls late at night. Haddon prided himself on having secured the first skull specimens from that region of Ireland, despite few of them being in good condition. Most were broken or weathered and, due to this, were probably a little smaller than they would have originally been.[69]

Residents of Inishbofin around the turn of the twentieth century.

Haddon then proceeded to read through his list of measurements. To the modern listener (and perhaps even to most Victorians), Haddon's research reads inexplicably as a seemingly unending list of monotonous, meaningless skull measurements. Every nook and cranny of the skulls had been subjected to some sort of measuring. Haddon speculated that the average Irish skull was typically long, low and narrow, with zygomatic arches not much expanded. The Irish were of average height (67 inches on average), and broadly similar to the population of western Britain.[70]

In these calculations, lives and personalities that had once been full and rich were reduced to a barely comprehensible rota of sizes and dimensions, dehumanising the people who once occupied them and stripping them of identity and personality. Haddon didn't want to get to know the humans behind the skulls in the same way that modern visitors to the National Museum of Ireland engage in an imaginative process of getting to know Clonycavan Man. This tedious quantification of human skulls tells us more about Haddon than the skulls' former owners.[71] Most puzzling is Haddon's lack of general conclusions or commentary upon these supposedly pure artefacts of Irish Celticness. The absence of any explicit interpretation dehumanises the skulls further still.[72] The impression given is that the measurements were being presented for reference only, but for who or what purpose remains unclear.[73]

More positively, unlike many other anthropologists, Haddon was less concerned with presenting the Irish skulls as primitive or 'apish' than were other craniologists operating in other parts of the world. Indeed, they spoke almost positively of the role of crossbreeding in human populations and the environmental adaptability of racial mixing.[74] He seemed fairly respectful towards this ancient Irish stock. Most people presumed that there had once existed an Irish Celtic past equivalent to the past of Greece and Rome and, for that reason, in the nineteenth century, the remote islands off Galway's coast became sites of cultural and scientific attention. They were imagined as places where the direct ancestors of the original Celts, of Clonycavan Man, still lived, relatively unaffected by modernisation and civilisation. Haddon wasn't entirely naïve and knew that some interbreeding with non-islanders must surely have taken place over time, particularly from the Early Modern period, for no place is altogether isolated from the world surrounding it.[75] Nonetheless, despite these nuances, the skulls were still seen as symbolising the true Irish Celt who existed before Britain's unwelcome intrusion.

Haddon's research took place in the context of a far broader cultural fascination with the western islands and their residents. The Gaelic Revival of the late nineteenth century encouraged a resurgence of interest in the Irish language and Gaelic culture, including sports, literature and mythology. Much of this was spearheaded by the Gaelic League, formed in 1893, led initially by Douglas Hyde, who gave a presidential address entitled 'The Necessity for De-Anglicising Ireland'.[76] Although the league claimed to be apolitical, it inevitably became bound up with a growing Irish nationalism, which in just a few decades would stage the Easter Rising and many other dramatic events that led to independence and partition. The argument for national independence was played out on a cultural level by forging a strong Irish identity, rooted in Celticness, not Britishness, and predicated on the ancient past that existed long before Britain's malign interference began. Cultural decolonisation was at work in the processes of remembering, or perhaps more accurately inventing, an indigenous Irish culture.[77]

For many leaders of the Irish cultural revival, ancient remnants such as the Inishbofin skulls symbolised this lost Celtic past. The skulls represented not primitive, brutish savageness or people not evolved into full human beings (a common trope in craniological studies of the time undertaken elsewhere) but, instead, a noble, refined, spiritual, even peaceful, people, who had evolved away from the impulsive life of the savage without being tainted, polluted and corrupted by British oppression, plantations and the intermingling of gene pools. The skulls represented a missing link between ancient and modern. Yet the theft of the skulls by English or Anglo-Irish anthropologists hailing from Dublin only intensified the antagonism felt towards British influence and the ongoing dehumanisation of the colonised.

In light of all of this, writers, artists and other cultural figures visited the islands off Ireland's barren west coast hoping to recover oral traditions of folklore and history, for here was the basis of an authentically Irish identity that might invigorate a newly independent country in the future. Prominent in the culture of these islands were old sagas, folk tales, myths and stories about exotic creatures such as fairies. The traditions and people of the west of Ireland were truly Irish. One great irony is that many of those leading the way in the cultural revival had elite Anglo-Irish backgrounds. But regardless, in these remote, desolate, rock-strewn islands, Ireland would be reborn. Geographically and spiritually, these islands were as far away from England as it was possible for Irish soil to be. The ruins and remains scattered across the islands provided a sense of continuity with an imagined Ireland that had existed before Viking and British conquest, places untouched by historical processes of disenchantment.[78]

Of course, a somewhat caricatured interpretation of Gaelicness was being created, one just as fictional as the craniologists' renderings of the ancients, but the reconstruction of ancient Irish life was just as much a political as a cultural project. Whereas Haddon reduced ancient people to dry lists of measurements, for more romantically inclined people, the skulls of Inishbofin brought to life premodern simplicity and ancient wisdom, a good model for the type of person who would populate a newly independent Ireland freed after centuries in British shackles.[79] More broadly in western counties, there was a growing cultural pessimism often directed at cities and a general feeling that the west was degenerating rather than progressing or evolving positively. This led to an idealisation of rural life, evident in much of the Irish cultural revival. In Ireland, these ideas intertwined with the urge for de-anglicisation.

John Millington Synge was a key figure in the Irish cultural, and specifically literary, revival. His best-known play, *The Playboy of the Western World* (1907), was angrily received due to its depiction of Irish peasants, so much so that during its initial run audiences famously rioted at the Abbey Theatre, Dublin, at the time the heart of the city's cultural life. Synge hailed from a wealthy, Protestant, Anglo-Irish family, landed gentry in Co. Wicklow. While living in France in 1895 he met William Butler Yeats, one of Ireland's foremost literary figures, who urged him to visit the Aran Islands. Synge arrived there in 1898 and for the next four years visited often, collecting stories and folklore while perfecting his Irish-language literacy. He found life on the islands to be the perfect antidote to modernity and began to publish regular accounts of life there in the *New Ireland Review*, later collated into a book, *The Aran Islands*, published

Residents of the Aran Islands around the turn of the twentieth century.

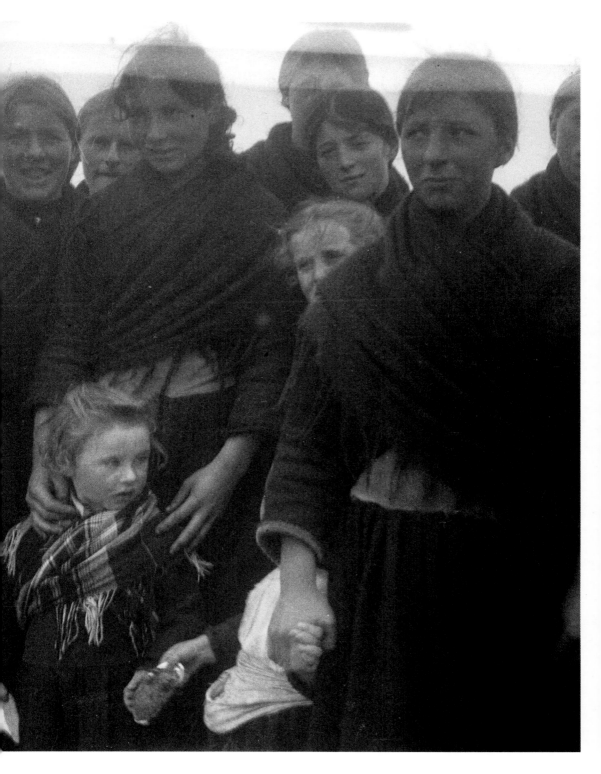

in 1907. Synge believed that beneath the islanders' Catholicism could still be discerned a substratum of the pagan beliefs of their ancestors. Many of his subsequent plays were based on his experiences in the Aran Islands.

Depicting the islanders as untainted by modernity, Synge wrote that in Inishmaan the 'absence of the heavy boot of Europe has preserved to these people the agile walk of the wild animal, while the general simplicity of their lives has given them many other points of physical perfection'. For him, it was a place where 'a touch of the refinement of old societies is blended, with singular effect, among the qualities of the wild animal'. Interestingly, Synge also wrote that 'few of the people, however, are sufficiently used to modern time to understand in more than a vague way the convention of the hours, and when I tell them what o'clock it is by my watch they are not satisfied, and ask how long is left them before the twilight'.[80]

The tone of these romanticised accounts could not have been further from the impenetrable calculations of the craniologists, who proved incapable of infusing their objects of study with much humanity or dignity, let alone romantic nuance. Perhaps this inspired Synge, in *The Playboy of the Western World*, to poke fun at the Dublin-based anthropologists' penchant for skull collecting. One character, Jimmy Farrell, asks his farmer friend Philly Cullen: 'Did you never hear of the skulls they have in the city of Dublin, ranged out like blue jugs in a cabin of Connaught ... They have them there making a show of the great people there was one time walking the world. White skulls and black skulls and yellow skulls, and some with full teeth, and some haven't only but one.'[81] The impression given is that Synge was not overly impressed.[82]

Of course, the islanders had stronger reasons than the cultural revivalists for disliking the anthropologists. In 1893, another anthropologist, Charles R. Browne, tried to steal more skulls from the monastery, although by then the islanders had grown wiser. Pre-empting the theft, they hid the skulls in a secret location. As an alternative, Browne was forced to rely upon taking photographs and surreptitiously observing passers-by. He commented upon the 'shyness of the people', 'the strong aversion shown by many people to having their portraits taken' and the problems identifying hair colour when all the women wore a shawl, 'which was drawn more closely on the approach of a stranger'.

In these comments, the reader gets the impression of considerable distrust towards the scientific visitors, although Browne seems oblivious to the repulsion felt towards him among the 'natives'.[83] For the skulls had formed part of those natives' personal heritage, something which the dry quantifications of the craniologists could never successfully capture and comprehend. It was these personal, cultural meanings attached to the Inishbofin skulls that remained of prime importance in the twenty-first-century debates surrounding their return from Trinity. This fascination with faces, heads and skulls remains evident in our captivation with the preserved features of Clonycavan Man, the presumptions we make about red-haired Irish people and our morbid fascination with historical beheadings. They are more than just heads and skulls and our ideas about this area of the body are deeply intertwined with our sense of identity – in this case, a strong sense of Irish identity.

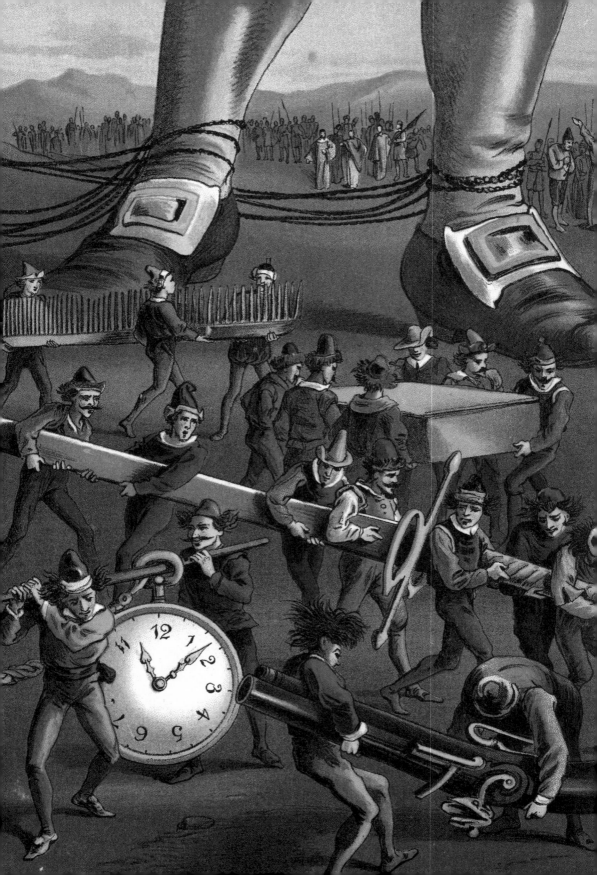

CHAPTER 2

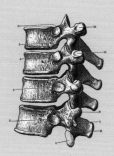

HEIGHT

People and beings of unusual height, whether small or tall, have played an important role in Irish popular culture and beliefs. The Giant's Causeway, Brian Boru's Harp, fairies, leprechauns – all feature prominently in the imagery that defines Ireland, whether that's the harp on the side of a pint of Guinness or the leprechaun outfits that bedeck the streets of Dublin every St Patrick's Day. Ireland has an international reputation as a land still enchanted, an island in which ancient mysteries and beliefs can be uncovered by visitors. Looking at Irish history through the lens of ideas about height reveals much about ancient Irish beliefs, the nature of being a king and warrior in premodern Ireland, how unusual bodies were both medicalised and put on display (alive or dead) in the eighteenth century and the persistence of folklore well into the twentieth century.

For millennia, the Irish have held strong beliefs that giants were responsible for building striking landmarks such as the unique rock formations that characterise the island's north coast. Such ideas made sense at a time before modern geological knowledge. Gradually, though, over time, as a new secular world came into being, driven by empiricism and science, people of unusual height became characterised as physically disabled. Concern about their poor health was not altogether unfounded. The giant Irish people of the eighteenth and nineteenth centuries did indeed tend to die at a young age due to height-related health complaints. Still, this pathologisation of unusually sized people, tall or short, contrasted sharply with earlier mythical ideas about strong, heroic giants and powerful fairies and dwarves.

GIANTS IN IRISH MYTHOLOGY

Was there an ancient world full of giants? Irish folklore abounds with tales of monstrously tall people believed to have built aspects of the natural landscape. Precisely how the Celtic Irish regarded their divinities is unclear, but it seems that they connected them with specific places considered worthy of reverence.

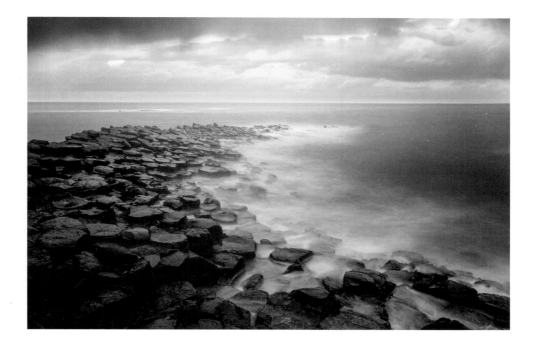

This is certainly the case for Irish folklore's most famous giant, Finn Mac Cuamhail (McCool), who, according to legend, built the famous Giant's Causeway in Co. Antrim.

The world-famous Giant's Causeway.

At the time, so the story goes, a bad-tempered Scottish giant named Benandonner was making a claim for Ireland. Enraged, Finn angrily threw boulders into the sea. Noting that their tips remained poking out of the water, Finn got the idea to use the boulders to pave a bridge (or causeway) leading from Ireland's northeast coast to Scotland's Isle of Staffa. When he landed in Scotland, he intended to challenge his rival to a duel over Ireland's fate. Finn was in for a surprise. Benandonner turned out to be exceptionally gigantic, even by giant standards. Violence and force were unlikely to work. Finn hastily retreated across the causeway.

Finn then came up with a plan which required his wife, Sadhbh, to disguise him as a baby in a cradle. This might seem like a strange request, but when

Benandonner arrived, he came across Sadhbh tending to her large 'baby' and asked himself: 'If that's the size of Finn's baby, just how big will Finn be?' In some accounts of the legend, Benandonner reached into the cradle to play with the 'baby', providing Finn with an opportunity to bite off four of his fingers. Benandonner raced back to Scotland, tearing away bits of the causeway as he fled, fearing that even more of these fearsome Irish giants might be following him. As Benandonner fled, Finn laughed, scooped out a large clump of land and flung this at his rival. After falling into the sea, this clump of land became the Isle of Man, and the void became Lough Neagh. Located 20 miles west of Belfast, Lough Neagh is the largest lake on the island of Ireland and in the United Kingdom.[1]

Walking along the Giant's Causeway today, it's easy to imagine why the ancient Celts believed that the site of natural beauty was the work of some kind of non-human. The Giant's Causeway consists of about 40,000 interlocking basalt columns. The tops of these columns resemble stepping stones that lead from the cliff foot and disappear into the sea. Most of the columns are hexagonal, having an order and logic to them which does indeed give the impression of being unnaturally created. The tallest of these is 12 metres (39 feet) in height. Identical basalt columns can be found at Fingal's Cave on Staffa, and it made sense to the ancient mind that the two natural wonders were created alongside each other. The modern explanation is that the Giant's Causeway is the result of an ancient volcanic explosion that occurred 60 million years ago. The volcanic lava quickly cooled, leaving the columns still spread across the northern Irish coastline.

Finn Mac Cuamhail is also associated with other natural Irish features. The Bog of Allen, located in the middle of Ireland, covers 1,000 square kilometres. It contains the Hill of Allen, thought to have been home to Finn and his band of warrior giants, the Fianna. In ancient Ireland, the Fianna were the protectors of the high king. Mythology depicts them as 50-foot-tall giants with long, flowing blond hair. In ancient times, the bog covered most of the Irish midlands, and even today it still stretches

An illustration of Finn Mac Cuamhail seated in a banquet hall, watching the Fianna fight.

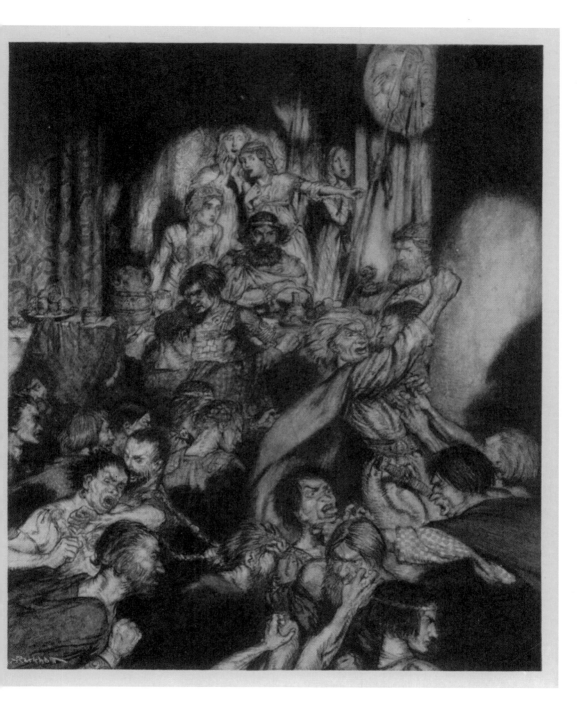

across counties Offaly, Kildare and Laois. (People from the midlands are still regularly nicknamed 'boggers', although calling them by this name causes considerable offence.)

Finn built a giant fortress on the Hill of Allen and used the surrounding raised boglands as a training ground for his Fianna warriors, who had acres of unused land to practise tossing giant rocks for miles. Nowadays, the hill is a few miles from Newbridge. If visitors travel north to Howth Castle, they might stumble across a huge dolmen (a stone megalithic tomb) rumoured to be one of the great rocks thrown from the Bog of Allen towards Dublin Bay. The capstone weighs 70 tonnes and dates from around 1500 BC. How the ancients transported such heavy rocks remains a mystery. Perhaps it was the work of a giant after all? Curiously, situated at the top of the Hill of Allen is a circular folly tower built in 1863. While constructing this tower, workers came across a large coffin containing gigantic human bones, which were subsequently reburied on the site. Some speculate that these were the remains of Finn Mac Cuamhail.[2]

When strolling along the banks of the River Lagan in Belfast, visitors encounter a strange statue: a large colourful blue fish. This is the Salmon of Knowledge. According to folklore, there once lived an ordinary salmon who happened to eat nine hazelnuts which had fallen into the Well of Wisdom. Much to its surprise, the salmon gained all the world's knowledge. This would be passed on to anyone who caught and ate the now highly intelligent fish. A poet named Finn Eces (or Finegas) spent seven years fishing for this salmon. When he eventually caught it, he instructed his servant, the young Finn Mac Cuamhail, to cook, but not eat, the knowledgeable fish. While cooking, Finn touched the fish with his finger to check if it was cooked and burned his finger on a drop of boiling-hot fish fat. Sucking his thumb to relieve the pain passed all of the salmon's knowledge to young Finn. Despite his seven wasted years of fishing, Finn Eces forgave Finn and told him he could eat the rest of the fish. His knowledge and wisdom later allowed Finn to become the leader of the Fianna.[3]

Finn is usually presented as a hero, but other giants, such as Balor of the Evil Eye, were malicious. Balor was the chief of a demon race of Fomorians.

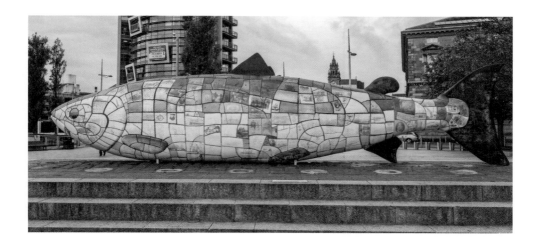

Monstrous, hideous-looking creatures, the Fomorians were a race of supernatural giants, and also one of the earliest races said to have invaded and settled in Ireland. It remains uncertain whether the Fomorians came from the sea or the underworld.

Statue of the Salmon of Knowledge, located in Belfast's city centre.

Some accounts depict them as having only one eye, leg and arm, while others depict them as having the bodies of human beings but the heads of goats. They took part in the mythical first battle of Moytura in Co. Sligo and then in a second battle in the same place which occurred 30 years afterwards. This is where the Fomorians were subdued and Balor met his fate.

While young, Balor happened to glance into a potion being brewed by his father's druids. The fumes caused him to grow a huge, poisonous evil eye, which could only be covered by seven heavy eyelids. It took four strong men to open the eyelids. The eye's gaze killed anything within its sight. For a while, Balor, afraid of no one, ruled tyrannically in Ireland. The only thing that scared Balor was a prophecy that he would one day be killed at the hands of his own grandson. To escape this fate, Balor imprisoned his only daughter, Ethniu, in a tower, banishing her and forbidding her from all sexual contact with men. Despite his staunch efforts to avoid the possibility of having a grandson, Balor's daughter fell in love with a man named Cian who first arrived at the tower to

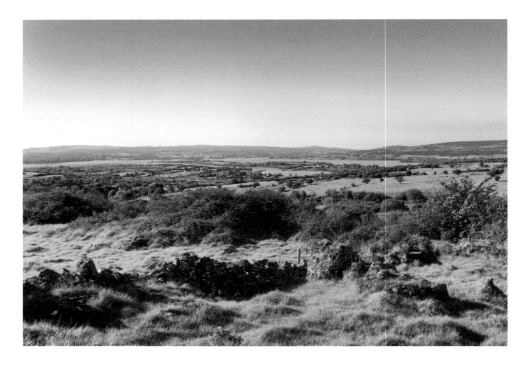

The Giant's Grave, Co. Sligo, at the site of the mythical Battle of Moytura.

take back a magical cow which Balor himself, sealing his fate, had stolen. They fell in love instantly and had three children, one of whom was named Lugh. Infuriated, Balor mercilessly ordered the children to be drowned, but Lugh survived by chance and was raised secretly. The prophecy came true, and Lugh eventually killed Balor at the Second Battle of Moytura with a spear through the evil eye. Still existing there is the Giant's Grave, built between 4500 and 2500 BC and said to hold the remains of a giant killed in this second battle. Perhaps Balor is buried here.[4]

Few people today would believe that all of this actually happened, but the stories, legends and tales clearly held meaning for the ancient Irish and their understanding of the world. The Celts were a deeply spiritual people. They believed the gods to be everywhere, presiding over every aspect of life. They associated particular rivers, springs, lakes, forests and mountains with certain gods. Each river was dedicated to a goddess to ensure the land remained fertile. The names of rivers like Shannon and Boyne refer to ancient fertility goddesses. Lugh became one of the greatest gods and was associated with justice, oath-keeping and nobility.[5]

Early Irish myths and stories probably originated in prehistoric times, stories that are now largely lost to us. For centuries, they were transmitted orally before eventually being written down in manuscripts by Christian monks. It's notoriously hard to figure out whether the characters featured in the stories are real or fantasy, gods or mortals. The two worlds are intertwined: reality, magic and fantasy all mingle. We have a richer record of Irish Celtic mythology than other strands of Celtic culture because Ireland, unlike most of Europe, was not colonised by the Romans, so its culture continued to thrive uninterrupted. Ireland remained characteristically 'Celtic' until Christianity arrived in the fifth and sixth centuries AD, and the stories seem to have been transcribed from the seventh century on.[6] The Irish body of myths is among the largest and best preserved of the various branches of Celtic mythology and is split into the 'mythological', 'Ulster', 'Fianna' and 'Kings' cycles.[7]

The scientists who discovered the gigantism gene in DNA centuries later speculated that the ancient belief in giants may hold a grain of truth after all. In ancient Ireland, some people really did tower above others.[8] In the twenty-first century, clinicians diagnose exceptionally tall individuals with acromegaly, or acromegalic gigantism, a hormone disorder that results in excessive growth of the human body. However, the belief in a world of supernatural beings, some god-like, allowed the ancient Celts to develop other explanations and to reflect upon those of exceptionally large build with wonder, linking them to anomalies and unusual structures in the natural world which surrounded them, such as the Giant's Causeway.

IRISH GIANTS

Those living in the eighteenth century felt a curious fascination with the world. Improved global transportation, the arrival of sophisticated printing presses (now powered by the efficient piston steam engine) and the introduction of newspapers and cheap books offered readers images and descriptions of all manner of people, creatures and places across the world.[9] A new genre of travel writing emerged in which voyaging authors recorded their impressions of the people and places whom they had encountered for readers back home.[10] The world became aware of the Giant's Causeway in 1693 when Richard Bulkeley, a fellow of Trinity College Dublin, presented a paper on his visits to the site. It acquired even more fame when Dublin artist Susanna Drury presented her watercolour paintings of the causeway to the Royal Dublin Society in 1740, which were later engraved. From here on, the causeway featured prominently in Irish travel writing. In the nineteenth century, it became a popular tourist attraction when a tramway opened connecting Portrush, the Giant's Causeway and Bushmills, and it remains so today.[11]

Unusual-looking humans prompted intrigue and fascination, and these included people of uncommon height. Born in 1761 in Littlebridge, a hamlet on the border of counties Derry and Tyrone, Charles Byrne was one such real-life giant whose extraordinary height attracted considerable public interest

As he grew up, it became apparent that something was unusual about his appearance. He kept on growing and growing and became exceptionally tall, towering above all the other boys of his age. The local community speculated that Byrne must have been conceived on top of a haystack, a traditional explanation for a person's great height. In the eighteenth century, people were generally smaller than us, but even by today's standards, Byrne was gargantuan. He was 7 feet 7 inches tall. (At the time, rumours circulated that he was closer to 8 feet 4 inches.)

Byrne died in 1783, at the tragically young age of 22. Nonetheless, he led a packed life. During his short lifetime, he met King George III and became a celebrity, and in the final year of his life, he lived in London entertaining large audiences in theatres in Piccadilly and Charing Cross. Londoners described him as a 'modern living Colossus' and a 'wonderful Irish giant'. His affable and likeable nature probably helped his reputation. He even inspired a hit London stage show: *The Giant's Causeway*. However, Byrne suffered from poor health. One fateful evening, while drinking in his local pub, the Black Horse, he was pickpocketed. His life savings of £700 were gone. The theft exacerbated his failing health; his drinking habits spiralled. Two months later, Byrne died in his home at Cockspur Street, Charing Cross.

This was not the end of Byrne's story. In fact, his death had only just begun. Also living in London at the time was a famed Scottish surgeon named John Hunter, one of a lineage of prominent medical men. Hunter owned a private museum and was always on the lookout for unusual specimens to display there. The two men had met and Hunter, noticing the friendly giant's precarious health, offered to pay Byrne (in advance) for his corpse. As his health declined further, Byrne suspected that Hunter was planning to snatch his body upon death, dissect it and display the remains in his museum. Considering this a deeply undesirable fate, Byrne arranged with his closest friends for his body to be sealed in a lead coffin, taken to Margate and buried at sea. Unbeknown to Byrne, Hunter caught wind of these plans and intercepted the coffin (measuring 9 feet 4 inches) en route to Margate. (Another story tells us that Hunter bribed one of Byrne's friends with £500 to replace the corpse in the coffin with heavy rocks.)

As Byrne had anxiously predicted, Hunter stripped his corpse of flesh and, four years later, displayed the skeleton in his Hunterian Museum for visitors to gaze upon. Byrne remained on display from 1799 until 2023.[12] In 1998, novelist Hilary Mantel published a fictionalised account of the fraught relationship between Byrne and Hunter, entitled *The Giant, O'Brien*. O'Brien is portrayed as a storyteller and lover of folk tales who transitions from speaking Irish to English throughout the novel, whereas Hunter is depicted as a rational, science-obsessed man with an insatiable desire for experimenting upon humans and animals, both living and dead.[13]

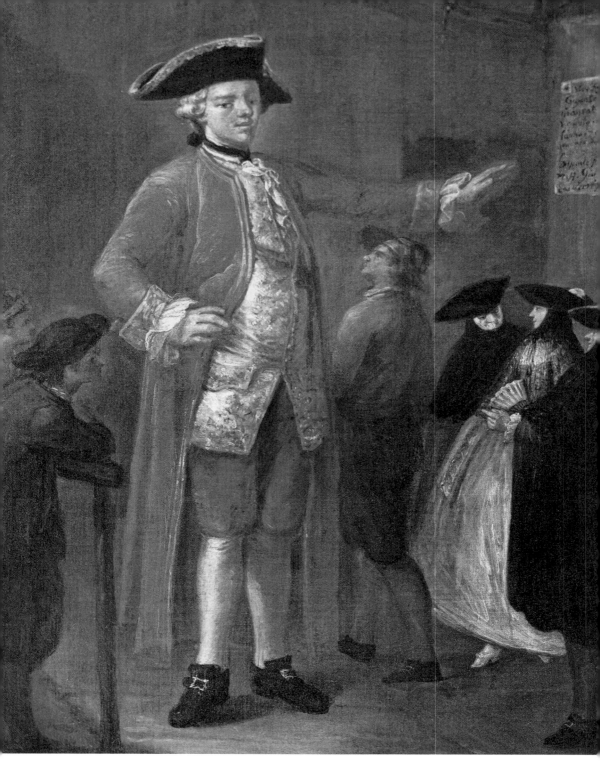

Cornelius Magrath, an eighteenth-
century Irish giant.

In 2011, a group of scientists investigated a sample of Byrne's DNA and discovered that he had an extremely rare mutation in his AIP gene that can play a role in causing pituitary tumours, the illness thought to have killed him.[14] The scientists had another reason for examining his body. A small number of people in Ireland still live today with this genetic mutation and share family histories of pituitary disorders. The scientists thought that investigating Byrne's preserved skeleton might help shed light on their predicament. They concluded that he and these families all shared a common ancestor who lived in Ireland sometime around AD 500. Interestingly, Byrne is sometimes thought to have been a relative of a number of other giants, including the Knipe twins from Magherafelt and Patrick Cotter O'Brien from Cork.

In contrast to ancient times, when giants were looked upon with wonder and marvel, almost as heroic individuals, people in the eighteenth century were more likely to view the very tall as sick, unhealthy people. A pathological language of sickness and weakness replaced heroic legends. A telling comment was made by encyclopedist Robert Chambers in 1864:

> Of the ancient giants it is said that they were mighty men of valour, their strength being commensurate with their proportions. But the modern giants are generally a sickly, knock-kneed, splay-footed, shambling race, feeble in both mental and bodily organisation.[15]

One of these sickly giants, Cornelius Magrath, was born near Nenagh, Co. Tipperary, in 1736. When he turned 15, Cornelius was seized with pains in his limbs. According to some rumours, he grew by 21 inches in the space of a year. (In reality, he was around 7 feet 5 inches.) As with Charles Byrne, the health problems associated with abnormal height struck in the teenage years. Writhing in agony, he travelled to Youghal, Co. Cork, in 1752 to receive saltwater treatments to alleviate the distressingly painful symptoms caused by his rapid growth. For a few months, he stayed at the home of Dr Berkeley, Bishop of Cloyne, until he recovered the full use of his limbs. According to contemporary accounts, 'his hands were as large as a middling shoulder of mutton, and the last of his shoe, which he carried about with him, measured fifteen inches'. One peculiar, and probably untrue, story is that the Bishop of Cloyne changed Magrath's diet from the despised potato diet into a more 'civilised' one, and his health greatly improved in the space of a month, by which time he was able to walk without pain once again.

When back on his feet, Magrath found that crowds of fascinated people were following him around. Surprised that so many people wanted to stand there and look at him, Magrath decided to make himself a living by exhibiting himself. Like Charles Byrne, he moved to England, and by 1753, Magrath was a huge star in London, described as 'the only representation in the world of the ancient and magnificent giants of that kingdom [Ireland]'. A contemporary description from London reads as follows:

> There is now in this city one Cornelius Magrath, a boy of 15 years 11 months old, of a most gigantic stature, being exactly 7 feet 9 inches three quarters high. He is clumsy made, talks boyish and simple. He came hither from Youghal where he has been a year going into saltwater for rheumatic pains which almost crippled him, which the physicians now say were growing pains for he is grown to the monstrous size he is of within these twelve months.

We have two images of Magrath. One depicts him as a well-built, well-proportioned, straight-limbed man, standing proudly tall. It was painted by Venetian artist Pietro Longhi in 1757 when Cornelius was aged 20 and entitled *True Portrait of the Giant Cornelio Magrat, the Irishman*. Longhi presented Magrath as a man with considerable physical dignity. However, D.J. Cunningham, a Dublin-based anatomy professor, later pointed out that in reality Magrath 'must have possessed a most repulsive face, while his limb bones indicate in the clearest manner that he was afflicted with the condition known as knock-knee and could not possibly extend his arm in the manner indicated in the drawing'. It has also been speculated that Magrath suffered severe sight loss due to his condition, possibly even blindness. A German engraving shows him comically towering above a smaller Prussian soldier. By this stage, Magrath was travelling across Europe.

Magrath's health declined, and he decided to return to Ireland. He had made friends with some students from Trinity College, but when he died aged just 23 from a fall (presumably because of his weak limbs), the students stole his body. Magrath was dissected, his bones were preserved and his skeleton was put on indefinite display at Trinity College. A fate all too common for giants, it seems. In the 1890s, Cunningham observed that 'it is questionable if there is a museum specimen in Dublin which is better known, or which has excited a wider interest, than the skeleton of Cornelius Magrath'. Cunningham was particularly interested in examining Magrath's skeleton, which had then been displayed for 131 years, as acromegaly had recently been identified as a growth-related disease, and Cunningham thought that the preserved giant skeletons might offer clues to aid diagnosis and treatment. He also visited Charles Byrne's skeleton.[16]

The skeleton had not been well cared for. Infuriated, Cunningham wrote that 'some museum assistant ... seems to have taken the skeleton particularly asunder and subjected it to shocking usage'. To mask the skeleton's shoddy treatment, the museum assistant had given Magrath a coat of paint followed by several coats of varnish. 'So thick was this covering that it completely concealed the essential features of the skeleton', complained Cunningham, who spent weeks carefully removing the layers of paint and varnish. Much to his chagrin, he discovered that many of Magrath's bones had been lost and a sloppy attempt had been made to replace them 'in the most reckless and ignorant manner'. Magrath's left thumb contained a foot bone that had once belonged to someone else. Fingers had been transplanted from other skeletons. The end of some of the longer bones had been sawn off. Cunningham removed the borrowed bones and replaced them with wood models. The skeleton was restored. To aid this process, Cunningham went over to visit Charles Byrne's skeleton, which he noted had fewer deformities.[17]

Another exceptionally tall Irishman, Patrick Cotter, grew over 8 feet tall. Born in Kinsale, Co. Cork, in 1761 to parents of ordinary height, he originally trained as a bricklayer, but at age 18, a showman bought him from his father. The showman promised to pay Cotter £50 per annum, but he found himself being exhibited in Bristol with no remuneration other than food, clothing and lodging. As a punishment for bitterly complaining, the showman accused Cotter of being in debt, and he was thrown unfairly into a debtor's prison. Until 1869, people could be imprisoned simply for being accused of being in debt. The showman hoped that Cotter would cave in and agree to work without pay. But Cotter's distressing situation came to the attention of a gentleman in the city, possibly William Watts, who sympathised and proved the contract to be illegal. Once again free, Cotter decided to exhibit himself for his own profit. In his first three days, he earned £30.

By the nineteenth century, the great fairs were in decline. Once glorious trading centres, they had degenerated into raucous, riotous places. (Donnybrook Fair in Dublin was among Ireland's most famous fairs.) Nonetheless, they still offered opportunities for individuals like Cotter, with their unusually shaped bodies, to self-exhibit as part of a so-called 'freak show'.

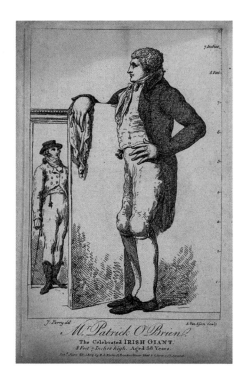

Above Patrick Cotter O'Brien, the Irish-born Bristol giant.

Opposite Patrick Cotter O'Brien and Count Burowlaski, a Polish-born dwarf and musician.

Cotter became a familiar figure at the St Bartholomew annual fair, which had thrived for 700 years. He appended O'Brien to his stage name, to become Patrick Cotter O'Brien. People with the surname O'Brien are believed to descend from Brian Boru, an Irish king who lived between

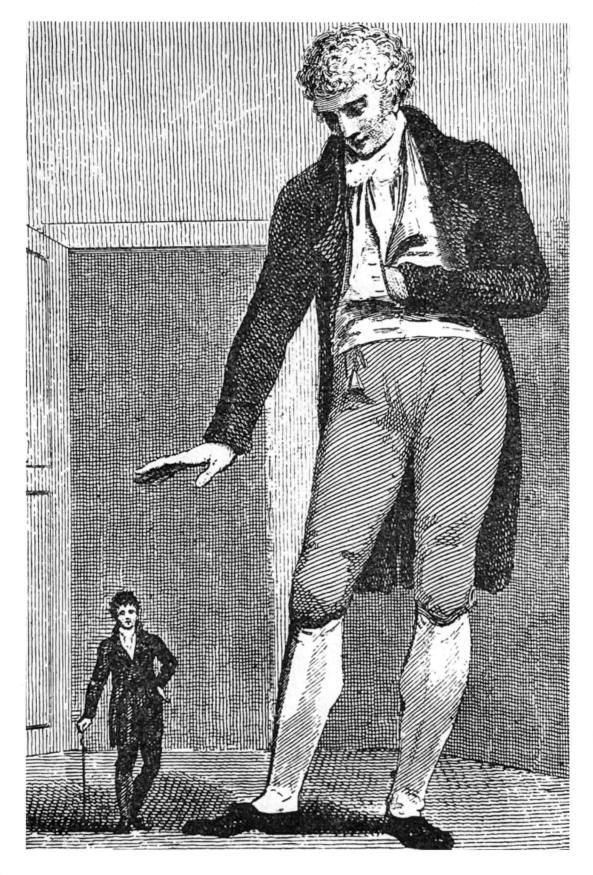

c.941 and 1014 and was known for many things, including being gigantic. Cotter claimed (falsely) that Brian Boru had been 9 feet tall and that his royal ancestry explained his own tall height. (Charles Byrne also claimed to be an O'Brien, although he reportedly resented Cotter's competitive presence as another 'Irish Giant'.) In his publicity, Cotter claimed to be a 'lineal descendant of the old puissant King Brien Boreau [sic] and has in person and appearance all the similarities of that great and grand potentate. It is remarkable of this family, that, however various the revolutions in point of fortune and alliance, the lineal descendants thereof have been favoured by Providence with the original size and stature which have been so peculiar to their family.'

Cotter became wealthy from his stage shows and spent his adult life living in Bristol. He was described as having 'less imbecility of mind than the generality of overgrown persons, but all the weakness of body by which they are characterised'. In his later years, he walked with difficulty and felt much pain when sitting down or standing up. When he died in 1806, aged 47, it proved impossible to find a hearse that could accommodate his 8-foot-4-inch lead-encased casket. Fourteen men were needed to carry his coffin to its grave. Cotter requested that his body be entombed in 12 feet of solid rock to prevent exhumation for medical research, fearing that his body, like those of other giants, would fall into the hands of the anatomists. His deep grave was cut beneath the floor of the Roman Catholic Chapel in Trenchard Street, Bristol. Up to 200 people reportedly attended the funeral. Iron bars were embedded in the concrete to help render the grave impenetrable.

Unusually for a giant, Cotter's grave remained undisturbed for a century until March 1906 when a group of workmen laying drains accidentally discovered it. Cotter's remains were measured and photographed and then reburied. In 1972, his remains were once again examined.[18] It was common for friends to collect the unusually large belongings of giants. Cotter's giant boots are still displayed at the Kinsale Museum. Other souvenirs taken included his enormous stockings, a large watch, an oversized pair of glasses and an enormously large gold ring, 1.75 inches in diameter, with an Irish harp pictured upon it. Household items were also collected from Patrick's home including an armchair measuring 25 inches across, a knife 24 inches in length, and an accompanying fork 19 inches in length.[19]

While the majority of famous Irish giants were men, Mary Murphy was the 'Portrush Giantess'. Over 7 feet tall, she was described as attractive and well-proportioned. Despite her gigantic height, Mary was not short of suitors. One local man fell in love with her, but she eventually settled for a French sea captain who passed through the local port and lured her with promises of silks, finery and a life of adventure. After marrying her, he gave up his life at sea and toured the countryside exhibiting Murphy as a freak show attraction. He dressed her in high heels and a hat to make her appear even taller. Murphy reportedly danced an Irish jig and sang a folksong for King William and Queen Mary of England, who paid her a guinea, a fee which her husband probably enjoyed spending. The last mention of Murphy in the historical record is of her being exhibited at a Paris show in 1701. By then, her husband had left her, and she died destitute in France. The young Portrush man who had once fallen in love with Murphy lived as a hermit in a hut near the Giant's Causeway and died of a broken heart.[20]

It's difficult to reach a firm opinion on the various tall Irish people who exhibited themselves in the eighteenth and nineteenth centuries. They were well-loved, charismatic individuals, immensely popular with the many people whom they met. However, the giants led tragically short lives diminished by poor physical and mental health. Nowadays, we would describe those in poorer health as suffering from physical disabilities, which raises questions about the unscrupulous nature of 'freak show' organisers, who actively sought out unusually shaped people and took advantage of their physical misfortune to accumulate profit. Yet, it's also possible to view the giants as individuals who became empowered, and sometimes very wealthy, by putting themselves on display in a society which usually hid disabled people away from public view.[21]

Questions still linger today about what to do with the large skeletons eagerly collected by the anatomists. Even today, Charles Byrne's exceptionally tall skeleton still fascinates. His remains are periodically examined by scientists hoping to find clues about height-related problems. They have confirmed, using modern-day insights, that Byrne had an enlarged pituitary fossa and probably died from a pituitary tumour. In the 2010s, a campaign was mounted to end the unethical display of Byrne's body and to bury it either at sea or at the Giant's Grave. The campaign was led by academic Thomas Muinzer, medical ethicist Len Doyal and Hilary Mantel, the aforementioned author of the novel about the giant man. There seemed to be little reason why a London museum would even want to continue hoarding the centuries-old skeleton of an unfortunate Irish man.[22]

On 11 January 2023, the Hunterian Museum officially retired the skeleton from public display and replaced it with an oil portrait of the bodysnatching surgeon, John Hunter, although even this portrait still featured the feet of Byrne's skeleton hanging above Hunter in the corner. Back in Ireland, Trinity College Dublin refuses to release Cornelius Magrath's giant skeleton as it continues to 'inspire scholarship' in its students, although many people question the value of retaining Cornelius's remains. Trinity's students' union favours the respectful burial of the remains.[23]

BRIAN BORU

So, who was Brian Boru, the tall man whose legendary height Patrick Cotter used so effectively in publicity for his shows? Brian Boru was an Irish high king who lived between 941 and 1014 – to the age of 73, a spectacularly long life by the standards of the time. Although Patrick claimed that Brian had stood 9 feet tall, this was probably an exaggeration.

'High king' was a royal title in Gaelic Ireland held by whoever claimed to be the lord of all Ireland. The high king ruled from the Hill of Tara, an ancient ceremonial site in Co. Meath which still contains the remains of 20 ancient monuments, the oldest of which is a Neolithic passage tomb built around 3200 BC.

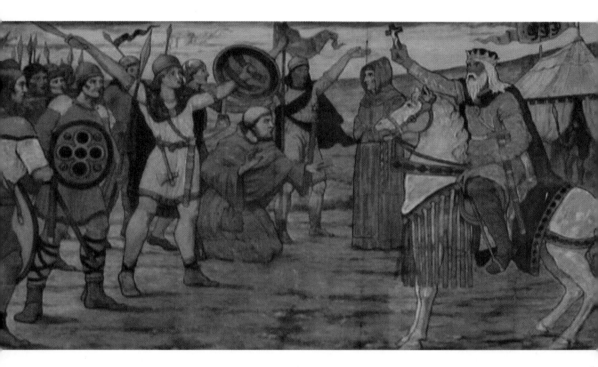

The idea of a national king of Ireland was first recorded in the seventh century, although in practice the king usually only held real power in his own region, lacking sufficient authority to dominate the entire island. The Uí Néill dynasty, which claimed descent from Niall Noígíallach, a king of Tara who died around AD 405, dominated the island until it was overthrown by Brian Boru. After making himself king of Munster, he subjugated Leinster and then declared himself high king. He founded the O'Brien dynasty, which produced around thirty monarchs between the tenth century and 1542.

The victory of Brian Boru.

Brian Boru is best known for defeating the Vikings after centuries of raids, plundering and attempts at conquering the island. The Vikings were a seafaring people from Scandinavia who raided, pirated, traded and settled throughout parts of Europe between the eighth and eleventh centuries. Ireland was not exempt, and Vikings started by plundering islands on the north and

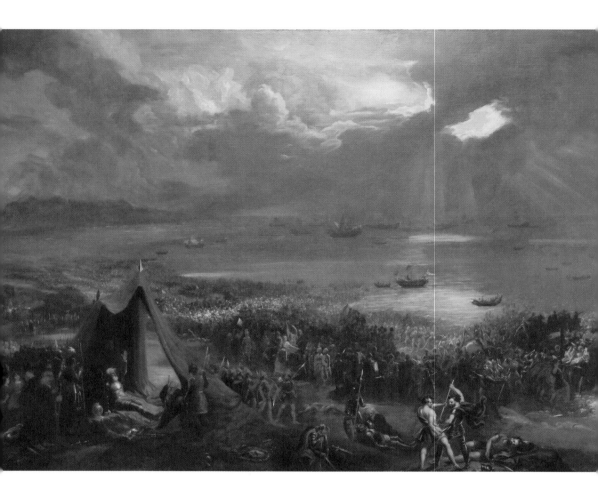

Painting of the Battle
of Clontarf.

west coast from 795. They had a reputation for targeting monasteries to steal their valuable treasures. Viking ships were fast, effective and manoeuvrable, with a small draft. Ireland is replete with rivers flowing into its surrounding seas, which allowed Viking fleets easy access even to inland areas.

As time passed, the Vikings decided to settle. In 841, Dublin was established as one of the Vikings' fortified bases or 'long-ports'. Under Olaf Guthfrithson, Dublin grew into a substantial commercial centre in the mid-tenth century, although it was constantly attacked by the Gaelic Irish. Other new settlements included Waterford, Limerick, Cork and Wexford, Ireland's first large towns. Most of Ireland remained primarily rural, but these impressive coastal urban centres served as important ports and international trading points.

Throughout the ninth century, the Vikings moved further inland using their increasingly large, powerful fleets. In 837, a fleet of 60 longships carried 1,500 Vikings up the River Liffey, while another of similar size traversed the River Boyne, attacking inland areas. Great monastic towns such as Armagh and Clonard were plundered. By 849, Vikings from Denmark were not only attacking the Irish but also the more established Vikings of Norwegian origin. Decades of fighting followed. The Vikings were forced to leave Dublin in 902. However, a new Viking fleet entered Waterford in 914, commencing the so-called Second Viking Age. The Vikings found it much easier to conquer countries such as England and France which had a strong centralised government. In contrast, Ireland was composed of over 150 different kingdoms, each ruling over small territories, making it impossible to gain full political control over the island.

It was during the Second Viking Age that Brian entered the story. It's fair to say that he had an axe to grind with the Vikings. While young, a group of marauding Vikings had plundered his own home and killed his mother. Brian's life took on a new direction when, shortly after this fateful incident, he was sent to a monastery on Innisfallen, an island in Lough Leane, near Killarney, to study Latin. While studying there, he became fascinated by Julius Caesar's battles and absorbed ideas on successful battlefield strategies. In 951, Brian's father, king of the Dal gCais (the tribe who dominated Munster), was killed by

Vikings, and his brother Mahon succeeded him as king. Brian was horrified when his brother formed a pact with the Vikings, although they later reconciled. Following Mahon's death, Brian assumed the title of king.

A reputation for being tall helped warring leaders instil fear among their enemies, and Brian's impressive height, combined with his military planning skills, must have contributed to his fearsome reputation. Brian could reportedly wield a sword over half his height, with a hilt of alloyed gold and set with jewels. He defeated the Vikings in Munster and reached an agreement with Máel Sechnaill II, king of Tara, that he would rule the south of Ireland, leaving the north to Máel. Brian and Máel collaborated on a raid against the Dublin Vikings in 998. In 1000, Brian put down a revolt by the Dublin Vikings, which forced Máel to acknowledge him as the high king of all Ireland.

A showdown between Brian and the Vikings eventually took place. Clontarf is nowadays an affluent coastal suburb of north Dublin, but on 23 April 1014 it was the site of a fierce battle. Brian's forces fought a Norse–Irish alliance of Sigtrygg Silkbeard (king of Dublin), Máel Mórda mac Murchada (king of Leinster) and a Viking army from overseas led by Sigurd of Orkney and Brodir of Mann. The fighting lasted all day and was so fierce that only 100 Connacht men and 20 Dublin men survived. The Vikings were better armed and wore mail for protection, but the Irish had the advantage of using smaller spears, which they could hurl at the enemy, and greater numbers. Towards the end of the day, forces from Dublin and Leinster fled to their ships but found that the tide had come in and carried their ships away to sea. Trapped with no way out, they were slaughtered or drowned.

In total, 6,000–12,000 people died in the Battle of Clontarf. Both sides suffered heavy losses, but the Vikings and Norsemen were defeated, signalling the end of Viking rule in Ireland. Brian himself was killed, along with his son Murchad and grandson Toirdelbach. Nonetheless, Brian was transformed into a national hero remembered for freeing the Irish from foreign domination. (In reality, the Vikings remained in Ireland long after Clontarf and the battle was between Brian and his rival king, but still the myth remains powerful.) According to some versions of the story, Brian was in his tent praying when Brodir found him and killed him. Other accounts insist that he died in action. His body was brought back to Swords, north of Dublin, and on to Armagh, where it was interred. Twelve days of mourning followed.[24] It's little wonder that Patrick Cotter O'Brien drew such inspiration from the reputation of this fearsome Irish military leader.

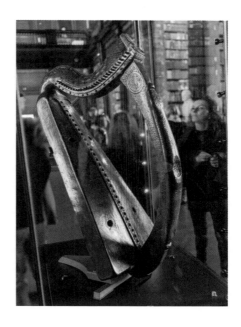

Brian Boru's harp.

At Trinity College can be found 'Brian Boru's Harp', a medieval musical instrument displayed in the beautifully eloquent Long Room. (The Book of Kells can be found on the floor below.) It has a small, low-headed design with 29 strings and is said to have a sweet, resonant, bell-like tone when played. Legend has it that the harp was once owned by Brian Boru, as the instrument's name suggests, although this seems unlikely. It was probably crafted in the fifteenth century, and probably for a member of an important family, possibly the O'Briens. Nonetheless, the myth helped give the harp its name. This harp is Ireland's national symbol and appears on national heraldry. If it looks strangely familiar, it has been used as the Guinness logo since 1862. Ryanair also uses the harp symbol. Interestingly, the harp was badly restored in the 1830s, and in 1961 it was sent to London to be dismantled and reconstructed by the British Museum into the wider shape which it originally had in medieval times. However, the heraldry and trademarks upon which it was modelled still feature the badly restored thinner version.[25]

THE SMALLER SIZED

In the small village of Slaghtaverty, not too far from Limavady, in Co. Derry there once lived a dwarf named Abhartach who was both a magician and a dreadful tyrant. The ancient Irish valued stature and size, and warriors such as Brian Boru were renowned and feared for their height. This was not the case for Abhartach, who was constantly ridiculed for being short. Seeking revenge and power, Abhartach visited a druid and learned to become far more powerful. He perpetrated great cruelties on the people who had mocked him, striking them down with blight and illness or crushing them with great stones.

Eventually, Abhartach was slain by a chieftain named Cathrin (although this has sometimes been accredited to Finn Mac Cuamhail). Being small in size, Abhartach was buried standing upright, but he reappeared the next day even more cruel than before. Cathrin slew and buried him a second time, but Abhartach escaped from the grave once more to terrorise the country. After consulting a druid, Cathrin killed the dwarf a third time but this time buried him with his head facing downwards to subdue Abhartach's magical power. This did the trick and the dwarf never appeared again.[26] Abhartach's grave is now known as the Slaghtaverty Dolmen and consists of a large rock and two smaller rocks under a hawthorn tree. In 1997, attempts were made to clear the land, but the workers who tried to cut down the thorn tree noticed that their chainsaws kept malfunctioning. While attempting to lift the great stone, a steel chain snapped, causing the hand of one of the workers to bleed into the ground.[27]

Evidently, the Irish have also been fascinated by humans (and other creatures) of smaller stature and, until relatively recently, these played an important role in Irish popular culture. Chief in importance of these small creatures was the fairy. Fairies have existed in most cultures, although they take on unique forms in particular countries. In Ireland, fairies are typically less malign than in some other cultures, but they can be very mischievous and even downright vicious when annoyed, so it's best not to cross them. Humans can accidentally wander into their world, just as they wander into ours, but this

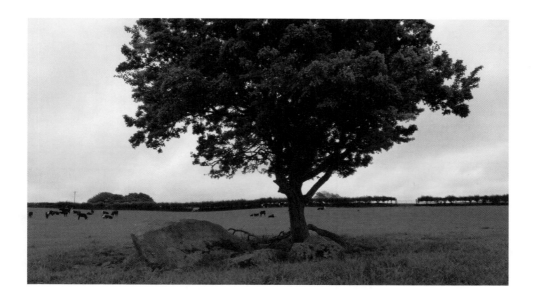

tends to enrage the fairies. In Ireland, fairies are generally split into two types: trooping fairies and solitary fairies.[28]

Abhartach's grave is still a site of local superstition.

Belief in fairies stretches back to ancient Ireland. Irish folklore describes a great ancient tribe known as Tuatha Dé Danann (which translates as 'people of the goddess Danu'). This tribe is thought to have ruled Ireland between 1897 and 1700 BC and is often referred to as the 'little people' (or the 'wee people' in the north). According to legend, they first arrived in Ireland from a great mist on the Connacht coastline. At the time, the Fir Bolg ruled Ireland and were displeased to hear about the new arrivals. After a mighty battle, Tuatha Dé Danann took control of Ireland and respectfully allowed the Fir Bolg to remain in Connacht.

The new rulers were civilised and cultured. They owned four great treasures. The first was the Stone of Fal. Placed on the Hill of Tara, this screamed when a true king of Ireland stood on it. The other treasures were the Magic Sword of Nuadha, the Slingshot of the Sun God Lugh and the Cauldron of Daghda. Tuatha Dé Danann took part in the battles at Moytura and helped shatter the power of

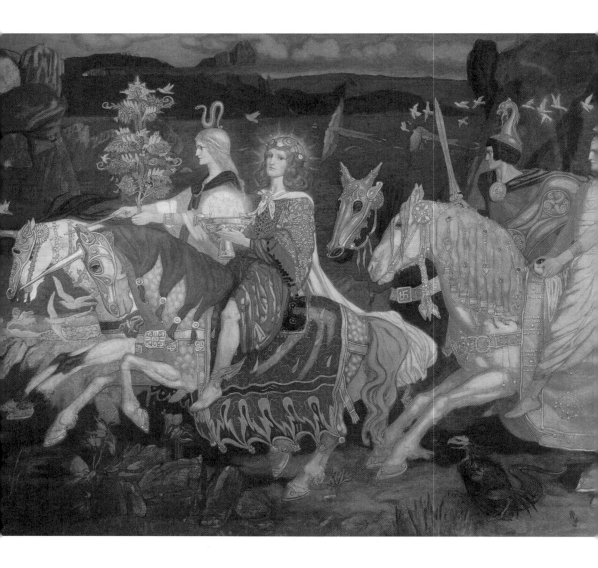

Tuatha Dé Danann (or the tribe of
Goddess Danu), who later became
fairies according to Irish mythology.

the Fomorians. However, their king, Nuadha, lost his life in the battle, and Lugh was instated as king. Tuatha Dé Danann were later defeated in battle, although they were allowed to live underground or in places such as hills. Fairies are the spirits of Tuatha Dé Danann, driven by their conquerors to the hills, caves and underground. Their artistic skill was still visible in sepulchral mounds, stone-inscribed spirals and bronze spearheads.

The ancient belief in fairies withstood centuries of Christian influence in Ireland. As Christianity gained influence, faith in the Celtic gods slowly vanished, but a popular belief in fairies withstood this broader socio-cultural change. Fairies were re-envisioned as fallen angels barred from heaven because of their indecision about whether to support God or Satan.[29] Well into the late twentieth century, many Irish people truly believed that fairies inhabited the sidhe (or hills).[30] They remained prominent in Irish storytelling. Whether or not fairies were nice was an uncertain matter. The fairies were cast aside from heaven for their unworthiness, but they were not considered evil enough for hell.[31]

Much of our knowledge of Irish fairy beliefs stems from the renewed interest in Irish traditions witnessed from the late nineteenth century. In an increasingly secularised, disenchanted world, those who still believed in folk myths and legends found themselves subject to ridicule. This happened to a man named John Mulligan, whose story was recorded in the early nineteenth century. John believed devoutly in fairies and angered quickly if anyone doubted him. His neighbours learned not to vex him, but one day some new neighbours arrived in Ballybeg to spend their summer break from Trinity College with their uncle. The students laughed at every story told by John, dismissing them as 'impossible' and as 'old woman's gabble'. It transpired that John had knowledge of fairies only through his grandmother's old tales and not through first-hand experience.

Enraged, John got drunk and rode off into the night. However, he paused along the way when he came across a 500-year-old oak tree which caught his attention. The moon was shining brightly on the aged tree. Each leaf seemed to be bathed in a mysterious, beautiful light. Jack then noticed some 'lovely little forms dancing under the oak with an unsteady and rolling motion'. 'Never did man see anything more beautiful', thought Jack, adding that 'they were not three inches in height, but they were white as the driven snow, and beyond numberless'. However, he accidentally distracted the strange little creatures by speaking. The fairies vanished; the night darkened. Jack returned and described to the Lord of Ballybeg 'their beautiful dresses of shining silver', 'their flat-crowned hats glittering in the moonbeams', 'the princely stature and demeanour of the central figure', the 'enchanting music'. He decided to take the young students to the site to see for themselves. However, they discovered nothing but shiny mushrooms under the tree. Jack was ridiculed for the rest of his life by the local villagers, who renamed him 'Mushroom Jack'.[32]

Jack's description of how fairies looked would have been unfamiliar to those living in earlier centuries. It is only in the past century that fairies have been depicted as dainty, little-winged, cute and Disneyesque.[33] As Elizabeth Andrews, who published her book *Ulster Folklore* in 1913, noted:

> We must not, however, think of Irish fairies as tiny creatures who could hide under a mushroom or dance on a blade of grass. I remember well how strongly an old woman from Galway repudiated such an idea. The fairies, according to her, were indeed small people, but no mushroom could give them shelter. She described them as about the size of children, and as far as I can ascertain from inquiries made in many parts of Ulster and Munster, this is the almost universal belief among the peasantry. Sometimes I was told the fairies were as large as a well-grown boy or girl, sometimes that they were as small as children beginning to walk; the height of a chair or a table was often used as a comparison, and on one occasion an old woman spoke of them as being about the size of monkeys.[34]

A child encounters a group of mischievous fairies.

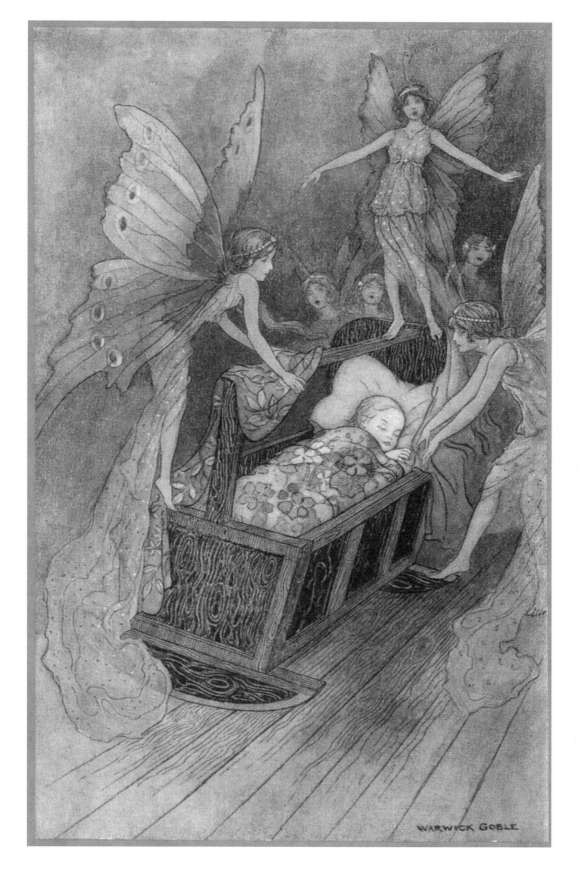

WARWICK GOBLE

Andrews was part of the Irish cultural revival, which took matters such as fairies seriously. Instead of ridiculing the peasantry, Andrews and others meticulously recorded the tales of fairies told by the people.

William Butler Yeats published a book in 1888 entitled *Fairy and Folk Tales of the Irish Peasantry*. In this, he wrote:

> These folk tales are full of simplicity and musical occurrences, for they are the literature of a class for whom every incident in the old rut of birth, love, pain and death has cropped up unchanged for centuries, who have steeped everything in the heart, to whom everything is a symbol.[35]

These curious beliefs were thought to serve as a portal into the minds and culture of the ancient Irish. Irish folklore was a central impulse behind the Irish literary renaissance. Yeats was obsessed with folklore and mythology and sought to develop a literary tradition based on the life of the Irish peasantry (a radical idea at the time). This was a discernible shift from deriding the Irish peasantry, as had previously been common, towards romanticising, and taking seriously, their lives, traditions and beliefs. Scholars and writers carefully recorded local tales of fairy sightings in ways that were objective and non-judgemental, with a focus on recording and describing. Yeats published two anthologies on fairies, the other one being *Irish Fairy Tales* (1892). His books on fairies are intriguing for the modern reader for their depictions of supernatural phenomena and for the empathetic depictions of the people whom the author met on his journeys. Their depictions contrast sharply with early nineteenth-century caricatures of the slovenly, drunken peasant with his beloved, but much disparaged, poteen, potatoes and pet pig.[36]

The Irish called upon the fairies to explain all manner of life occurrences. People who died suddenly had died from a 'fairy stroke'. People who found themselves unexpectedly crippled had fallen asleep near a fairy fort.

In older images, leprechauns were far less jovial than they are today.

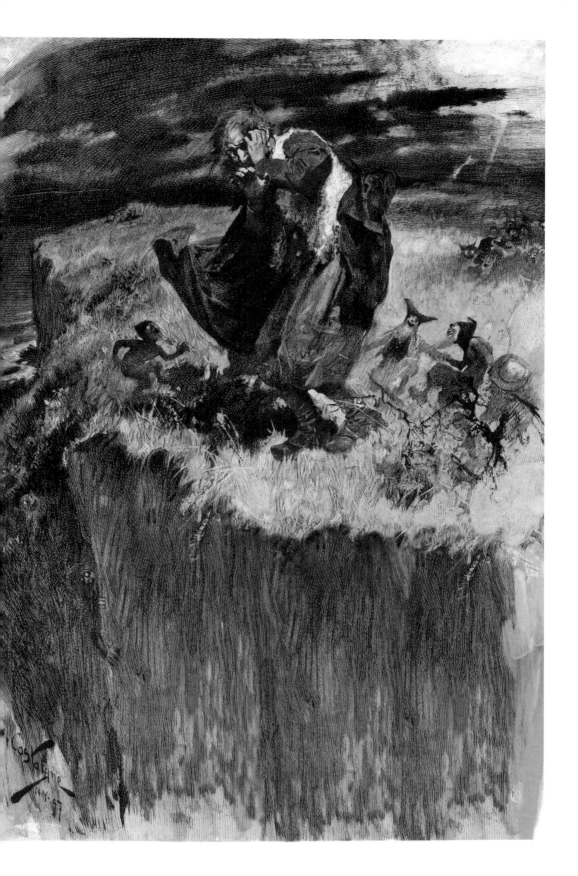

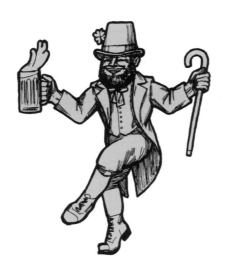

A stereotypical depiction of a
leprechaun holding a pint of stout.

Fairies could carry away living people and leave substitutes in their place: corpses or changelings. One popular tale told of a woman who had accidentally found her way into a fairy fort and spent the rest of her life blinded in one eye. In these tales, perhaps, were the remnants of ancient Irish Celtic culture.[37]

Fairies and music are often associated in Irish folklore. Fairies enjoy dancing, singing and playing music. Fairy music and dancing tend to be spotted by humans late at night, usually at midnight or in moonlight. Fairies are good at playing the pipe, fiddle or harp. For a human to hear fairy music might be an omen of good fortune or, on the other hand, a portent of great evil, sorrow or even death. Fairy music can be so powerful that humans find themselves compelled to dance to it without rest, for hours, or even for a whole week. When the fairy music finally stops, the mortal dancer is exhausted and usually dies soon afterwards. If a person suspected of being a changeling was able to play unusually beautiful music, this was taken as a sign that they were indeed a substitute.[38]

Many different types of fairies exist in Irish culture, and the most famous is the leprechaun. Nowadays, a leprechaun is depicted as a cheerful man with flowing ginger hair and beard, of small height and dressed in a green coat and hat. In reality, though, leprechauns aren't particularly nice fairies. They enjoy causing harm and damage. Unsociable and solitary creatures, they sit on their own making and mending shoes and avoid contact with both humans and other leprechauns. Their manner is dour. Ugly and stunted in growth, they wear dull clothing and are quarrelsome and foul-mouthed.[39] On a more positive note, leprechauns hide pots of gold at the end of rainbows. Like other fairies, the leprechaun can grant wishes, and if a human happens to catch one, he will be obliged to grant three wishes before being free to go. The earliest known reference to the leprechaun appears at the end of the medieval tale Echtra Fergus Mac Léti (Adventure of Fergus Son of Léti) and contains a scene in which Fergus, the king of Ulster, falls asleep on the beach and is dragged into the sea by three leprechauns whom he subsequently captures. Fergus was granted three wishes in exchange for their release.[40]

Over the centuries, the leprechaun has often changed its appearance. Before the twentieth century, leprechauns were depicted as wearing red, not green. This is confirmed by many sources, including Yeats. The modern image of the leprechaun bedecked in green is a more recent invention. As Ireland secured independence in the twentieth century, and showcased green as its new national colour, the leprechaun's appearance changed. Where the hat came from around the same time remains a mystery. (Whether or not female leprechauns exist is yet another mystery.)

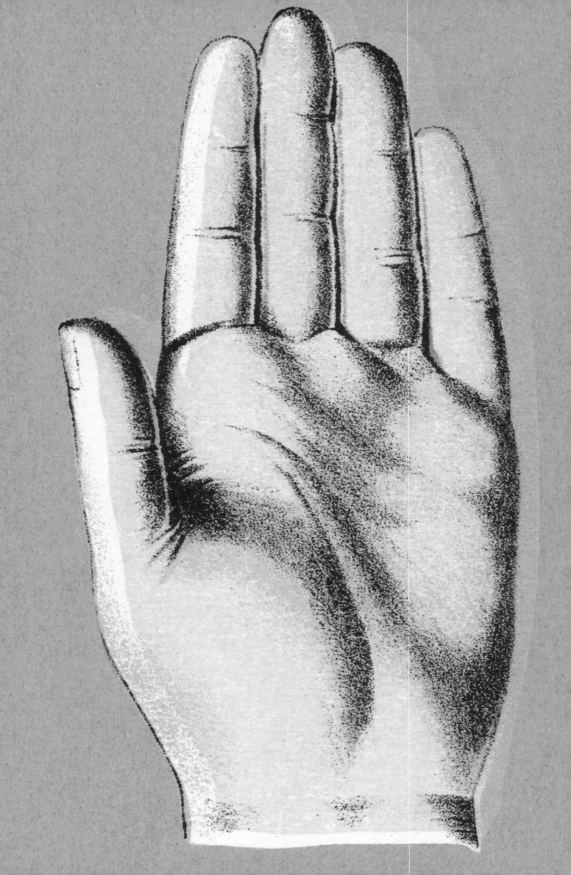

CHAPTER 3

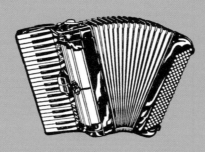

HANDS

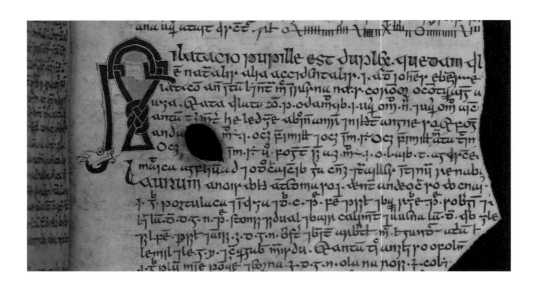

Ogham script in early
Irish medieval tradition.

Only primates such as humans, chimpanzees, monkeys and lemurs possess hands. Human hands contain dense clusters of nerve endings that enable us to use touch as one of our most important senses. Touch is useful for many reasons. It helps us gauge the temperature of objects which we might be tempted to touch and locate items in the dark when sight is restricted. As anyone who owns a pet will confirm, almost all other animals, upon spotting some food, move their mouth towards that food before eating it. In contrast, we pick up food with our hands and lift it towards our mouth, allowing us to keep a close watch on our surroundings, with our head held upright, while we busily eat. In our evolutionary past, this might have helped us keep watch for enemies; in more recent times, it encourages us to socialise at mealtimes. Also in our distant past, hands proved useful for climbing trees to hide from enemies and secure nutritious foods from elevated treetops and branches.

The human hand is a surprisingly sophisticated tool compared with the claws and paws owned by many other animals. We can turn our hands 180 degrees with ease, ball them into a fist and create all manner of unusual shapes.

As human civilisation developed, the flexibility of our hands led us to learn how to make and use tools, create weapons, grab, gesture, throw, club things, carry food around, gather material to build shelters and, eventually, play music, write down words and create works of art ranging from the basic to the eye-droppingly intricate. Much of our knowledge of the past is available to us only because people decided to write it down. The advent of Christianity in Ireland saw the arrival of monks who served as scribes, writing down ancient knowledge in their impressive books and preserving them for posterity. St Patrick, Ireland's patron saint, was among these scribes who helped save ancient writings from the marauding barbarians. Our hands have also served other purposes. Historically, the Irish bedecked their fingers with rings to symbolise marriage or engagement, but other symbols, such as the Red Hand of Ulster, symbolise a bloody military victory.

SCRIBES

In AD 476, the mighty Roman Empire finally fell. In truth, it had been declining for centuries. Having ruled large swathes of Europe, Asia and Africa since Rome's birth in 753 BC, the empire was ravaged by 'barbarian' Germanic and Celtic tribes: Ostrogoths, Visigoths, Franks, Angles, Saxons and Vandals. During the Sack of Rome in AD 455, Vandals besieged the empire's capital. The barbarians took over Europe, destroying the very essence of cultured, civilised life. Following on from the empire's end, Europe slipped into a so-called Dark Age, a morose era of economic, intellectual and cultural decline. The barbarians actively destroyed all that remained of the classical world, roaming across Europe, burning cities and destroying libraries. Literacy. Political theory. Mathematics. None of these interested them. Ancient Greco-Roman intellectual and cultural achievements risked being forever lost.[1] Civilisation itself seemed to be ending.

Meanwhile, the Irish Celts continued to be an unruly bunch. Even the fearsome Romans had avoided trying to rule Ireland. Its inhabitants remained divided in a seemingly endless rota of small kingdoms populated by constantly warring tribes. The Irish Celts were considered barbarians themselves. Unlikely candidates, then, for coming to Europe's rescue by collecting and preserving ancient European knowledge and wisdom. But save it they did, and all by hand. Starting from the fifth century, scribes in Ireland mastered Latin, Greek and even some Hebrew. As if that wasn't impressive enough, they devised an Irish grammatical system and wrote down Ireland's native oral literature. European culture, including that of Celtic Ireland, was preserved for posterity in magnificent books adorned with illuminated, animated capital letters and sweeping Celtic patterns imaginatively decorating art, jewellery and sculpture. Books, a relatively new invention, were far easier to handle than the cumbersome rolled-up scrolls they replaced.[2] Through the painstaking task of writing down all the knowledge they could find, the Irish 'saved' what was left of Greco-Roman and Western Christian civilisation. But how did such a disparate, militant, arguably still prehistoric, groups of islanders manage this feat?

The ancient ways of the Celtic Irish had flourished largely untrammelled by the Roman Empire's bureaucratic tendencies and its official conversion to Christendom in AD 323.[3] Christianity only truly arrived in Ireland during the fifth and sixth centuries, when monasteries sprang up across Ireland. Christianity was introduced in Ireland without bloodshed, which makes the country unique. There are no prominent Christian Irish martyrs of this time. What became known as 'green martyrdom' took place, an alternative to bloody or 'red' martyrdoms. Green martyrdom refers to Christians who, rather than wage war, left behind society's comforts and retreated to self-imposed lives of solitude and abstinence in isolated mountain regions, lonely islands or remote woods. Quiet reflection, not brutal warfare, was the order of the day.[4]

Green martyrdom formed the basis of monasticism, and geographical isolation allowed monks to pray and work without distractions. Ireland still had no major towns or cities (until the Vikings arrived), and the monastic establishments which sprang up, from around AD 500, grew into the first major population centres. Monasteries

Scribes in Ireland toiled over the preservation of ancient and medieval manuscripts.

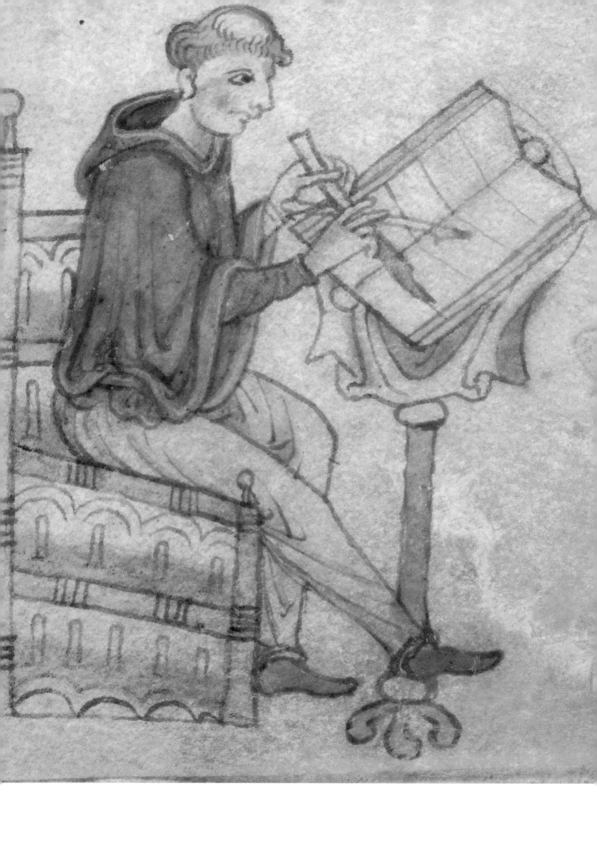

were remarkable places. The largest resembled small villages replete with high stone walls, small churches, accommodation huts and graveyards.

Wherever they went, the monks built monasteries by dragging logs, timber and wattle from the nearest forest. Most of them had a tract of land attached, granted to the founder by the local king or lord, allowing agriculture to become a chief means of employment. A hospice, or guest house, might be attached to monasteries to house visitors needing shelter. Some monasteries kept a fire perpetually burning in a little chapel. This was usually the case when a monastery was situated on the banks of a large river with no bridge. The monks would ferry people across free of charge. The perpetual fire of Kildare was kept alive from the time of St Brigid for many centuries. Similar fires were lit in Kilmainham, Seirkieran and Inishmurray. A bishop was attached to each monastery to provide spiritual direction.

In the monasteries, discipline was strict and useful work needed to be performed at all times. Aside from teaching, reading and transcribing, monks engaged in metalwork or developing herbal remedies. Monks usually had a sleeping cell but no other personal space. Food was simple and scanty. Notwithstanding their insistence on abstinence, monasteries acquired considerable wealth and power. Visitors to old monasteries often encounter a round tower, where the monks kept their valuables: chalices, jewellery, scriptures, paintings and suchlike. In later times, this treasure would set them up as targets for Viking raiders, who destroyed many of the monasteries, but those days were still to come.[5]

The monks had a pronounced missionary ethos that encouraged them to spread the gospel elsewhere, most commonly to Scotland, England and Wales. Between 550 and 1300, hundreds of monks departed from Ireland to spread the gospel to the pagans. The Hiberno-Scottish mission was a series of expeditions made in the sixth and seventh centuries by Gaelic missionaries which originated in the Dál Riata region (roughly encompassing the western seaboard of Scotland and the north-eastern tip of Ireland) before spreading the word across Scotland, Wales, England and Merovingian France. As those living

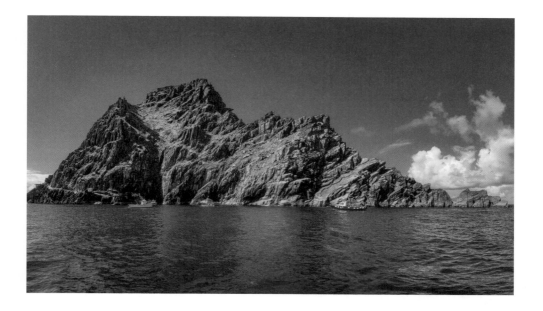

in the Dark Ages were mostly illiterate, monks taught them
by reading sections of the Bible out to any willing to listen.
Images such as those adorning Celtic crosses also helped
people understand Christ's teachings.[6]

Skellig Michael was
once home to a group
of Irish monks.

Despite their self-denying lifestyles, some monks had marvellous
adventures. In 565, Colmcille is said to have encountered and frightened
away the famous Loch Ness Monster, impressing locals so much that they
immediately converted to Christianity. St Brendan, who was born around 489
near Killarney, Co. Kerry, founded many monasteries, including at Ardfert,
Co. Kerry, and Clonfert, Co. Galway. He undertook many sea voyages around
Ireland, Wales and Scotland before making his most legendary journey, while
in his seventies, to (what is now) Canada. With a band of 17 monks, Brendan
sailed around the North Atlantic for seven years before eventually reaching 'the
Land of Promise of the Saints', which they explored before returning home with
fruit and precious stones. While there is good reason to doubt that a boat made
of ox hides, navigated by a man well into pension age, could have truly made

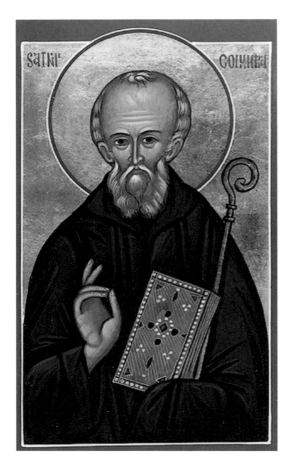

Irish scribe Colmcille, who spent much of his life on the island of Iona, Scotland.

the long journey across the Atlantic Ocean, a sailor and geographer named Tim Severin recreated the voyage in 1976 and 1977, and sailed to Newfoundland.[7]

Christianity survived by clinging to remote places such as Skellig Michael, an island off the coast of Co. Kerry, famous nowadays for being used as a location in the *Star Wars* series. However, in the sixth century, a group of warrior-monks lived there cut off from the world, voluntarily stranded on a small, treacherous island. Choosing the harshest, most remote places to live added to the sense of penance. By all accounts, the monks believed they were locked in a battle against Satan, or the world's 'dark side', using a life of self-denial as a weapon to aid their endeavours. Skellig Michael is notoriously inaccessible. It's only possible to reach in the summer months; even then, visitors must climb 600 steps to access the monastery. An unforgiving environment indeed. The monks survived by living off their vegetable gardens, bird's eggs and whatever else they could find.

Unusually for the time, monks were highly literate. Ireland's monasteries were renowned for their excellent teaching of poetry, literature and the arts, as well as the gospel. It is for this reason that Ireland became known as the Land

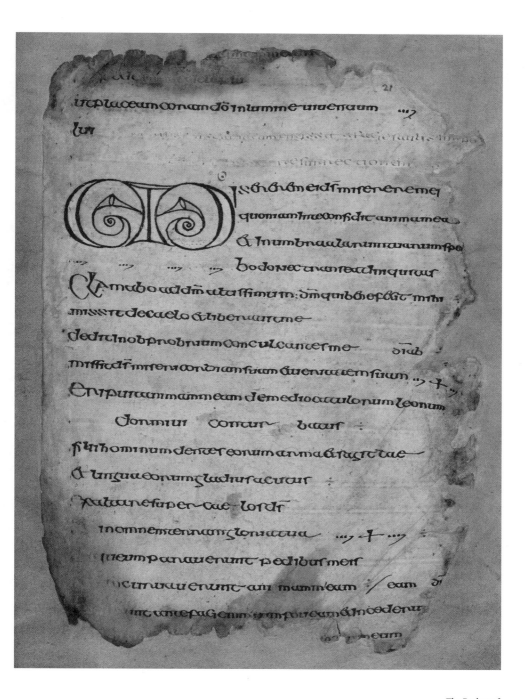

The Psalter of
St Columba.

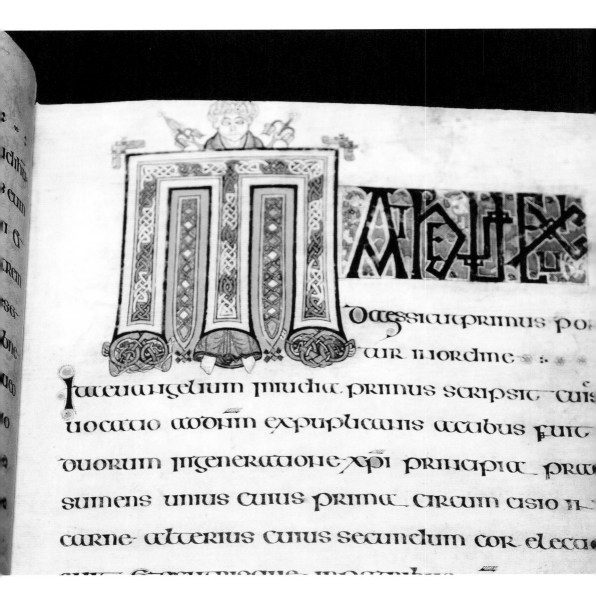

A page from the Book of Kells,
currently housed at Trinity
College Dublin.

of Saints and Scholars, a description still used today. Reading was an important activity for monks, and all monasteries contained libraries of varying sizes. Before the invention of the printing press in the fifteenth century, books had to be written and copied entirely by hand. In the context of the cultural destruction that followed the decline of the Roman Empire, the Irish monks, intentionally or otherwise, played a crucial role in preserving ancient, Christian and Irish lore. Labouring entirely by hand, the Irish monks worked in freezing cells to preserve ancient texts and save Western culture from the barbarians. Through these books, knowledge could be transmitted among the various monastic schools throughout Ireland and beyond.[8]

The remote island of Iona is also famed for its monastic activities. It was founded by one of Ireland's three patron saints, Columba (later known as Colmcille), born in Co. Donegal in 521 to a family connected to local royalty. (Colum means 'dove', and the 'cille' later appended to his name means 'church' in Gaelic. Colmcille was the Church's dove.) He studied under St Finnian at Clonard Abbey, Co. Meath, and was later ordained as a monk. By the still tender age of 30, Colmcille had founded around 20 monasteries. The walled city of Derry is thought to have been founded by Colmcille, who established a monastery there (although this has been contested).

Colmcille loved books. As a student, he adored St Finnian's coveted psalter (a volume containing the Book of Psalms), so much so that he decided to covertly make a copy of it. Working in the dark of night to conceal his surreptitious replicating, Colmcille faced a problem. He had no candle. According to legend, though, his five left-hand fingers shone brightly while his right hand assiduously copied. Upon discovering the copied book, King Diarmait was enraged and demanded that Colmcille return the unauthorised duplicate to Finnian, and Colmcille found himself embroiled in the world's first-ever copyright case. Some years later, Diarmait killed some of Colmcille's followers, forcing Colmcille to declare a war in which he proved victorious against Diarmait's followers. Colmcille claimed back the contested facsimile, which was known from then on as the Cathach (meaning 'battler').[9]

This was not the end of the story. In 563, the high king exiled Colmcille to Iona, a desolate rock only 3 miles long and 1.5 miles wide. Despite its cramped size, Colmcille made a home there, and Iona became a centre for Christian learning for the next three centuries. Colmcille devoted every moment of his spare time to transcribing and writing in a small wooden hut. Entirely by hand, he transcribed around 300 copies of the New Testament, a notably lengthy book, which he presented to the various churches that he founded. Colmcille also wrote several hymns and recorded Ireland's famous events, battles, legends and stories. Much of our knowledge of ancient Ireland stems from Colmcille's painstaking efforts to preserve so much literature.[10] Colmcille died in 597 and was buried in Iona.

Colmcille laboured at the very same time that Europe's great continental libraries were being decimated. Rome's first public libraries had been founded at the time of Augustus (who reigned between 27 BC and AD 14). Three hundred years later, the number of libraries had grown to 28. However, by the fifth century, the libraries had all but disappeared. The few books still being copied tended to be in the hands of private collectors – nobles, for instance, who owned small libraries. The invading barbarians were largely illiterate and had no qualms about destroying books. But even as continental Europe became increasingly illiterate, a vibrant literary culture quietly persisted along its isolated Celtic fringe.[11]

The scribes made book pages from mottled parchment (or dried sheepskin), which was abundant in Ireland, a land with no shortage of lambs and sheep. Calfskin was reserved for the most honoured texts. Scribes transcribed their text onto separate pages and gathered these together in a booklet (or quire) which was stitched with other quires into a larger volume.[12] Once collated together, the books produced by Colmcille and others were lavishly adorned with a protective metal cover bedecked with jewels and other valuables.

The Book of Durrow is Ireland's oldest extant manuscript and consists of texts from the Gospels of Matthew, Mark, Luke and John. Its origins are unclear. It seems to have been created in

Illustrated pages from the Book of Kells.

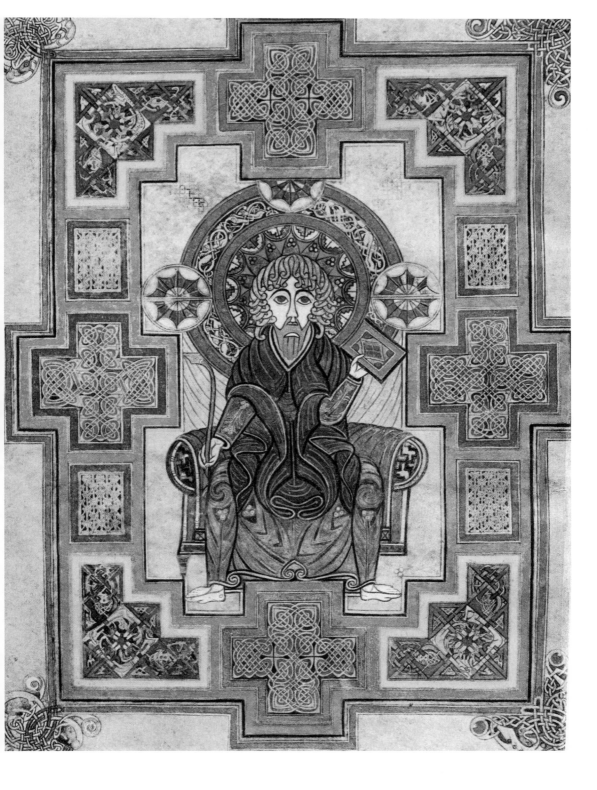

Durrow Abbey, Co. Offaly, a monastery founded by Colmcille around AD 700 (although legend insists that Colmcille himself copied the book while still alive). After the abbey was dissolved in the sixteenth century, the book went into private ownership. It survived somehow even despite horrified sightings of a seventeenth-century farmer immersing it in water, hoping to create holy water to cure his cows of sickness. Eventually, what was left of the Book of Durrow was given to Trinity College Dublin.[13]

Also found in Trinity College's impressive Dublin city centre grounds is a far more famous book, now a major tourist attraction: the Book of Kells. An illuminated gospel written in Latin around AD 800, it was kept in the Abbey of Kells, Co. Meath, where it acquired its popular name, though it was created in an unknown Columban monastery. It is also sometimes known as the Book of Columba. Having somehow survived the pillaging of Kells Abbey by Vikings, it remained in Kells until 1654, when Oliver Cromwell's cavalry decided to station themselves in the church. The governor of Kells sent the book to Dublin for safekeeping, and it now remains in Trinity College Dublin on permanent display. Famous worldwide for its extravagant illustrations and ornamentation (by this stage, the monks were really showing off their artistic talents), the Book of Kells presents a curious mix of Christian imagery, Celtic knots and mythical beasts. Most important of all, it was part of a broader effort to preserve ancient Latin and Christianity's core texts from the savage barbarians, all performed painstakingly by hand.[14]

ST PATRICK

Visitors to the town of Kells might notice an array of Celtic crosses erected to commemorate various prominent Irish people. The oldest of these dates from the ninth century. It marked a design shift away from ornamental Celtic patterns to scriptural references. The 3-metre-high cross contains a Latin inscription: *Patrich et Columbae Crux*, which translates as the Cross of Patrick and Columbia. Alongside Colmcille and Brigid of Kildare, Patrick is one of Ireland's three patron saints. Though, technically, Patrick was never formally canonised as he lived before the Catholic Church developed laws on such matters. Regardless, the Irish venerate him as a saint. He is credited with converting all the Irish to Christianity and is known as the Apostle of Ireland.

Patrick was unusually literate for his time, and we know of his life largely through his handwritten Confessio (or Confession), a text contained in the ninth-century Book of Armagh. According to this, at age 16 Patrick was taken captive from Britain by Irish pirates who forced him to live as an animal herder working for the chieftain Miliucc (or Milchu) near Slemish Mountain, Co. Antrim. Patrick became deeply unhappy. Shepherds worked in isolated conditions and rarely encountered other people. He found solace in prayer and came to believe that his life of solitude had been granted by God as a time when he could have his sins forgiven and convert to Christianity.

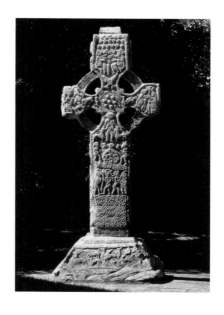

The Cross of St Patrick and St Columba (South Cross) in Kells.

Legend tells that after a lonely six years a mysterious voice spoke to Patrick informing him: 'Your hungers are rewarded. You are going home. Look, your ship is ready.' Good news indeed, the only problem being that Miliucc's farm was nowhere near the sea. Patrick walked for 200 miles across unfamiliar land and eventually arrived on Ireland's south-eastern coast, somewhere near Wexford, where he saw his ship. Its sailors were loading a cargo of Irish hounds which they hoped to sell for a large bounty on the continent. Initially, the sailors were wary of Patrick's request to travel with them. After Patrick prayed, the sailors changed their mind and offered him the opportunity to suck their nipples. (While this might seem strange, it was an ancient Irish way of making up with someone.) Patrick declined the offer but nonetheless went on board with the repentant sailors.

Three days later, the party arrived in a strange land to discover only devastation and destruction around them. For a fortnight, they trudged across deserted land where they came across not one living person. A few dogs lay half-dead by the side of the roads. The travellers walked for 28 days in this wilderness, and their food supplies soon began to run out. 'What use are your prayers when we're starving to death?' asked one of the sailors. Patrick reassured him that God would send food that day and, after praying for sustenance, the travellers heard the sound of a stampede. Miraculously, it was a herd of wild boar, rushing down the road towards them.

Some years later, after he returned to Britain, legend also tells that Patrick saw a vision of a man named Victorius handing him countless letters. One of these was headed 'Vox Hiberionacum', a Latin phrase which translates as the 'Voice of the Irish'. A moment later, Patrick claimed to have heard a multitude of voices begging him to 'walk among us once more'. Over time, the intensity and frequency of these visions increased, and after a period of study in Europe, Patrick returned to Ireland. Receiving a lukewarm welcome in Wicklow, he travelled instead to the Skerries coast of Dublin. Patrick went on to establish bishops in northern, central and eastern regions of the island. He appointed himself primatial bishop at Ard Mhacha (now Armagh), close to Emain Macha, seat of the Ulster kings. He also set up a bishop near the Hill of Tara. By placing bishops close to the kings, Patrick hoped to keep an eye on the powerful rulers and limit their depredations.

Having been kidnapped as a youth, Patrick missed out on a formal education while herding sheep in Antrim. Throughout his life, he struggled to communicate directly in Latin. However, he was literate, if not perfectly so, and wrote a number of works which are often described as a curious mix of elementary Latin and older forms of Irish. As an adult, Patrick spent time in Gaul to receive a more thorough classical education. There, he was ordained priest, and then the bishop of Hippo. As well as his Confession, another

St Patrick, the patron saint of Ireland.

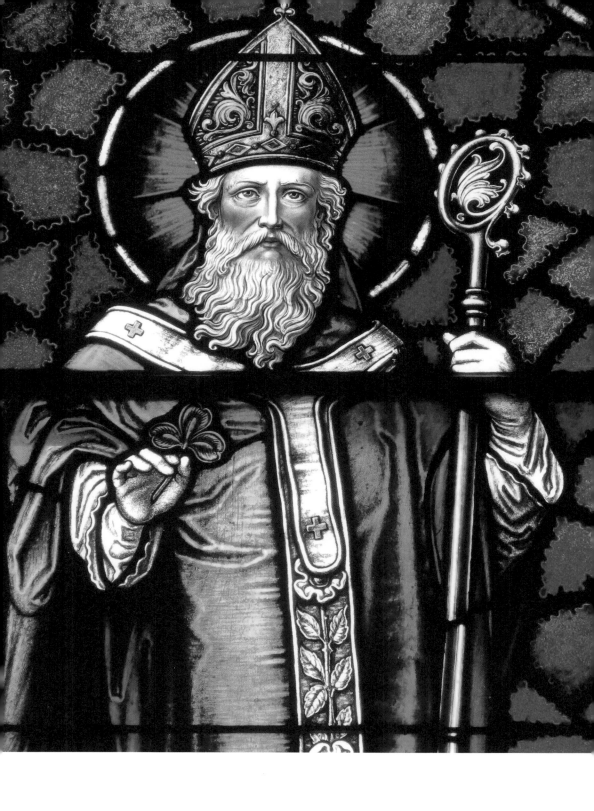

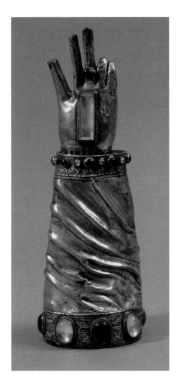

Shrine of St Patrick's hand.

Latin work survives which is accepted as having been handwritten by Patrick: the Letter to the Soldiers of Corocticus. We know more of Patrick's life through two seventh-century writings by Tírechán, a bishop in north Connacht, and the Vita sancti Patricii (Life of St Patrick) of Muirchú moccu Machtheni. Both drew from a lost work called the Book of Ultan.

Patrick is considered a largely successful leader. In his lifetime, the Irish slave trade ground to a halt, intertribal warfare decreased and Patrick established many monasteries and convents. But he struggled to transform Irish sexual mores, which were fairly open at the time, and also had strained relations with British Christians, who refused to recognise the Irish as fully fledged Christians because they had never been Roman. By the end of Patrick's life (probably 461), the Roman Empire was in chaos and the death of the last Roman emperor was just 15 years away. However, largely thanks to Patrick, Ireland was moving away from chaos into peace.

Many myths surround Patrick. What's fact and fiction is often unclear. Most famous is the claim that Patrick chased all the snakes out of Ireland. In fact, existing literature from the seventh and eighth centuries attributes this feat to Colmcille, and it's only from the twelfth century that the historical record credits this instead to Patrick. The story goes that a group of snakes attacked Patrick while he was fasting on a mountain. Angered, he chased them all into the sea. (Interestingly, Ireland does not have any native snakes – they were probably kept out by rising seas after the last Ice Age.) In another tale, Patrick used the shamrock, a three-leaved plant famously associated with Ireland, to explain the Holy Trinity – he is depicted clutching a shamrock on coins from the 1680s. In fact, the Celtic Irish had many triple deities, which might have helped Patrick's evangelisation endeavours. Patrick is also said to have met two members of Finn Mac Cuamhail's band of warriors, the Fianna, who had somehow survived to Patrick's time and attempted to convert the two men, Caílte mac Rónáin and Oisín, unsuccessfully.[15]

St Patrick's Day is celebrated raucously on 17 March, the supposed date of his death sometime between 463 and 493. From as early as the ninth century, monasteries and churches marked his passing each year. Made an official Christian feast day in the seventeenth century, the Church treats 17 March as a solemn and holy day of obligation, marking it with a good meal and a lengthy sermon. In contrast, Irish people nowadays treat St Patrick's Day as a day of excessive drinking, a global celebration of Irishness in which they show pride in their national identity by drinking copious amounts of Guinness until they drunkenly collapse. Other secular celebrations include public parades, festivals, the wearing of green attire and the fixing of shamrocks to clothes. Historically, Church Lenten restrictions on eating and drinking were lifted for the day, explaining why this holy day became so closely associated with drunkenness, enjoyment and revelry. In Ireland, St Patrick's Day is a public holiday, but it is also widely celebrated unofficially around the world, particularly in places the Irish emigrated to from the nineteenth century. Indeed, until the late twentieth century, the diaspora celebrated St Patrick's Day far more vigorously than those remaining in Ireland.[16]

St Patrick's official colour is actually blue, but most Irish people unknowingly wear green on St Patrick's Day. Green was only associated with Ireland from the eleventh century, long after Patrick lived. Yet another interesting fact is that there might have been two Patricks. This controversial theory was first proposed by Thomas Francis O'Rahilly, a prominent scholar of Celtic languages and an esteemed member of the Royal Irish Academy. His book *The Two Patricks*, published in 1942, suggests that the mission of the first Patrick lasted from 432 to 461 and was followed by a second mission and Patrick between around 462 and 490. This was an intellectual earthquake. It caused a scholastic civil war. Perhaps the most important question of all was which Patrick the saint was. Had the Irish been accidentally praying to the wrong Patrick for centuries? Which Patrick did what exactly? Arguments on the matter rumbled on for decades.[17]

But what if the scribes, and Patrick too, hadn't meticulously spent their lifetimes scribing and writing? What if the Irish had joined the barbarians at the gate and decided to destroy the knowledge being scrupulously preserved? Would we still know much of Patrick and the various myths surrounding him, as well as the broader ancient world in which he lived? Would Ireland ever have become so closely associated with Christianity? Would we still celebrate St Patrick's Day?

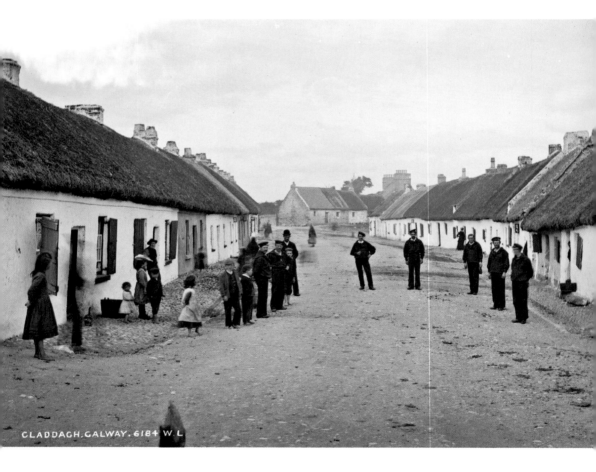

The Claddagh community
of Co. Galway.

Interestingly, it is possible to visit what some people believe to be the very hand that Patrick wrote with. Patrick's bodily remains are said to have been enshrined by Colmcille in 553 and rediscovered centuries later in Downpatrick Cathedral. It was customary for relics (such as bodily remains or objects that had touched the body of a saint) to be placed in small shrines made of wood or metal, or in sturdy containers. We have seen this already with St Oliver Plunkett's head. Patrick's relic is thought to have been removed by Robert Bruce in 1316, a Scottish king who waged a three-year military campaign in Ireland. Until the eighteenth century, the shrine was looked after by the Magennis family of Co. Down. It changed hands a few times until 1840, when it was acquired by Bishop Denvir. The relic itself has long disappeared, although the shrine remains. Hollow and made of gilt silver, the shrine depicts a sleeved right forearm and hand, cut off just below the elbow. Three of the fingers stretch fully outwards, while the other two are concealed behind the rest of the hand, representing the hand in the attitude of benediction. The hand is attractively jewelled and appears thicker than the normal size of a man's hand.[18]

WEDDING RINGS

The Irish have a famous kind of ring – the Claddagh ring – which features a heart representing love, a crown signifying loyalty and two clasped hands symbolising friendship. Its motto is 'let love and friendship reign' and its name comes from a fishing village of that name in Co. Galway, which dates to the fifth century and the arrival of Christianity in Ireland. Claddagh translates as 'stony shore'. Victorian visitors wrote regularly of the Claddagh region. One described 'a typical collection of low thatched cottages, built without much regard to system, the inhabitants of which for many generations have preserved their individuality amidst the surrounding population'. For generations, Claddagh's residents actively discouraged outsiders from settling in the region and intermarrying, all of which helped preserve their unique cultural identity.

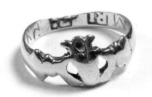

The oldest known
Claddagh ring, reportedly
created by Richard Joyce.

This identity appeared to have withstood centuries of influence from the Vikings, Anglo-Saxons, Normans and Spanish who regularly visited Galway. Unlike most other Irish people of the time, they had little interest in politics. A deeply moral and religious people, they never travelled on a Sunday, and they observed all Christian festivities. The traditional dress for women consisted of a blue mantle, red body gown and petticoat, with a handkerchief round the head and the feet bare, and the famous Claddagh ring, handed down through the generations from mother to daughter. Claddagh culture was dominated by fishing, and it was rumoured that anyone caught fishing in their waters risked a bloody end at the hands of the Claddagh fishermen.[19]

Although these types of rings have been produced for several centuries, the name 'Claddagh ring' was adopted only in the nineteenth century. According to local legend, a seventeenth-century silversmith, Richard Joyce (1660–c.1737), invented the modern Claddagh design. Joyce was a member of the so-called 'Tribes of Galway', a group of 14 merchant families who dominated life in Galway city between the thirteenth and nineteenth centuries. Twelve of these families were of Anglo-Norman descent. Although the Tribes prided themselves on being a cut above the Gaelic people of Galway, they shared a common faith in Catholicism, which fuelled their opposition to Cromwell when he conquered Ireland. Displeased, the English government besieged Galway in April 1652. The city surrendered and the New Model Army confiscated all property belonging to the Tribes. It was Cromwell who first described the families as 'tribes', and they adopted the name themselves in defiance. But they never fully recovered their sociopolitical influence in Galway.

In 1675, Joyce was on his way to the West Indies when his ship was besieged by Algerian pirates, who were notorious for seizing both goods and passengers, whom they enslaved. Joyce became a slave apprentice to a successful goldsmith in Algiers from whom he learned his trade. During his captivity, he made a ring as a symbol of his love for a woman back home in Claddagh. Finally released in 1689, after King William III, newly anointed King of England, demanded the release of British prisoners, Joyce returned to Rahoon, a small town outside Galway. His master, used to having Joyce around, had tried to entice him to stay by offering him his daughter's hand in marriage and half his wealth.

But Joyce was in love. He returned to Ireland with his Claddagh ring and, with it, proposed to his sweetheart. She said yes, and the couple married, according to the legend. Some historians credit other goldsmiths with coming up with the design – Bartholomew Fallon and Dominick Martin, for instance. However, Joyce's designs were particularly popular at the time, displaying a curious charm steeped in North African influence, and his name became synonymous with the Claddagh ring, even if he may not necessarily have created its design. Joyce's initials are carved into the earliest surviving Claddagh rings, although some bear the mark of goldsmith Thomas Meade. The Claddagh ring proved hugely popular in Galway, the Aran Islands, Connemara and beyond, and it received international recognition from the nineteenth century.[20]

Claddagh rings are sometimes still used to symbolise friendship, and some mothers continue to gift a ring to daughters on their coming of age. Typically, though, their chief use is as an engagement or wedding ring. Claddagh rings are worn in ways that convey the wearer's relationship status. A single woman, looking for love, places the ring on her right hand with the heart pointing towards her fingertips. Turned the other way, heart pointing towards the wrist, the wearer makes others aware that someone has 'captured her heart'. She is in a relationship. Wearing the ring on the left hand signals that she is either engaged or married.[21]

In the nineteenth century, the Irish peasantry generally thought that only a marriage involving a gold ring was legally binding. Not everyone could afford gold, and it was common for a gold ring to be borrowed and then returned. The very same ring might be used for many marriage ceremonies. However,

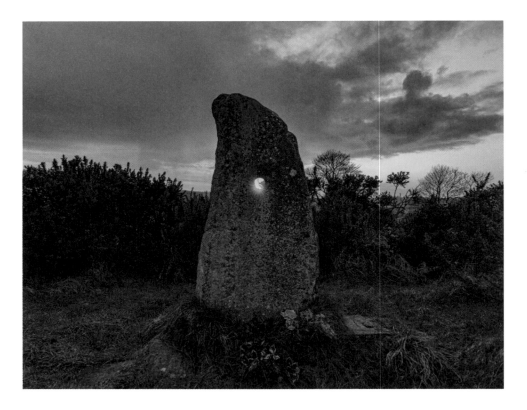

The Holed Stone at Doagh was once used as a substitute for a wedding ring.

the Claddagh system differed, with the ring being passed through the generations. Those wearing a ring in the nineteenth century, while looking at the old patterns and designs that adorned it, could imagine the marital life of past generations all the way back to the 1700s. Although weddings were now Christian in nature, it has been speculated that sacramental rings were also used by the Celtic Irish.[22] In the absence of a ring of any description, some couples sealed an agreement to marry at the Holed Stone at Doagh, Co. Antrim. Bride and groom would position themselves at either side of the stone and join their hands through a circular hole carved through the stone, which acted as a proxy for a real ring. This custom was still being performed as recently as the 1960s.[23]

Marriages have served various purposes in Irish history. In medieval times, marital alliances among the elite were essential for politics, society and the economy. Christian approaches to marriage were formalised in the twelfth and thirteenth centuries, but Gaelic traditions lived on across much of Ireland, particularly in non-anglicised regions. Traditional Irish law allowed a man to keep a number of concubines, encouraged permissive attitudes towards divorce and remarriage and was even unconcerned with cousins marrying each other. Having several spouses allowed aristocratic men to build large families, perhaps even a dynasty. Co-habiting and trial marriages were also common among the Gaelic Irish.[24] The Protestant state that emerged in Early Modern Ireland did not approve of marriages between Catholics and Protestants. From 1726, Catholic priests faced execution if caught presiding over a mixed marriage. The harsh penalty was removed in 1883, although such marriages remained prohibited.[25]

By the eighteenth and nineteenth centuries, firmer preconditions were in place before a marriage could take place. A couple could no longer be closely related by blood or affinity (e.g., in-laws and step-siblings), an earlier marriage or engagement was considered undesirable, and consent was crucial. Once these conditions were met, the bride and groom would declare their intention to marry to the family and community. The 'reading of the banns' took place on three consecutive Sundays in a couple's home parish. In these small communities, marriage was a very public affair. Engagement periods were typically short. The wedding was performed by an ordained clergyman, preferably before witnesses, and the marriage had to be consummated.[26]

Marriages typically took place when the bride and groom (particularly the bride) were young. Until 1972, Irish girls could marry as young as 12, and boys at age 14. While many marriages were arranged, marriage divination practices were popular. One of these involved a girl placing a piece of wedding cake under her pillow to induce dreams of her future husband. Crumbs from a wheaten bannock, a type of bread known as bride's cake, would suffice. Halloween was seen as a particularly powerful night to attempt marriage divination.[27]

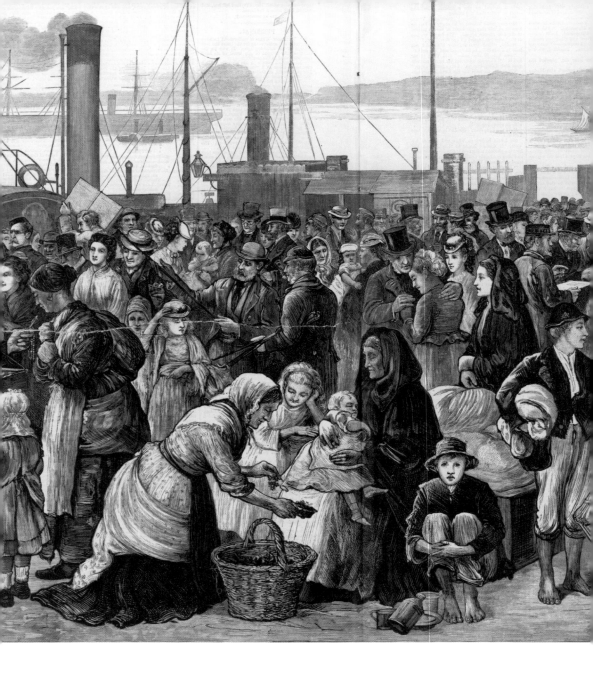

From the nineteenth century
on, Irish women emigrated en
masse to countries including
America and Australia.

Brides were thought to be exceptionally vulnerable to being carried off by fairies, but men too were known to kidnap potential brides for a few days usually to compel them into marriage. Often, this granted the man access to the dowry, money, land or property tied to the woman. Once a young woman was known to have been in the company of a man, it was presumed that her virginity was no longer intact, and it would prove almost impossible to find another man willing to take her on. Sometimes, a couple in love would connive against their parents by staging a kidnapping, a rebellion against the imposition of arranged marriages with partners towards whom they had no amorous feelings. In the eighteenth century, there were at least 200 such abductions, with a further 900 between 1800 and 1850.[28]

Abductions ranged from playfully consensual to shockingly brutal. From the seventeenth century, Protestant heiresses were sometimes kidnapped and assaulted by Catholic men to force them into marriage and restore lands confiscated from their families. The problem became so threatening to Protestants that abduction was made a capital offence in 1707 and remained so until 1842. At least 150 abductors were transported to Australia. One particularly notorious incident occurred in March 1822 in Aughrim, Co. Cork, when 12 armed men, led by James Brown, entered the house of Richard Goold, the son of a prosperous farmer, looking for Richard's older sister. She happened to be out, but 16-year-old Honora, another sister, was at home. Mistaking Honora for her older sister, the kidnappers absconded with her. After realising his mistake, James proposed anyway, but Honora declined. Over the next week, James repeatedly raped Honora. She was found in a 'most pitiable condition'. The incident caused a national scandal.[29]

In a predominantly rural society, land was a crucial resource. Marriages were planned and organised carefully in light of this. In Anglo-Irish traditions, a woman brought her dowry with her to the marriage and also any property she may have acquired. When she married, the property passed into the hands of her husband, who became her guardian. Dowries were typically land-based or involved the exchange of valuable cattle. This contrasted with older, and more equitable, Gaelic marital customs which granted a wife far more freedom in looking after goods or property which she brought into the marriage. Under Gaelic law, married women were comparatively free and independent. This was less so in later marriages, which often resembled an economic arrangement.[30] This raises an intriguing question. Were Irish marriages loveless? Perceptions exist that many nineteenth-century Irish people were locked in arranged marriages, devoid of compatibility, companionship and intimacy. In reality, just as today, the happiness, or otherwise, of married couples probably varied immensely. Nonetheless, this caricature of the loveless nineteenth-century marriage persists.

Earlier in the century, relatively few women left Ireland. Their contributions to family life were valued and recognised. Actively engaged in important aspects of rural life such as dairying, Irish women were relatively content. During the famine, large numbers of Irish people emigrated to America, Britain and Australia, fleeing the death, disease and starvation surrounding them in those dark years. Afterwards, the small holdings that had once been scattered across Ireland were consolidated and replaced by large farms, often refocused on cattle rearing. The wage-earning capacities of rural Irish women decreased.

This income decline restricted women's choice of marriage partners. From the 1850s, the inheritance of the family farm by only one son and the dowering of only one daughter became the norm, especially in western regions. Since siblings no longer shared their parents' prosperity equally, marriage was delayed, if it happened at all. Men married when their farm required a wife. Romantic love was not a top priority. Many women were dispossessed, had no property and lived as celibate dependents on family farms, with little prospect of ever marrying.

Facing limited employment opportunities and a loveless single life, around 700,000 young women emigrated between 1885 and 1920, usually alone, seeking a more fulfilling life outside of Ireland. No other country but Sweden historically witnessed such a large, sustained migration of single women. It's an anomaly in the history of European emigration. The women who left did so because they felt superfluous in their home communities. Rather than accept the celibate life of a spinster, they simply opted to leave. Women's emigration was acutely common in the west and south west. Some people consider this widespread emigration a powerful act of female self-determination, but it could equally be thought of as a sign of desperation. The loss of so many Irish women further contributed to nationwide population decline. Between the 1880s and 1920s, Ireland's population fell by about one-fifth.[31]

Around this time, marrying one's cousin also fell out of fashion. The arrival of social Darwinism, eugenics and, later, genetics, forced a rethink of the consequences of consanguineous marriage (between relatives) for the national gene pool. Doctors debated whether such marriages were responsible for seemingly rising levels of deafness, scrofula, tuberculosis, 'mutism' and 'insanity' across the island. Cousins who procreated, scientists and doctors feared, produced children with weak bodies, muscles and brains. Close inbreeding was thought to deteriorate the stock of animal species, and humans seemed no different.[32]

In 1883, prominent Irish public health official Charles A. Cameron read a paper to the Academy of Medicine in Ireland about consanguineous marriages, which he described as 'barbarous and savage'. According to the 1881 census, Ireland had 5,136 'mutes'. One hundred and thirty-five of these were the children of first cousins, ascertained Cameron, who believed the practice to be more common among Protestants than Catholics.[33] Debates about the consequences of procreating with a cousin continued well into the twentieth century and became closely linked with concern about recessive genes causing various forms of disability. A 1955 clinical study suggested that 1 per cent of Northern Ireland's population was married to a first cousin, with the problem of 'inbreeding' being worsened by disinclination among Catholics and Protestants to procreate with members of the other denominations.[34] However, dating as an Irish person still carries a high risk of accidentally matching with a cousin or relative of some description. In 2018, genealogists worked out that the average Irish adult has more than 14,000 living cousins scattered across the world.[35]

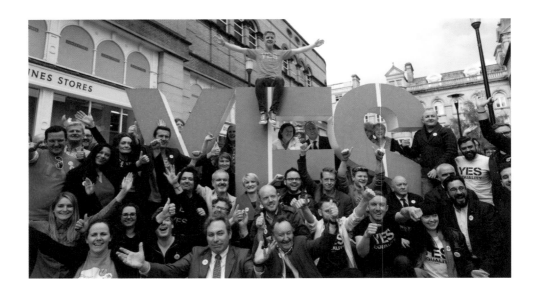

On 22 May 2015, a referendum took place in Ireland to legalise same-sex marriage.

In more recent times, the Republic of Ireland became the first country in the world to extend civil marriage to same-sex couples via referendum, which took place on 22 May 2015. While marriage equality had been granted in some other countries, nowhere else had legislative change been put to a public vote. Ireland likes its referendums. At the time of writing, there have been a massive 38 referendums for amendments to the Constitution of Ireland. The marriage equality referendum was hugely symbolic. Record numbers registered their votes, and Irish emigrants returned from across the world to ensure they had their say. Sixty-two per cent voted yes, and thirty-eight per cent no. The constitution was then amended, with the following sentence added to Article 41: 'Marriage may be contracted in accordance with law by two persons without distinction as to their sex.'

The huge majority revealed shifting Irish attitudes towards LGBTQ+ communities in modern Ireland, as well as a more general shift away from basing marriage on stark economic considerations towards love, companionship and compatibility. The overwhelming support for same-sex marriage also provided an opportunity to express mounting objections to the power and social influence of the Church. In the twentieth century, Church and State interests grew remarkably entwined in both Ireland and Northern Ireland. Religious morals influenced policy, which led to a range of legal restrictions being placed on abortion, divorce, pornography and all matters sexual. In the years immediately leading up to the referendum, harrowing revelations emerged about widespread sexual, physical and emotional abuse in Ireland's religious institutions: mother and baby homes, for example. The national mood shifted towards distrust of churches, whether Catholic or Protestant, and a desire to limit their sociopolitical influence. The legalisation of same-sex marriage signalled a confident move towards demanding sexual freedom, in line with most other Western countries, and the exchange of wedding rings among couples regardless of their sexual orientation.[36]

RED HAND OF ULSTER

Between 1952 and 1973, the government of Northern Ireland used as its flag the Ulster Banner, popularly referred to as the Red Hand Flag. The creation of this new flag coincided with Queen Elizabeth II's coronation in Britain, though the right to display arms on a flag had been granted in 1924. In 1953, the banner was flown over the Parliament Buildings at Stormont for the first time to honour Elizabeth's visit. That year, the Minister of Home Affairs announced that those wishing to have a distinctive Ulster flag could use the Ulster Banner instead of the Union Flag (more commonly referred to as the Union Jack). The Red Hand Flag remains in use for sporting purposes today. This flag, with a stark white background, features a red hand in a white star-shaped badge with six points representing the six counties. (The province of Ulster has nine counties and has a

The Red Hand of Ulster is the symbol of Northern Ireland.

separate provincial flag.) As its name suggests, the symbol contains an open hand which is coloured red, with fingers pointed upwards and palm facing forwards.[37]

The hand is red because it is bloody. As such, it provides a suitable metaphor both for the centuries of armed conflict that have stricken Ireland and, more specifically, for the 30-year period of conflict in Northern Ireland known as the Troubles (1968–98), which directly caused 3,500 deaths and ruined the lives of countless other people. The Red Hand is a rare example of a cross-community symbol used in Ireland. Its roots as a Gaelic Irish symbol allow republicans and GAA clubs to use it, and loyalists also use it due to its association with the province of Ulster.

The Red Hand of Ulster originally denoted the northern Uí Néill, several dynasties in medieval Ireland which claimed descent from Niall of the Nine Hostages. (A southern Uí Néill also existed.) Niall Noígíallach, as he was also known, was a legendary, semi-historical Irish king. While details are blurry, he reigned in either the fourth or fifth century AD and is credited with being one of the high kings of Ireland. Medieval texts claim that three sons of Niall (Eoghan, Conal Gulban and Enda) invaded north-western Ulster, reducing the territory owned by the Ulaid, and divided the land between them. (A cautionary note: these details are obtained from potentially untrue propaganda created by the Uí Néill family in subsequent centuries to cement their political supremacy.)[38]

The oldest surviving mention of the Red Hand of Ulster dates from the thirteenth century. In 1243, Walter de Burgh became the first Earl of Ulster and combined his family cross with the Red Hand to create a new flag. The O'Neills adopted the symbol in 1317. In medieval Irish literature, several real and legendary kings were described as 'red-handed' to signify their status as great warriors, including Lugaid Lámderg (Lugaid the Red-Handed). The O'Neills believed that a red-handed king named Aodh Eangach would help them drive the English out of Ireland. Between 1594 and 1603, a Nine Years' War took place against English rule in Ireland, and the war cry 'The Red Hand of Ulster to victory' was associated with the O'Neill family. According to a more gruesome

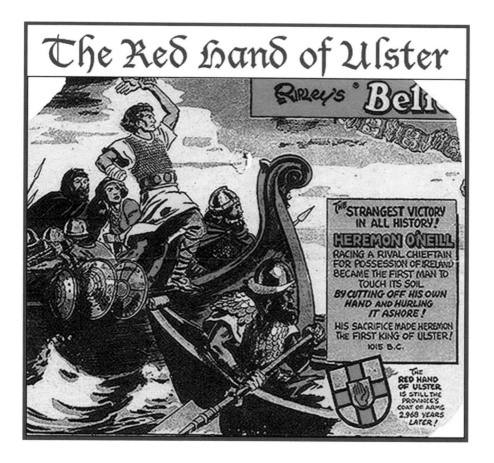

The Red Hand of Ulster

A historical depiction of
the Red Hand of Ulster.

legend, it was once believed that the first man to lay his hand on the province of Ulster would have claim to it, encouraging numerous warriors to rush towards it. One chopped off his hand, threw it over his comrades and won the land. Other variants of this story depict a boat race, with the victor being the first to touch the shore. Some believe this handless person to be an O'Neill or even Niall of the Nine Hostages.[39]

Residents of Northern Ireland today are said to never be more than 100 feet away from a Red Hand of Ulster. Loyalist communities, who march every 12 July, have distinctive banners, uniforms and flags, many of which are adorned with the Red Hand, even despite its Gaelic associations. The symbol is used to endorse their vision of their own ethnic identity.[40] In Northern Ireland, identity is of utmost importance, and the Troubles was an extended conflict between those who identified as British and those who identified as Irish. From its inception, the Northern Irish state was designed and maintained in ways that sustained the sociopolitical dominance of the Ulster Protestant majority while marginalising the needs of the minority Catholic community, many of whom refused to recognise the new state. This situation eventually culminated in the Troubles.

One loyalist group named itself the Red Hand Commando. Contradictorily, it used an Irish-language motto, Lámh Dearg Abú (meaning 'red hand to victory'). This was a highly secretive organisation and was the only major loyalist

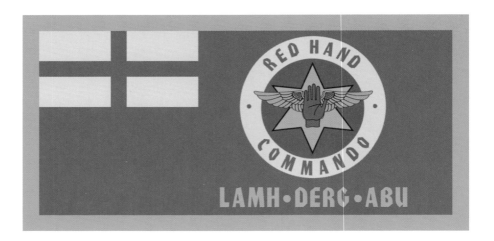

The Red Hand Commando was a loyalist paramilitary group active during the Troubles.

paramilitary group whose ranks were not penetrated by supergrasses (informants). In the early 1970s, the Red Hand Commando was particularly popular around the Shankill Road, Sandy Row and parts of East Belfast. In 1972, it became part of the Ulster Volunteer Force. Membership is thought to have been at least 1,000. A number of its senior figures helped form the Progressive Unionist Party

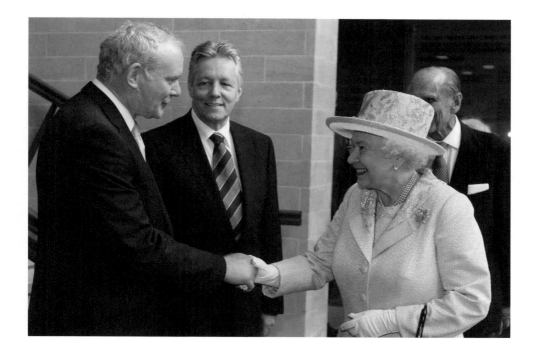

in 1979. Controversially, the group is associated with random drive-by shootings of Catholic civilians and no-warning bombs left in pubs frequented by Catholics.[41]

In 2012, Martin McGuinness and Queen Elizabeth II shake hands.

The world knew that the Troubles were truly over in 2012 when an unexpected handshake took place. It lasted only four seconds but was a moment of historical significance. At a charity event in Belfast, Queen Elizabeth II and Martin McGuinness famously shook hands. McGuinness was the former commandant of the IRA, who for decades had been planting bombs on the British mainland. In 1979 the IRA assassinated Lord Mountbatten, the uncle of Prince Philip, husband of the queen. This was a hugely symbolic moment. A hand of friendship was extended between two countries that seemed to have been forever warring. The two looked oddly relaxed, even smiling openly at each other.

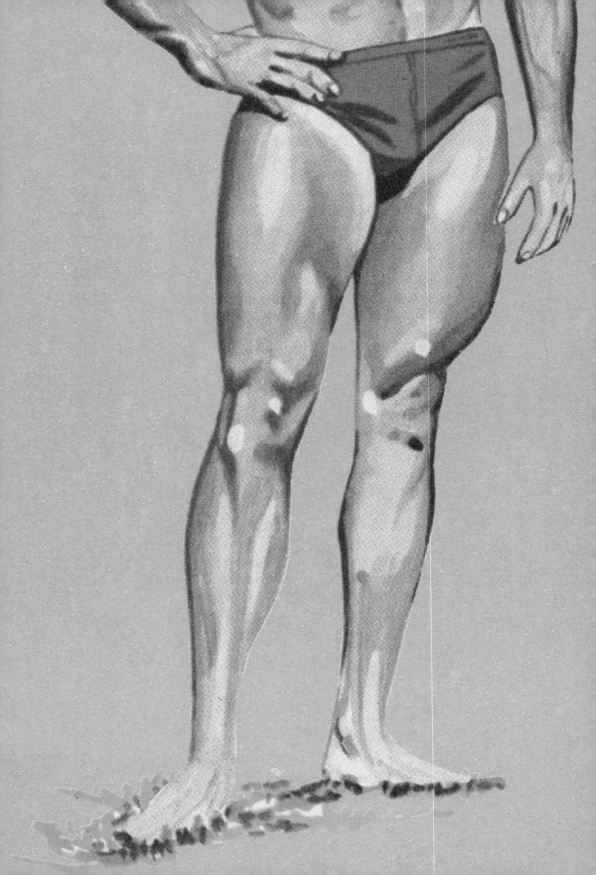

CHAPTER 4

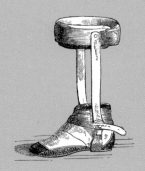

LEGS

How humans move, with one leg protruding ahead of the other, propelling us onwards, is incredibly rare in nature. We can even walk backwards if we wish (although this isn't recommended). A handful of dinosaurs walked on two legs. Nowadays, other than humans, only a small number of birds and animals walk. Ostriches and kangaroos, for example (although kangaroos can't walk backwards because they would trip over their large tail). At some point in our evolutionary past, humans became less adept at climbing and instead decided to stick closer to the ground. Over time, we developed surprisingly complex feet. Arched upwards, these support our weight, aided by knee joints that fully extend and lock. When other animals stand up, it tends to be for specific reasons, usually to try to reach something. Compared to more graceful humans, their efforts at standing upright look clumsy, ungainly and unsteady. In contrast, our upright human skeletal frame helps us maintain balance.

Around 1.8 million years ago, our ancestors developed long legs and a striding gait which made travelling longer distances easier. Learning to walk and run made humans more mobile. Our feet and toes evolved into stable platforms that spring us off the ground. Our pelvis, spines and lower limbs reshaped to help us maintain the bodily balance required to stay upright. Being bipedal also raised our heads, offering us a broader field of vision for detecting danger or resources.[1] Learning to walk and run was a useful skill indeed. In the twenty-first century, humans take advantage of this impressive evolutionary advantage by kicking a ball around a pitch while others stand around and cheer them on. In Ireland, Gaelic football (and many other sports thought to have ancient Celtic origins) has become hugely popular since the late nineteenth century. Dancing is another entertaining use of Irish legs. Both Gaelic football and Irish dancing are intrinsically bound up with national identity. However, a significant number of people in Ireland ended up losing the use of their legs for various reasons, including war and conflict.

GAELIC SPORTS

Football is big business. Curiously, many Irish people support English teams, especially Manchester United and Liverpool, even despite the often-mentioned 800 years of oppression. Ireland has its own football team, although it has made only three World Cup appearances (1990, 1994 and 2002). Northern Ireland also has a team, although it has made a similarly unimpressive number of World Cup appearances (1958, 1982 and 1986). The Irish are much better at another English game: rugby.

Some critics have lambasted this Irish fascination with English sports as evidence of anglicisation and British cultural imperialism. In 1884, the Gaelic Athletic Association (GAA) was founded. Much of the impetus came from a Clare man: Michael Cusack. Born in 1847 at the peak of the nationally devastating Great Famine, Cusack became a teacher later in life at Blackrock College, Co. Dublin. In his 1884 article published in the *Irishman*, Cusack declared that he wanted an end to 'the tyranny of imported and enforced customs and manners' and suggested that Ireland could advance, socially and politically, and far more fruitfully, without foreign (or British) influences. Cusack added that 'voluntary neglect of such pastimes is a sure sign of national decay and of approaching dissolution. The strength and energy of a

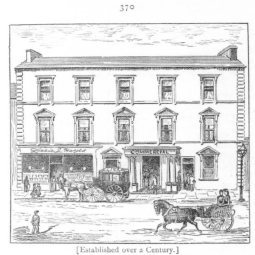

370

[Established over a Century.]

THE COMMERCIAL AND FAMILY HOTEL,

AND POSTING ESTABLISHMENT

The GAA was founded at a meeting in Hayes Hotel, Thurles, Co. Tipperary, in 1884.

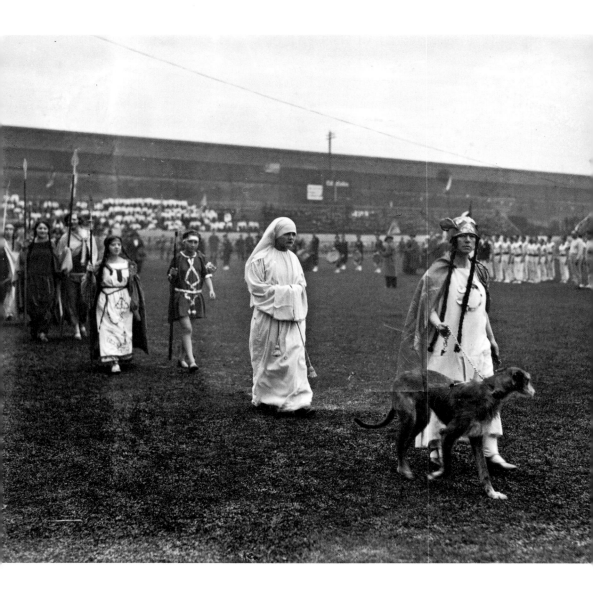

The GAA attempted
to revive the ancient
Tailteann Games.

race are largely dependent on the national pastimes for the development of a spirit of courage and endurance.'

For Cusack, the neglect of national games signified an Irish race in decline. Fearing that modernisation was destroying traditional ways of life, Cusack warned that 'foreign and hostile laws, and the pernicious influence of a hated and hitherto dominant race [the British], drove the Irish people from their trysting places at the crossroads and hurling fields back to their cabins where but a few years before famine and fever reigned supreme'. In these cabins, Irish peasants now wasted away their lives smoking and card-playing instead of triumphantly taking part in Irish sports. Cusack took issue with Irish athletic meetings having to follow the rules of the Amateur Athletics Association of England. 'Every effort has been made to make the meetings look as English as possible,' he grumbled.[2]

Cusack wanted Irish athletes to take control of their own affairs. One of his initial ideas involved reviving the ancient Tailteann Games of Celtic Ireland. According to the handwritten, eleventh-century Lebor Gabála Érenn (or Book of Invasions), these games were founded to honour the dead, proclaim laws and provide entertainment. According to folklore, the Tailteann Games started around 1600 BC, although the GAA claimed the later date of 632 BC. Evidence exists that the games were still played through the sixth to twelfth centuries AD until the Normans invaded and put an end to everyone's fun. Held annually during the last fortnight of July, games included the long jump, the high jump, running, hurling, spear throwing, boxing, sword fighting, archery, wrestling, swimming, chariot racing and horse racing. Traditionally, the games also featured a mass arranged marriage where couples met for the first time, married and were given a year to decide whether they wanted to stay together or divorce on the hills of separation. These trial marriages, as we might think of them, remained legal until the thirteenth century.[3]

In the nineteenth century, the GAA contemplated reviving the Tailteann Games, although without all the marriages. It settled instead for re-establishing hurling as a national pastime, a game of ancient Irish origin for men with a female equivalent called camogie. Players use a hurley stick to hit a small ball (a sliotar) between an opponent's goalposts, either under or over a crossbar. The sliotar can also be caught by hand and carried a short distance. Players wishing to run with the ball for more than four steps have to bounce or balance the sliotar on the end of their stick. We know that hurling has been played in Ireland since at least the fifth century and some historians date the game back as far as 1200 BC, when it was apparently played around the Hill of Tara, Co. Meath. There are stories of Finn Mac Cumhail and the Fianna enjoying hurling matches. According to Irish legend, the first Battle of Moytura was preceded by a fierce hurling match between two teams drawn from the opposing forces, with many casualties involved. As a prelude to a battle, the Fir Bolg and Tuatha Dé Danaan tribes are said to have played a game near Cong, Co. Mayo.

The ancient Brehon Laws mention a sporting game similar to hurling because compensation needed to be paid for hurling accidents and for deaths, deliberate or otherwise. The Statute of Kilkenny (1366) prohibited English people from playing hurling in case they picked up degenerative habits from the Irish (in many ways, a mirror image of Cusack's arguments about the harmful impacts of British culture on the Irish). Through the centuries, the British continued to look down upon hurling, viewing it as grossly inferior to archery and fencing. However, in the eighteenth century, the so-called 'Golden Age of Hurling', the Anglo-Irish landed gentry kept teams of players on their estates who challenged each other to matches.

In light of this cultural reappropriation, Cusack and his associates sought to reclaim the ancient Irish game for their own. Their endeavours formed part of the broader Irish cultural revival taking place around the turn of the twentieth century that self-consciously rejected British influence and revered an imagined Celtic past. The first meeting of the Dublin Hurling Club took place in December 1882, and weekly matches began to be played in Dublin's sprawling Phoenix Park. Hurling remains popular and players have never been required to wear protective padding. Wearing a protective faceguard only became mandatory in 2010,

Hurling is an ancient Irish sport revived in the late nineteenth century.

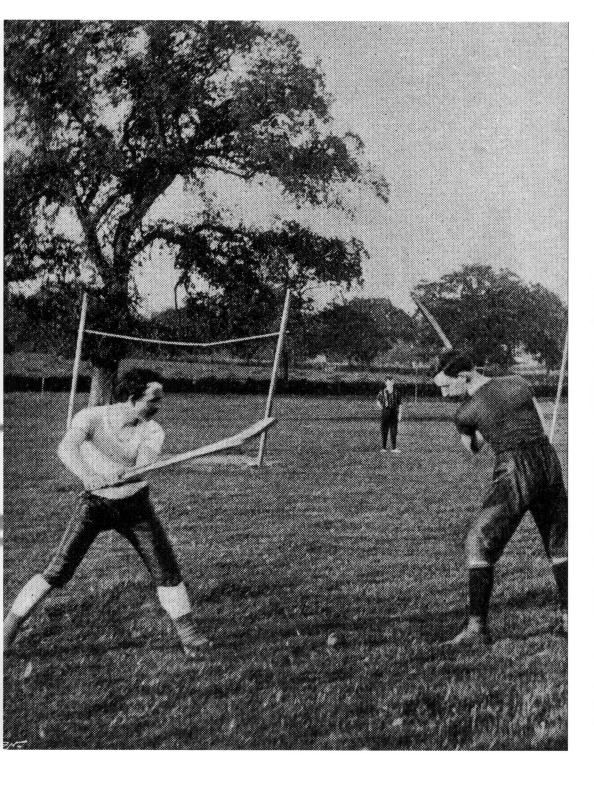

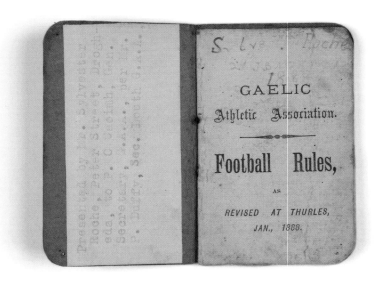

The rules for Gaelic Football are deliberately different from the rules for English football.

despite the sliotar being able to move at 100 miles per hour. All manner of injuries can occur. In 1997, one of goalkeeper Joe Quaid's testicles exploded after he was hit in the crotch by a sliotar. Half of the other one needed to be surgically removed. Surprisingly, he returned to the sport after recovering.[4]

Cusack formally inaugurated the GAA on Saturday 1 November 1884, in Thurles, Co. Tipperary, a date chosen deliberately for its mythological significance. This was the anniversary of the day that the Fianna's power died, according to Irish mythology. The choice of day was a symbolic Irish rebirth. From the outset, the GAA actively strove to counter national decline, which they blamed upon an unhealthy mix of emigration, poverty and tyrannical British neighbours. The inaugural meeting was poorly attended, but that didn't stop Cusack from reading out letters of support from some of Ireland's most prominent public figures and ambitiously emphasising the movement's future importance. Thomas Croke, the archbishop of Cashel, was its first patron, soon followed by land reformist Michael Davitt and nationalist politician Charles Stewart Parnell. Cusack was an excellent organiser but was less adept at getting along with people. He resigned after just 18 months. During his leadership, he introduced a rule that banned GAA members from playing 'foreign' games: tennis, cricket, polo, croquet and the like. Not coincidently, these were hugely popular games in Britain and had become increasingly popular among the Irish too. Within six months of the first meeting, GAA clubs had sprung up across Ireland.

Gaelic football, in particular, became associated with the campaign to rid Ireland of Britain. Football, of some description, had been played in Ireland since at least the 1300s. By the seventeenth century, it was widely played across the island and, as with hurling, enjoyed the patronage of the gentry and the enthusiasm of landlords. The 1695 Sunday Observance Act imposed a fine of one shilling for anyone caught playing sports, although it proved difficult to enforce. By the nineteenth century, various games involving kicking a ball were being played across the country.

The trouble with football (as with rugby) was its association with Britain, the country where professional teams were first created. So-called Gaelic football was reinvented in the 1880s, with new rules devised to distinguish it from the English form of the game. In 1884, the GAA formally codified its football rules as part of its broader agenda of promoting Irish sport and rejecting all British varieties. GAA football uses a slightly smaller ball, has teams of 15 players, is played by hand as well as foot (with broadly similar rules as hurling on this matter) and lasts for only 70 minutes. Gaelic football was faster, more thrilling and often more violent than its British counterpart. In the decades that followed, it began to be played around the world.

Perhaps unsurprisingly, given its shared interests in forging a strong, proud Irish identity, the GAA became associated with the Irish Republican Brotherhood (IRB) (later to evolve into the IRA). These close links made the GAA a target of opprobrium for the British authorities. IRB members had attended the very first GAA meeting of November 1884, although Cusack professed himself far

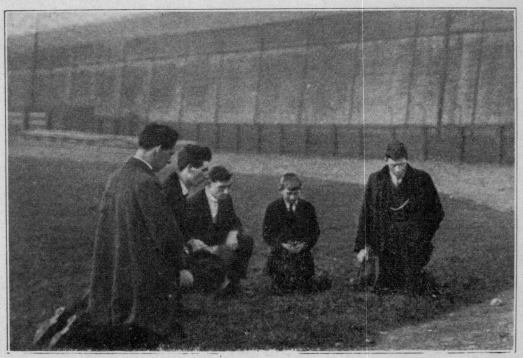

Photo   EXHIBIT 10   *W. D. Hogan, Dublin*

CROKE PARK. MOURNERS PRAYING FOR M. ROGAN, FULL-BACK, TIPPERARY FOOTBALL, TEAM, AT SPOT WHERE HE WAS SLAIN.

On 21 November 1920, the British Army opened fire on crowds at Croke Park, a day which later became known as Bloody Sunday. (Note: the caption on this image is incorrect: the name of the player who was killed was Michael Hogan.)

more interested in sports than revolutionary politics. Initially, the GAA was keen to stress its non-sectarian nature, and several Protestants were involved in the early days, but by 1887, only one member of the central committee of the GAA was not in the IRB. Officers of the Royal Irish Constabulary (RIC) were barred from joining, although they did infiltrate meetings, further testifying to the politicisation of Irish sport in this period. It was common knowledge now that the GAA was about more than simply sports.

Throughout the 1890s, the Catholic Church condemned the IRB and encouraged priests to demonise the GAA from their many pulpits. The number of GAA clubs swiftly dwindled. The GAA's central committee then decided to publicly support Charles Stewart Parnell, who had been controversially caught having an adulterous relationship with a married woman, Katharine O'Shea. At Parnell's funeral, 2,000 GAA men followed the cortège to Glasnevin Cemetery. With hindsight, this was not a good idea at all. Members left in their droves. But having survived the 1890s (just about), the GAA's fortunes picked up once more as ideas about national independence gained momentum in the twentieth century. Dublin Castle kept a close watch. During the 1916 Easter Rising, GAA members were among the rebels who fought to overthrow British rule.

Events culminated in a tragic day known as Bloody Sunday. Irish history features four Bloody Sundays, but this particular one took place on 21 November 1920. It began with an IRA operation, led by the revolutionary Michael Collins, to assassinate a number of British intelligence agents around Dublin. Fifteen members of the authorities were killed or fatally wounded. Most were from the British Army or RIC. A Gaelic football match was organised to take place that afternoon, which had raised suspicion. Proceeds from ticket sales were scheduled to go to the Republican Prisoners' Dependent Fund. At least 5,000 spectators attended, and some estimate the total to be closer to 10,000.

Around five minutes into the game, an aeroplane circled the ground of Croke Park twice and shot a red flare, a signal intended for the British authorities, who stormed in and opened fire on the crowd. Panicked spectators rushed to all four exits. The army prevented them from leaving the ground,

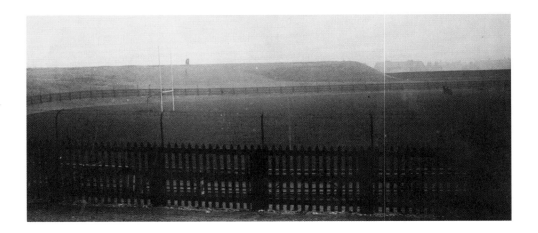

Croke Park one day after the incident.

causing a sequence of crushes around the stadium. Fearing they were about to be murdered, hundreds of people braved a 20-foot drop along the Cusack Stand side, convinced that the authorities intended to kill everyone there. The shooting lasted for less than two minutes. Fourteen people died. The police claimed that the shootings were provoked, but witnesses denied this. Even a military inquiry concluded that the military's actions were indiscriminate and excessive. A massacre had taken place on Irish soil at a seemingly harmless Gaelic football match.[5]

WAR AND LEG AMPUTATIONS

During the First World War, a British Army officer, Major Jocelyn Lee Hardy, gained fame for his battlefield courage and repeated escapes from prisoner-of-war camps. Hardy had been born in 1894 to a prominent Belfast family of wool merchants, although he grew up in London. On 2 October 1918, only a few weeks before the war ended, he was shot in the stomach and suffered a leg wound of such severity that amputation was required. The war had seen major investment in prosthetic limb technologies and, after being evacuated back to England,

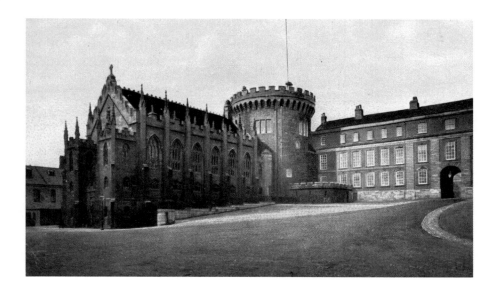

Hardy was fitted with one of these. Displeased with the results, he developed a rapid walking style, hoping to disguise his disability. From here on, he became known as 'Hoppy'.

Hoppy Hardy was seconded as an intelligence officer based at Dublin Castle in April 1920.

Hoppy Hardy had served in the Connaught Rangers and was employed after the war by the Military Intelligence Directorate. In April 1920, during the War of Independence (1919–21), he was seconded as an intelligence officer based at Dublin Castle. Despite his physical disability, Hardy led raids on various IRA locations. He became despised in IRA circles for his brutal interrogation of prisoners at Dublin Castle. Reportedly, he would trick suspects into providing information by using a revolver loaded with blanks to stage fake executions or by threatening to burn suspects with a hot poker.

The IRA shadowed Hardy. On one occasion, he evaded them at London's Euston Station, jumping into a taxi to escape an ambush. On another occasion, he evaded a group of assassins waiting on a Dublin dockside for him to return from a trip to England. The IRA intended to assassinate Hardy on the morning of Bloody Sunday, but he escaped death once again simply by not being in his room when the assassins arrived. The night before Bloody Sunday, three IRA prisoners had been captured: Conor Clune, Peadar Clancy and Dick McKee. On Bloody Sunday itself, all three mysteriously died while in custody, and it is rumoured that Hoppy Hardy was involved.

Accusations abound about Hoppy Hardy, and he is thought to have helped torture Kevin Barry, a young teenager who joined the IRA at age 15, who was threatened with a bayonet in his stomach and back. When this failed to have the desired effects, his interrogators threw Kevin to the ground, repeatedly kicked him and twisted his arm around his back. Kevin, who required hospitalisation, was then found guilty of murder and hanged in Mountjoy Prison, where he was also buried. (He was finally exhumed and given a state funeral in 2001.) Hoppy Hardy is also rumoured to have orchestrated the death of Seán Treacy, one of the men responsible for the Soloheadbeg ambush, which marked the starting point of the War of Independence.[6]

During the First World War, soldiers on all sides of the conflict were maimed and injured. Many lost limbs, including legs, creating a generation of disabled veterans dependent upon some degree of care for decades to come. However, the status of Irish soldiers who fought with the British was ambiguous, controversial and contested. Between 1918 and 1920, over 100,000 war veterans returned to Ireland. Around 30,000 Irish men had died. Four years of brutal warfare left behind many physical and psychological scars.

When the first batch of soldiers left Ireland in 1914, they were celebrated as heroes. By 1918, times had changed, and Irish veterans returned to a country now at war with Britain. At worst, the veterans were branded traitors to Ireland, having fought for the British. Some historians describe this as a 'collective amnesia' of Irish people choosing to forget their huge national sacrifice between 1914 and 1918. The shunning of the First World War veterans led to men who fought being erased from family histories and deliberately forgotten about in nationalist interpretations of twentieth-century Irish history.[7]

The British government initially awarded a disability pension for wounds, injuries or illnesses caused directly by wartime service. The pension bill was passed on to the

The British Army actively recruited in Ireland during the First World War, but returning soldiers often faced a frosty welcome home.

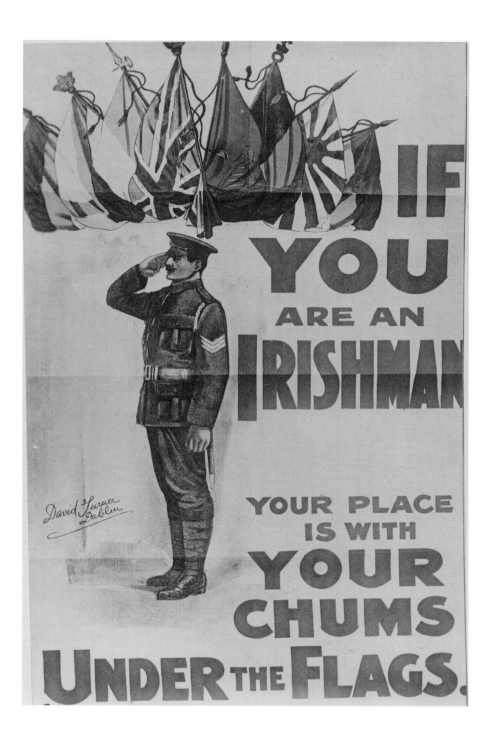

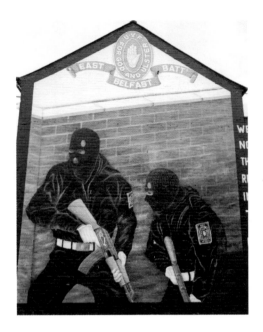

Kneecappings (or punishment shootings) were used during the Troubles to punish drug dealers and other miscreants.

Irish Free State in 1922. The new Irish government promised to continue providing pensions until the last surviving disabled veteran died. If a soldier lost two legs and seemed likely to need constant care for life, he was eligible to receive 100 per cent of the pension. If one leg had been amputated at the hip, he received 80 per cent. For a leg amputated below the knee, the former combatant was able to claim 50 per cent, as this injury was not considered severe enough to prevent him from working. Many complaints were raised about the stringency of the pensions, although they did come with highly desirable free medical care, availed of by around 27,000 men.[8]

Although the new Irish state formally supported ex-servicemen through pension schemes, in reality, the new Ireland placed little value on the physical sacrifices made by war veterans. In some areas of Ireland, admitting that one was an ex-serviceman guaranteed unemployment. During the War of Independence, reprisals, violence and employment discrimination against ex-servicemen were common. They were a major IRA target between 1920 and 1921. At least 82 were killed. The nationalist movement maintained a long-standing prejudice against Irishmen who had fought for Britain.

Some ex-servicemen, perhaps through disillusionment or a change of heart, decided to support Sinn Féin or join the IRA. Their contributions were no doubt welcome as they brought military experience with them. However, many other ex-servicemen openly criticised the IRA and found themselves targeted. Intimidation techniques aimed at ex-soldiers included death threats, kidnapping, beating, burning of houses and murder. Sometimes, former soldiers were denied entry into social occasions such as dances, refused employment or even refused hospital treatment.[9] To complicate matters further, after the Irish Civil War, around 55,000 ex-servicemen joined the new British Army. They might have been viewed with suspicion as 'traitors', but at least they were experienced. Even after independence, many Irish people signed up to the British, instead of the Irish, army, often finding work as army doctors, attracted by the better pay being offered over the Irish Sea.[10]

As conflict persisted long after the First World War in Ireland, the Irish government also had to pay compensation and pensions for those injured or bereaved during the War of Independence and Irish Civil War. The Army Pensions Act of 1923 provided pensions for Irish army soldiers who had been wounded or disabled during the Civil War, fighting against the anti-treaty IRA, and also for widows and children of soldiers. Even members of groups such as the IRA, Irish Volunteers and Irish Citizen Army were eligible to claim pensions if they had been injured between 1916 and 1922. The idea of granting pensions for those formerly engaged in guerrilla warfare was unusual at the time. To be eligible, applicants had to prove that they had been injured while taking part in an act of war (and not just injured coincidently while the conflict was going on or while doing something unrelated).[11]

The Bureau of Military History archives (an oral history of the revolutionary period collected by the Irish state between 1947 and 1957) contains a wealth of personal accounts, from all sides, of being injured and maimed. IRA member Patrick Ormond recalled receiving his life-changing injury:

> It was on 3 February 1925 when close to a roadblock at Ballylemon, I was fired on from a lorry of Free State troops, accompanied by an armoured car. I tried to escape to the shelter of Ballylemon Wood but was badly wounded in the right leg and unable to move. The Free State troops made an improvised stretcher from a barn door, placed me on it and brought me to Dungarvan Hospital where I

was a patient for ten months. After leaving the hospital, I returned to my home in Dungarvan. Since then, my right leg has been three inches shorter than my left leg. I am permanently incapacitated and able to walk only with difficulty.[12]

Men interested in joining the RIC were often intimidated by the IRA, and this account by IRA man Bernard Sweeney is suggestive of a warning that got out of hand:

> About March 1920, a local man named McCabe was going to join the RIC who were then very anxious indeed to get recruits and were holding out inducements to young men to join the Force. It was the object of the Volunteers to prevent men from joining that Force. One night, as McCabe was going home, he was taken off his cycle by the Volunteers and questioned about his joining the RIC. One of our men who was armed fired a shot accidentally, hitting McCabe in the leg. As a result of this, he had to have his leg amputated and that finished his attempt to join. The RIC made every endeavour to trace the people engaged in this incident. It was a dark night and McCabe did not identify anyone. The police made no arrests.[13]

Another interview contains this unusual story of the problems caused by the corpse of an ex-serviceman who had lost one of his legs:

> There was a man named Maher who was an ex-British officer living in Irishtown. He had a wooden leg but travelled extensively throughout the country. He was under suspicion of spying for the British for a long time, and we had been keeping him under observation. He was arrested by George Adamson and Ned Doolan in Carrickbyrne and court-martialled and sentenced to be shot.

He had a small pension from the British government, but claimed that he lived principally by begging, but our information, which was backed up by the evidence of the men who had been keeping watch on him, was that he was never known to have done any begging. He was found guilty by the court-martial and sentenced to be shot.

He was shot and his body was thrown into the Shannon. We did not want his execution to become known so as to avoid reprisals by the enemy on Carrickbyrne, and that was why his body was given to the river. We forgot about the wooden leg, and this kept the body afloat in the river where it remained for a considerable time. It was then hauled in and buried on the bank of the river by some of our men. I personally took charge of the execution party.[14]

The problem of floating bodies was surprisingly common, and another account states:

A man, whose name I do not know, but who was known as 'Slickfoot', was shot as a spy in the Carrickbyrne area. He had a cork leg and that was the reason he was called 'Slickfoot'. When he was shot, he was thrown into the river, but the cork leg made him float, so he had to be weighted down with sandbags.[15]

In the twenty-first century, the issue of paying pensions to those affected by the Troubles (typically due to participation, imprisonment or injury) is a much-discussed topic. One standout feature of the Troubles was the eagerness for kneecapping among paramilitaries, that is, shooting victims in the knees, and sometimes the elbow too. In Northern Ireland, 129 people had their legs amputated because of these punishment shootings, and many others were left with a disfiguring limp for the rest of their lives. Paramilitary groups saw themselves as law enforcers in their areas, having lost all faith in the police and state to protect them. Kneecappings were usually intended to punish drug dealers and other people considered guilty of antisocial behaviour. In total, around 2,000 people suffered punishment shootings through the 30 years of conflict. The characteristic limp was intended as a warning to others to behave themselves.[16]

An unexpected positive came from all of this. During the Troubles, surgeons encountered so many injured and missing limbs, through kneecappings or bomb blasts, that they became world-leading experts in orthopedic surgery. Most patients with limb problems were sent to Belfast's Musgrave Park Hospital, which developed extensive resources for fitting prosthetic limbs and rehabilitating patients with serious leg injuries.[17]

The sheer extent of conflict in Ireland throughout the twentieth century had a major impact on the physical well-being of those involved in, or caught up in, armed conflict, whether that was British intelligence agents such as Hoppy Hardy, IRA men fighting during the War of Independence and Civil War or, more recently, participants in, or victims of, the Troubles. These major events in modern Irish history were experienced by a significant number of people through severe disability or loss of limb. But, depending upon Irish society's perspectives on the nature of particular conflicts, those who went through life missing a limb were not always guaranteed sympathy and compassion.

IRISH DANCING

In 1999, Michael Flatley insured his legs for $40 million. Born to Irish parents who had emigrated to America, Flatley spent his adult life enjoying international renown for his Irish dancing skills. A serious leg injury would have ended his illustrious dancing career. His mother, Eilish, had been a gifted step dancer from Co. Carlow, and his grandmother, Hannah Ryan, was a champion dancer. Flatley's parents met at an Irish dance in Detroit and had five children. At the young age of 11, Flatley began attending dance classes at the Dennehy School of Irish Dance, Chicago, where the family were then living. Aged 17, he became the first American to win a World Irish Dance title at Oireachtas Rince na Cruinne (Irish Dancing World Championships). Flatley was also adept at boxing and flute playing but decided to earn his living through dancing. Some called him 'the white Michael Jackson'.

It was the Eurovision Song Contest that took Flatley's career to an international stage, an event Ireland has won an impressive seven times. The winning country is expected to host the contest the following year. In the 1990s, Ireland became so good at providing winning entries (1992, 1993, 1994 and 1996) that concerns arose about whether the country had enough finances to keep on hosting the contest so regularly. For the 1994 Eurovision Song Contest, Flatley was invited to perform a seven-minute show, which

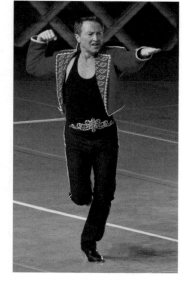

Michael Flatley became world famous in the 1990s with his *Riverdance* show.

he named *Riverdance*, during an interval. The Eurovision had never seen the likes of such a performance. It began with the haunting vocals of a choral group, Anúna, before dancer Jean Butler arrived on stage, emerging from a traditional Irish cloak. Flatley, the so-called 'Lord of the Dance', then burst on stage, followed by an energetic troupe of Irish dancers. Never before had Irish dancing been choreographed in such a mesmerising way.

Given its sudden popularity, *Riverdance* was swiftly expanded to a full stage production that debuted in Dublin in February 1995. One hundred and twenty thousand tickets were sold. By 2022, there had been 12,340 performances across the globe. In 1995, Flatley entered into a dispute with the *Riverdance* producers about salaries and royalty fees and soon found himself fired. Infuriated, he created his own show, *Lord of the Dance*, which premiered in Dublin before enjoying a long run in London, where it remained immensely popular for decades. Later in his career, Flatley produced the show *Celtic Tiger Live*, which traced the history of the

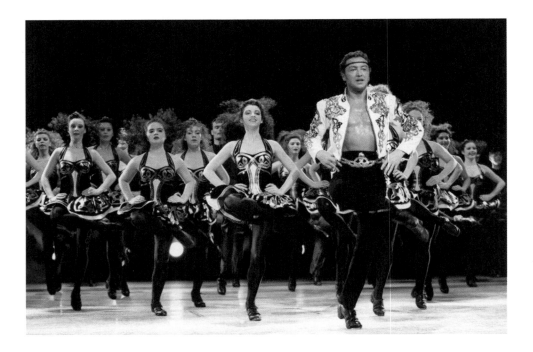

Riverdance remains hugely popular today.

Irish, focusing on their nineteenth-century emigration to America. 'I will be a dancer until the day I die,' he proclaimed in the programme.[18]

Irish dancing, as we know it today, evolved from dances of the seventeenth century and was a curious mix of Irish, English and continental dancing. The Normans are thought to have introduced round dances to Ireland. Presumably, dancing had long been popular in Ireland, but we have few historical records predating the seventeenth century, when sources begin to mention country dances and the famous Irish jig, accompanied by music played on the fiddle, a recently imported instrument, as well as bagpipes and the harp.[19] Solo or step dances are rarely mentioned until the eighteenth century, which suggests that they could be relatively modern.[20] The introduction of quadrilles changed the style of Irish dancing. Originating in France, quadrilles were brought in as 'square dances', possibly by Irish soldiers returning from the Napoleonic

Wars shortly after 1815. This gradually evolved into set dancing. Couple dances introduced in the nineteenth century included the waltz and polka.[21]

Dance was taught by travelling masters, wandering teachers who roamed around Ireland teaching French dancing etiquette and technique. The dancing master first appears in the historical record in the late eighteenth century. He was a whimsical figure who considered himself a gentleman, his arrival in a village was usually hailed with delight, as six weeks (at least) of music and dancing was to follow. The dancing master received a quarterly fee from his pupils. An unused house or building would be used for lessons. Dancing masters usually operated within a 10-mile radius. While friendly rivalry existed between the various masters, they seem to have respected each other's territory. Should two of them meet at a fair or sporting event, a 'dance-off' took place.[22]

By all accounts, dancing masters were flamboyant, brightly dressed characters who carried staffs. They taught group dances to less talented students and solo dances to the most gifted. Solo dances were usually demonstrated on tabletops, or the top of barrels, as local venues were often small. As a result, a peculiarly Irish form of solo dancing is thought to have developed involving arms being held rigidly to the side and with a lack of lateral movement. Only when larger dance venues became available could more body movement be realistically incorporated. Another variant of this story is that priests once considered the ritual hand movements evil and sinister and encouraged dancers to move only their legs, keeping their hands on the belt.[23] In 1779, English agriculturalist and traveller Arthur Young, in his travel book *A Tour in Ireland*, noted that 'dancing is very general among the poor people, almost universal in every cabin'. He mentioned 'the Irish jig which they can dance with a most luxuriant expression'. (On the same page, he also dismisses hurling as 'the cricket of savages'.)[24]

Like most things in twentieth-century Ireland, dancing became politicised. A debate ensued about which dances were acceptably Irish and which looked suspiciously English. The Gaelic League, formed in 1893 by Douglas Hyde to preserve the Irish language and de-anglicise Ireland, involved itself heavily in

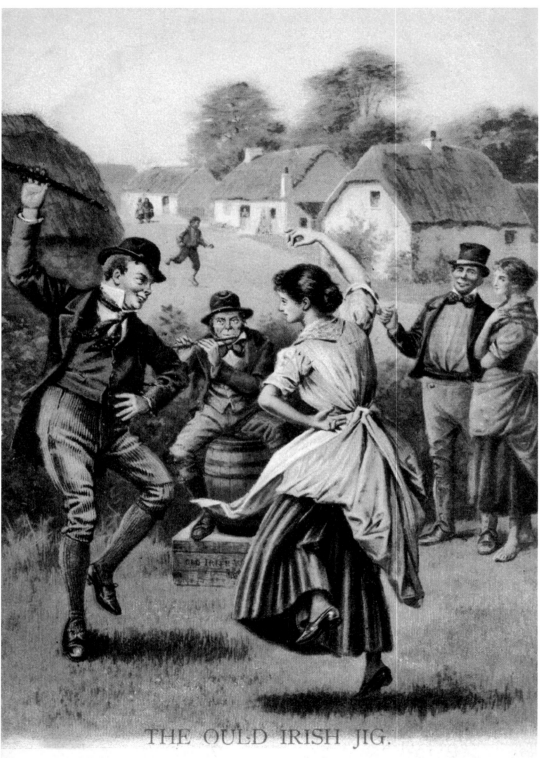

THE OULD IRISH JIG.

"Then a fig for the new fashioned waltzes
Imported from Spain and from France,
And a fig for the thing called the polka,
Our own Irish jig we will dance."

this discussion. The year 1897 saw the first public céilí, which took place (not without irony) in Bloomsbury Hall, London, organised by the Gaelic League. Sets, quadrilles and waltzes were danced to the characteristic sounds of Irish music.

In the 1920s, the Gaelic League set up dancing schools for children, an attempt to exert control over Irish dance. Only acceptably Irish dances were included in the Gaelic League's dance handbooks, and the league sought to ban many popular dances of the time if they seemed too foreign, including round dances, country dances and quadrilles. In 1929, the league formed An Coimisiún Le Rincí Gaelacha (CLRG) (the Irish Dancing Commission) to codify and standardise step-dancing. Over the decades, CLRG helped popularise its variety of Irish step dances around the world.[25]

Between the 1930s and 1970, céilí dancing became immensely popular and deeply associated with Irishness. In the Mansion House, Dublin, huge céilí dances were organised weekly and attracted thousands of people. Céilí bands were in great demand. At many events, the Gaelic League insisted that the Irish language be spoken, and no foreign dancing was allowed. Irish dancing teachers were forbidden to attend any form of modern, or non-céilí, dances. Céilí dancing isn't quite as popular nowadays, but there has nonetheless been a resurgence of interest in Irish music of all kinds.[26]

The Church has proven perpetually unhappy about dance-related gatherings, particularly any which brought together young people of the opposite sex. In 1670, one West Cork priest wrote: 'Women dancers are the cause of many evils, because it is they who bear arms in the devil's army. The devil compels them to gather on holidays for dancing, a thing which leads them to bad thoughts and evil actions.' Little changed over the centuries, and in 1875, the bishops of Ireland issued a pastoral address in which they denounced improper dances – an occasion of sin, so they argued.

In 1924, Dr O'Doherty, the bishop of Galway, warned anyone who would listen that the dances being indulged in were not clean, healthy dances, and added: 'Fathers of this parish, if your girls do not obey you, lay the lash upon their backs.' Some

Irish dancing has been popular for centuries despite being traditionally frowned upon by the Church.

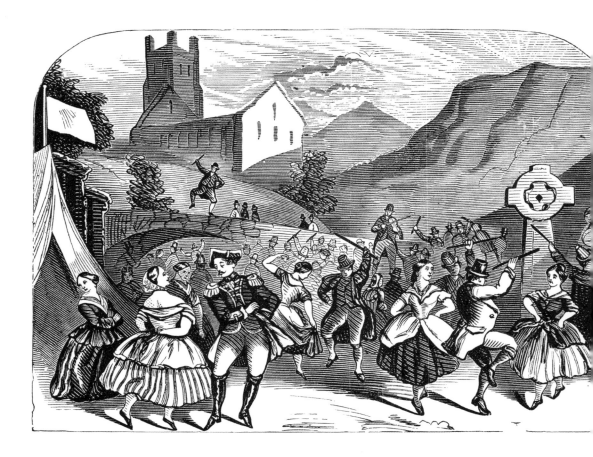

Dancing at a pattern fair at a holy well in the late eighteenth century.

priests burst into dances, beating attendees and musicians with sticks and marching girls home to their fathers for a further beating with a belt. Young courting couples were particularly prone to receiving a good whipping. Each week, Sunday Mass was infused with warnings about the evils of dancing. Set dances were targeted. The Gaelic League replaced these dances with 'traditional' dances which they had in fact recently invented themselves. Fortunately, the Gaelic League didn't entirely manage to kill off set dancing, and it would subsequently enjoy a renaissance, particularly from the 1970s onwards.[27]

After independence, the Catholic Church, which had increasing influence over state policy (the so-called 'confessional state'), clarified its views on popular entertainment. In the 1924 Lenten pastorals, the bishops condemned women's fashions, theatre, cinemas, 'evil literature', cars, drink and indecent dancing. Anything fun, essentially. In the 1920s, jazz was globally popular but the Catholic clergy in Ireland, and also the Gaelic League, saw jazz as sexualised, degenerate, corrupting and morally indecent. Jazz was certainly not an appropriate dance for a recently independent country, they argued, and nor was it particularly Catholic or Irish. The powers that be projected their anxieties and fantasies about immoral youthful behaviour onto jazz dancing.

An anti-jazz campaign was launched, and the government capitulated in 1935 by passing the Public Dance Hall Act, which banned all unlicensed public dances, ending long-standing traditions in rural Ireland of dances being organised in private houses. The clergy had recently built commercial public dance halls and hoped that the act would pressure everyone to attend dances organised instead under its watchful eye. Unsupervised dance halls were depicted as sites of vice, prostitution, sexual encounters, degeneration and 'giddy girls'. Presumably, the Church feared the rise of the 'modern woman' of the interwar period – one who was independent, outspoken and sexual. These debates also reveal anti-modernist tendencies in post-independence Ireland. The act was draconian. Dances could only be held with permission from the clergy, police or judiciary. Admittedly, enforcement was patchy in practice but the implementation of such an act raises problematic questions about the nature of the Irish state that replaced the British one and the extent of power which it sought to hold over the day-to-day behaviour of people living in Ireland. Could it have been that colonial tyranny had been replaced with the tyranny of the confessional state?[28]

CHAPTER 5

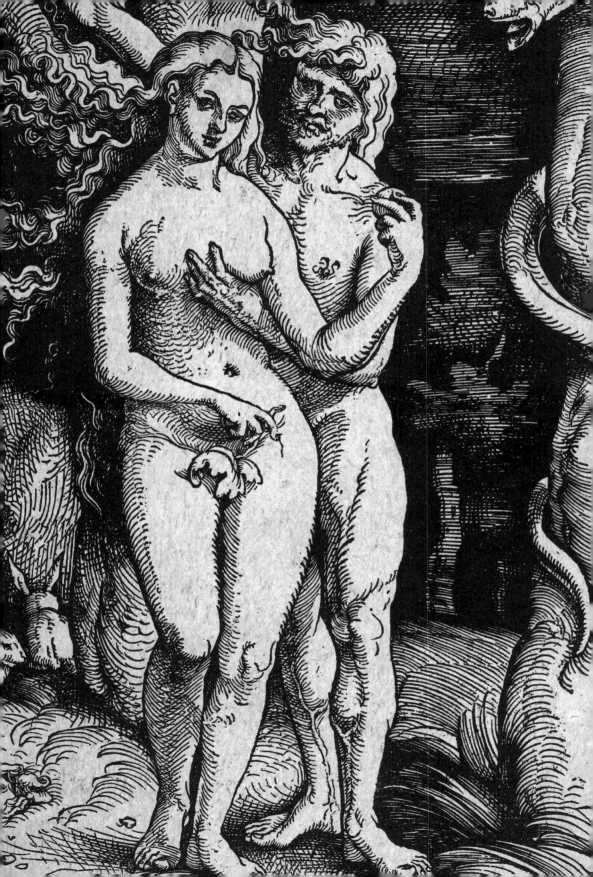

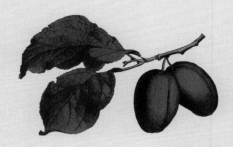

SEXUAL ORGANS

If we still lived in twentieth-century Ireland, the Church and State would almost certainly have banned this book for including this chapter. The Committee on Evil Literature (yes, really) which sat in 1926 would have considered its content far too obscene for the readers' delicate eyes. Its risqué content might have corrupted the readers' morals, undermining the very fabric of the new confessional state that emerged from the 1920s. This attitude was clearly illustrated in 1966, when Fine Gael politician Oliver J. Flanagan

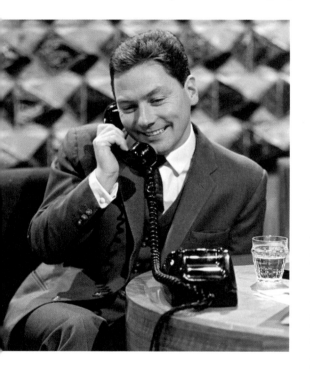

The Late Late Show is a popular Irish television show which occasionally caused controversy in the 1960s when airing sexual content.

famously criticised RTÉ's immensely popular programme *The Late Late Show*, claiming that 'sex never came to Ireland until Telefis [sic] Éireann went on the air'. The phrase is usually misquoted as the much catchier: 'There was no sex in Ireland before television.'

But was Ireland's sexual history really as chaste and pure as Flanagan believed? Absolutely not. In this obscene chapter, readers' morals risk being harmed by tales of sordid, illicit sex throughout Irish history and the mysterious Sheela-na-gigs (sexually explicit medieval carvings found across the country). The lives of some of Ireland's most notorious sexual partners will be explored, including Charles Stewart Parnell and Katharine O'Shea, Maud Gonne and W.B. Yeats, and Oscar Wilde and Alfred Douglas. Until quite recently, the consequences of becoming pregnant out of wedlock were very severe for women, with harsh social attitudes existing towards abortions and illegitimate births. The reality of people's sex lives was much more intricate and varied than religious authorities would have preferred.

SEX BEFORE IRISH TELEVISION

According to a 2004 documentary broadcast in Australia, the Romans were shocked by the Celts' hedonistic celebration of sex. The documentary featured a mix of academic talking heads and soft-porn re-enactments of the sexually voracious Fianna, all set against a clichéd musical backdrop of Enya-esque music. The documentary also presented homosexuality and bestiality as remarkably common and blamed the Church for crushing the libido of the sexually permissive Celts on its arrival in Ireland. Another of its key messages was that the Irish in the 1960s had the misfortune of being the most sexually repressed people in the world, also thanks to the Catholic Church.[1]

While it is notoriously hard to find much out about the private sex lives of the ancient Irish, it does seem that pre-Christian Ireland was a land of comparatively permissive sexual mores. Celtic Ireland was governed through the Brehon Laws, and their rules on sexual matters shocked the Christians, who replaced the ancient laws in the twelfth century. Brehon Law treated women comparatively favourably and allowed divorce on various grounds including infidelity, impotence, infanticide, attempted abortion, disclosing information on private sexual matters to others, theft and obesity. Polygamy was allowed. There is less of a sense that pre-Christian rulers used sexual behaviour as a means of asserting social control.[2]

The medieval Church insisted that intercourse should only take place between married couples. Even then, it was prohibited on holy days and during Lent and a woman's menstrual flow. Missionary was the only sexual position allowed. Men were not supposed to ejaculate anywhere outside of the vagina as this was considered a form of contraception. (The pulling-out method, as we call it today.) Ideally, married couples would have sex only to produce children, and not for fun or pleasure.[3]

In practice, premarital sex was always commonplace in Ireland, regardless of the Church's moral pronouncements. Up to 10 per cent of seventeenth- and eighteenth-century Irish brides were pregnant. Communities tolerated these scenarios if they involved an established couple scheduled to be married. Nonetheless, while women were expected to remain pure, chaste and faithful, the same did not apply to Irish men. Men from the landed classes commonly kept a mistress for sexual purposes, paid her attractive annuities and left provisions for any illegitimate children in wills. So long as this was out of public view, families generally turned a blind eye. An unfaithful wife, in contrast, faced divorce and never seeing her children again.[4]

After Christianity was established, Ireland was rocked by numerous sex scandals. The imposition of rigid sexual standards failed to deter many people from doing what came naturally to them. Medieval society was full of illicit affairs and sexual encounters, and we know about only a small minority of these: those people who were caught and exposed. In 1307, merchant John Don left his new wife, Basilia, at home for lengthy periods while travelling overseas on business. His sexually frustrated wife soon caught the attention of a man named Stephen le Clerk and the two became 'friends' while John was away. Upon returning, John warned Stephen to stay away from his house. However, while John made a trip to Cork, the lustful couple resumed their sordid affair.

This time, John meant business. He pretended to be on a visit to Youghal and persuaded the keeper of a tavern frequented by Basilia and her lover to act as spy. Believing John to be far away, the couple met in the tavern, and the keeper informed John. The enraged husband captured Stephen, beat him, bound him from head to foot and put an end to his wife's affair by castrating her lover.[5]

Details of same-sex sexual relations are almost impossible to find in the medieval historical record, given their clandestine nature, but these were no doubt common too. King Edward II and his lieutenant of Ireland, Piers Gaveston, are rumoured to have been lovers given that they seemed inseparable.[6]

Some of the most notorious sex scandals implicated the same men of the cloth who went around preaching to others about sexual morality. In 1366, Bishop Richard O'Reilly broke his chastity vows by having an affair with Edina O'Reilly, a married woman and also his first cousin. After Richard was caught in the act, he was excommunicated by Archbishop Milo Sweetman, who was far from impressed. Three months later, Richard promised to end his illicit sexual affair and the excommunication was lifted. However, within a few months, Richard had returned to his lover. A couple of centuries later, in the 1690s, residents of east Ulster started to notice something curious about young children in the area. Many of them looked suspiciously like the local dean. Dean Ward, the dean of Connor, was brought to trial for many matters including numerous sexual infractions and fathering several illegitimate children. Although most of his sexual encounters were consensual, a number of women accused him of rape.[7]

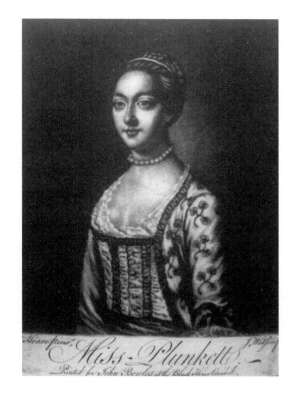

Peg Plunkett was a famous eighteenth-century Dublin prostitute who controversially wrote her memoirs.

Prostitution featured prominently in public discussion of sexuality. In the eighteenth century, Dublin's Temple Bar area was a disreputable den of street prostitutes, brothels and high-class courtesans. One well-known brothel owner, Peg Plunkett, published her three-volume memoirs (later republished as *Peg Plunkett: Memoirs of a Whore*), revealing much about the sexual preferences and perversions of the men who frequented her premises.[8] Another Temple Bar brothel keeper, Dorcas 'Darkey' Kelly, was known for being a serial killer. After being convicted of killing shoemaker John Dowling on St Patrick's Day 1760, Kelly was partially hanged and then burned at the stake on Gallows Road (now Baggot Street).[9]

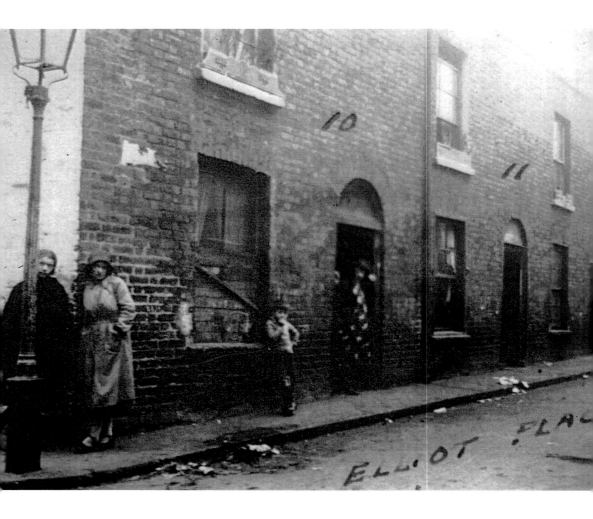

The Monto was an area of
Dublin once notorious for the
sheer number of prostitutes
who worked there.

Prostitutes set up shop wherever the army or navy went. The opening of the Royal Barracks (now Collins Barracks) in 1702 meant that sex work also proliferated further up the River Liffey from Temple Bar. The Monto was another area of Dublin which became known as a red-light district, further downstream. In what is now the area around Connolly Station on Dublin's northside, up to 1,600 prostitutes worked at any given time of night between the 1860s and 1950s, reportedly Europe's largest red-light district. King Edward VII is rumoured to have lost his virginity in the Monto. In the 1920s, the Church and police staged a major clampdown in the area.[10]

Many women turned to prostitution from poverty and desperation, but State and Church viewed these women as fallen, immoral wretches more deserving of punishment than support. Doctors agreed as they blamed prostitutes for spreading sexually transmitted diseases. The Contagious Diseases Acts of the 1860s granted public health authorities permission to detain any woman suspected of selling her body and force her to have a vaginal inspection for disease. The men who paid for their services were not sought out or tested against their will for venereal disease. The acts caused considerable anger. Women's groups led by Anna Haslam in Dublin and Isabella Tod in Belfast campaigned vigorously against such intrusive state measures that targeted desperate women.[11]

A few male prostitutes gained notoriety, including Dublin-born Jack Saul (popularly known as Dublin Jack), born in 1857 in a filthy, grim Dublin tenement slum. His parents did not marry until he was six months old because Elize, his mother, was still underage. Starting out as a teenager, Jack made money as a rent boy. In 1884, a huge national scandal erupted when Irish nationalists alleged that homosexual orgies were taking place among staff at Dublin Castle. One man charged with gross indecency was Martin Oranmore Kirwan, a captain in the Royal Irish Fusiliers. One of Kirwan's sexual partners when he was a young lieutenant had been none other than Dublin Jack. Kirwan was acquitted, but with his reputation in tatters, he resigned.

By then, Jack had moved to London and found employment at Drury Lane Theatre. In 1887, he moved into a male brothel at Cleveland Street in north

London. After a teenage boy working at the brothel turned up at a post office to lodge a significant sum of money, the Cleveland Street scandal broke out. Prominent people including Lord Euston were accused of frequenting the brothel to secure the sexual services of teenage boys. Jack was called as a witness and delivered his evidence with brazen effrontery. Less is known about Jack's later life, but it appears to have been quieter. He returned to Dublin at some point and is known to have worked as a butler there.[12]

SHEELA-NA-GIG

Above the doors and windows of numerous medieval buildings across Ireland are found carvings of an unseemly looking woman: Sheela-na-gig. Puzzled visitors who cast their eyes upward might wonder what drove the medieval Irish to create such ugly, visceral sculptures. Naked, squatting, cackling, bald,

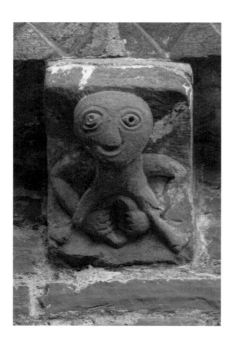

thighs spread wide open, watching and listening with her comically large eyes or ears, flaunting her withered sagging breasts, Sheela-na-gig greets onlookers by invitingly pulling apart her vulva. An exhibitionist, she unabashedly offers sexual pleasure to men wandering by, although her monstrous appearance makes this indecent proposal feel deeply disturbing, even menacing.

These sexually explicit carvings were created all over Europe, but Ireland has the greatest number of any country, with at least 100 having survived. By comparison, Britain has only 45. No two Sheela-na-gigs are the same. The carvings are reminiscent of the better-known gargoyles that ominously

The Sheela-na-gig is an explicit statue that was popular across Ireland in the medieval period.

decorate medieval buildings. First carved in France and Spain, the oldest known Sheela-na-gigs date from the eleventh century. They became popular in twelfth-century Ireland, especially in rural areas occupied by the Normans. None has been found in areas governed by the high king of Ireland, suggesting that Sheela-na-gigs were an English import. Their crude design hints that local amateur carvers or stonemasons carved them, and not sophisticated, skilled craftsmen.[13]

From the sixteenth century, the clergy actively destroyed Sheela-na-gigs or removed them from public view. This angered the rural Irish, and even some priests, who went to great lengths to preserve their precious carvings. Still today, hidden Sheela-na-gigs are discovered in wells, riverbeds and shallow graves. The tradition was largely forgotten about until the 1820s when the British were conducting an ordnance survey across Ireland. One outraged surveyor, John O'Conor, encountered a number of these hideous carvings and wrote about his livid disgust upon finding one carved into a church in Co. Tipperary. How could such an unholy, immoral carving have found a place on the walls of a sacred place, he fumed?

Hands shaking with rage, O'Conor wrote the following scathing passage in his notes:

> A shockingly crude naked female with splayed legs and fingers holding open a gaping vulva. Two odd breasts, one with two nipples, a triangular Celtic head and a pipe-stem neck ... whose attitude and expression conspire to impress the grossest idea of immorality and licentiousness.

Infuriated by the pornographic spectacle before his eyes, and unimpressed by its open invitation of sexual delight, O'Conor described the carving as 'an ill-executed piece of sculpture' created by 'the wantonness of some loose mind'. It was 'very bad taste to exhibit such a fixture on a Christian chapel', he concluded. After making some investigations, he discovered that locals called the carving 'Sile ni Ghig'.[14]

Johann Georg Kohl, a German writer travelling in Ireland during 1842, wanted to examine one of these provocative sculptures for himself and scoured the island in search of a Sheela-na-gig. Kohl was fascinated by the descriptions of the carvings which he had heard, although he never revealed who had divulged these. Discussions with locals revealed that Sheela-na-gigs were still used as antidotes to the evil eye and that priests tolerated them, feeling that carvings were a lesser evil than the real thing. Puzzled, Kohl asked what was meant by this, and he was told that living Sheela-na-gigs exist: women who can heal any person caught under the spell of an evil eye by lifting their skirts and exposing their genitalia, much to the annoyance of the local clergy.[15]

Throughout the nineteenth century, more offensive Sheela-na-gigs were discovered. Clergymen and churchgoers frowned upon this renewed interest in such lewd artwork; archaeologists regarded them as undesirably lascivious; museum curators locked the pornographic filth away from impressionable public eyes. Only in the twentieth century were Sheela-na-gigs taken more seriously as artefacts that might enrich understanding of Irish social traditions.[16]

That said, scholars disagree on their meaning. Explicit, erotic and enticing, but simultaneously monstrous and sexually unappetising, Sheela-na-gig remains an enigma. To intensify the inherent ugliness of their carvings, Irish sculptors added facial scars, saggy breasts and ribs protruding through the torso. The most widely accepted explanation is that the grotesque figures, and their placing on church walls, deliberately presented female sexuality as sinful and corrupt. Sheela-na-gig's repulsive, contorted features were intended to warn against lust and remind viewers of the creatures lurking in hell ready to torture sinners, particularly those with carnal knowledge, for the eternity to come.[17]

This denigration of sex was a peculiarly Christian obsession, and other theories propose that the Sheela-na-gig tradition stretches back to more liberal Celtic times. Sheela-na-gig is reminiscent of the Cailleach, a hag-like Celtic goddess associated with rugged landscapes, horned beasts and stormy, wintry weather. Many of Ireland's bleakest landscapes are named after her. The Hag's Head is a craggy, prominent mountain in the Cliffs of Moher, Co. Clare. Leaba

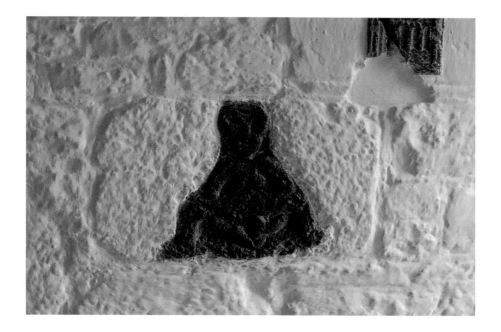

Chailli ('the Hag's Bed'), in Glanworth, Co. Cork, is rumoured to be the former site of a hag's house, now her grave. Sliabh na Cailli ('the Hag's Mountain') in Co. Meath contains a number of megalithic tombs and a kerbstone known as the Hag's Chair.[18]

Sheela-na-gigs were carved in various places including outside churches.

These interpretations hardly cast feminine sexuality in a flattering light. Unlike most other Celtic goddesses, the hag is neither sensual nor beautiful. Her unsightliness suggests malevolence. However, some ancient myths tell of the hag's shape-shifting abilities. In these, the hag appears in an elderly, lustful form. Because of her ugliness, men refused the hag's sexual advances, except one man who bravely accepted. After the man and hag finished their sexual union, she transformed into a stunningly beautiful maiden. As if that were not good luck enough, the lady then conferred royalty upon her satisfied partner and blessed his reign as king.[19]

In reality, Sheela-na-gig probably served some purpose in both Celtic and Christian culture. After all, Christianity did not simply arrive in Ireland and replace Celtic traditions overnight. Indeed, one way of persuading the Celtic Irish to convert was to incorporate pre-Christian figures, including goddesses, into Catholicism, a process of cultural assimilation which had previously worked well for the Roman Empire.[20]

Feminists developed more complimentary explanations after noticing that ancient Irish iconography and literature contained several powerful female figures, of which Sheela-na-gig was one. Refusing to reduce Sheela-na-gig to a monstrous whore whose features were intended to put people off having sex, they note that the carvings have many Celtic predecessors. Evidence for this includes Celtic sculptures found around Lough Erne, Co. Fermanagh, which have similar bodily proportions. Travellers can visit two stone carvings in a remote Victorian graveyard on Lough Erne's Boa Island which clearly feature Sheela-na-gig's characteristic posture and enticing sexual gesture.

In feminist reinterpretations, Sheela-na-gig emanates great power from her gaping, open vulva. While transmitting sexual energy, she bestows sovereignty on future kings and prowess on male warriors. This fits well with other tales in Irish mythology. Queen Medb married, or at least slept with, various men who became king of Connacht. Sovereigns must be sexual and fertile to produce heirs and guarantee the land's fertility, revealing the close links between power, kingship and sexuality, and yet it is female sexuality which drives all of this.[21]

PARNELL AND O'SHEA'S ADULTEROUS AFFAIR

Despite its preferred identity as a chaste, moral country, Ireland has been rocked by several sex scandals. One of the most well-known involved Charles Stewart Parnell. Born into a wealthy Anglo-Irish Protestant landowning family in Co. Wicklow, Parnell founded the Irish National Land League in 1879 and later became leader of the Home Rule League. After a spell of imprisonment in 1882, he renamed the league the Irish Parliamentary Party.

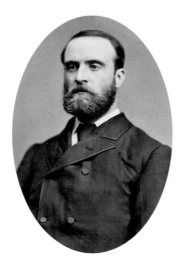 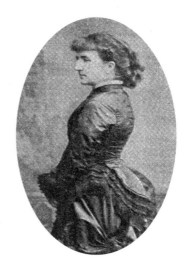

In 1887, Parnell was accused of supporting the Phoenix Park Murders of 1882. Chief Secretary Frederick Cavendish and Permanent Under-Secretary Thomas Henry Burke had been fatally stabbed in one of Dublin's busiest parks. Parnell's support was later disproved.[22] His downfall came

Towards the end of the nineteenth century, the love affair of Charles Stewart Parnell and Katharine O'Shea (a married woman) caused huge controversy.

soon after. In 1880, Parnell met Katharine O'Shea and fell immediately in love, but there was a problem. Katharine was married to Captain William O'Shea. O'Shea had only married Katharine to allow him to ascend into a new social milieu. Their marriage was not particularly happy. Less than a year after the wedding, O'Shea had run up significant debts and turned to gambling, hoping to recoup some of his finances. He was declared bankrupt in 1870 shortly after the birth of their first child. The captain separated from Katharine in 1875 but refused to divorce her as he hoped to obtain a substantial inheritance from her rich aunt. Unusually for the time, the pair lived separately.

Given all of this, it is unsurprising that Katharine responded enthusiastically when a better catch came her way. Katharine's heart began to race the very second she first encountered Parnell. As she later recalled:

> He came out, a tall gaunt figure, thin and deadly pale. He looked straight at me smiling, and his curiously burning eyes looked into mine with a wondering intentness that threw into my brain the sudden thought: 'This man is wonderful and different.'[23]

She also wrote:

> Turning more to me, he paused, and as the light from the stage caught his eyes, they seemed like sudden flames. I leaned a little towards him … and his eyes smiled into mine.[24]

Despite having been separated from Katharine for six years, in 1881 O'Shea challenged Parnell to a duel and forbade his estranged wife to see her lover ever again. This didn't work out as planned, and Parnell fathered three of Katharine's children: Claude Sophie (1882), Claire (1883) and Katharine (1884). The gossip mill having been fuelled, the affair became an open secret. Parnell also committed the ultimate Victorian sin of moving in with Katharine.

By 1886, Captain O'Shea had grown tired of his wife's shenanigans and filed for divorce. Katharine's rich aunt left her money to her cousins. The divorce proceedings, which took place in 1890, were a messy, sordid public affair. Katharine alleged that in her marriage she had suffered cruelty and neglect and O'Shea's adultery. Parnell never denied his role in Katharine's adultery, which did not help his cause. O'Shea was victorious and won custody of Parnell's two surviving children. Parnell's enemies renamed Katharine 'Kitty', a slang term for a prostitute. Parnell, at the peak of his political power, was scandalised. Katharine then broke the vows of her first, Catholic marriage by remarrying. She and Parnell were wed on 25 June 1891 (although not in a church). The Catholic Church was shocked and also feared that Parnell might wreck the Home Rule cause. Parnell refused to step down from the Irish Parliamentary Party, and the party split in two. Even some of his closest political allies deserted him to join the anti-Parnellite faction of the party.

His career and health in ruins, Parnell died later that year, in Katharine's arms, of pneumonia, aged just 45. Katharine lived the rest of her life in relative obscurity. She lost most of her fortune to fraud. Parnell's campaign for Home Rule was set back by the affair for much of the 1890s and early 1900s. There was a slight twist in the love story. Captain Henry Harrison had been Parnell's bodyguard and devoted himself to Katharine's service after Parnell died. In 1931 and 1938, he published two books which aimed to restore Parnell's tainted reputation.[25] Parnell and Katharine's affair had changed the very direction of Irish history, so it is surprising that Katharine never actually set foot in Ireland.

SEX IN A MAUSOLEUM

Another controversial romance involved a heated love triangle between Maud Gonne, William Butler Yeats and John MacBride. Gonne was born in England in 1866, although she spent much of her youth in France. Her father was a captain in the British Army, and she spent some of her childhood living in Ireland while he was stationed there. When barely out of her teens, Gonne became the mistress of a French politician 16 years her senior: Lucien Millevoye.

Yeats was born in 1865 in Sandymount, Co. Dublin. He studied poetry from an early age and became fascinated with Irish legends and the occult. In 1889, he published his first volume of literary work. That same year, he also met Gonne for the very first time in Bedford Park, London. Gonne and Yeats spent days together discussing literature and Irish affairs, before she departed for France, having refrained from mentioning to Yeats that she had given birth to Millevoye's son just three weeks earlier.

Gonne's son, Georges, tragically died from meningitis aged two. Yeats, still unaware of Gonne's status as mistress and grieving mother, met with her again in 1891 in Kingstown (now Dún Laoghaire), coincidentally on the same boat used a few weeks earlier to transport Parnell's body. Gonne was grief-stricken for Georges but pretended that she was mourning for Parnell. In her

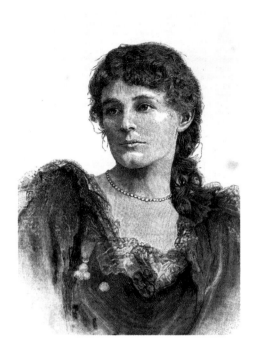

William Butler Yeats was infatuated with Maud Gonne, but his love was unrequited. After years of failed marriage proposals, he proposed instead to her daughter Iseult.

grief, Gonne sought solace in occultism and spiritualism, interests which she shared with Yeats. That same year, Yeats proposed to Gonne three times, but his love was unrequited. Gonne did not feel the same way for him and was put off in part by Yeats's reluctance to get fully involved in Irish nationalism.

Despite the constant rejections, Yeats continued to court Gonne over several years in France, England and Ireland. Her affair with Millevoye had ended, but in 1893, she suggested to Millevoye that they should attempt to reincarnate her son by having sex in the mausoleum beside her dead infant's coffin. Gonne believed that conceiving a baby with the same father would cause Georges' soul to transmigrate into a new child. As a result of this encounter, her daughter Iseult was born on 6 August 1894, though Gonne pretended that the child was her niece. In the meantime, Yeats, still infatuated, had become a well-known literary figure and Gonne his famous muse. Only in 1898 did Maud begin to confess some of her secrets to Yeats, who was nauseated and horrified.

In 1903, Maud married the penniless Major John MacBride, much to her family's disapproval. Her sister, Kathleen, begged her to instead marry the far more reliable Yeats. By then, Maud had also taken on responsibility for Eileen Wilson, the illegitimate teenage daughter of her father. Yeats was immensely hurt by her marriage, which was a complete disaster. Problems surfaced during the miserable honeymoon as the extent of MacBride's drinking problem became apparent. Two years later, Gonne requested a divorce on the grounds of drunkenness, an assault on the cook and, most seriously, alleged adulterous relations with Gonne's half-sister Eileen. Maud got custody of her son. Yeats's hatred of MacBride continued to grow.[26]

In the years that followed, Gonne involved herself in various political initiatives including Inghinidhe na hÉireann (Daughters of Ireland), Cumann na mBan (Women's Council) and campaigns for free school dinners for Irish children. Yeats became ever more famous and influential. Gonne stayed in Paris when MacBride was visiting Dublin and vice versa, carefully avoiding one another.

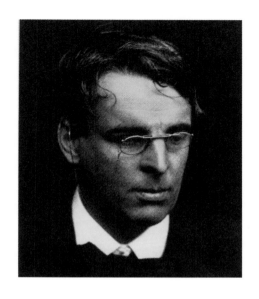

W.B. Yeats, one of Ireland's most prominent literary figures.

Yeats was staying in Gloucestershire, England, on Easter Weekend 1916. He was taken aback by the news from Ireland of an uprising and equally slighted that the rebel leaders had not confided in him about their plans, given his close friendship with some of them. In one of his most celebrated poems, 'Easter, 1916', he outlines his torn emotions. It contains the famous line, 'All changed, changed utterly: A terrible beauty is born'. Never missing an opportunity to besmirch his former rival in love, Yeats called MacBride, one of the Rising's executed leaders, a 'drunken, vain-glorious lout' who had 'done the most bitter wrong' in the poem. Gonne was not impressed and seems to have resented the slurs directed towards her now-deceased former husband. She wrote to Yeats: 'No, I don't like your poem. It isn't worthy of you and above all it isn't worthy of your subject.'[27]

In 1916, Yeats was 51 and decided to marry and produce an heir. He tried his luck once more by proposing to Gonne, who turned him down again, before changing his tactic. Yeats shifted his amorous intentions to 21-year-old Iseult. Iseult had in fact proposed to him when she was 15, and Yeats to her when she was 17. Aged 21, she said no. In September 1917, Yeats finally proposed to someone who said yes: 25-year-old Georgie Hyde-Lees. Their marriage was a success.

THE LOVE THAT DARE NOT SPEAK ITS NAME

At the time, a man falling in love with a married woman was considered controversial but paled in comparison with the thought of two men falling in love or having sexual relations. One of the most famous literary lines penned in relation to an Irish person vaguely describes 'the love that dare not speak its name'. It was written by Lord Alfred Douglas in September 1892 and published in a literary magazine, *The Chameleon*, in December 1894. The line is widely regarded as a euphemism for homosexuality.

Douglas was an English poet and journalist, educated at Oxford University, where he edited an undergraduate journal, *The Spirit Lamp*, which carried a homoerotic subtext. High up in the social world, Douglas was the third son of the Marquess of Queensberry (who is himself famous for inventing modern boxing rules). In 1891, Douglas was introduced to Oscar Wilde, who was 16 years older. Wilde was born in Dublin in 1854, the son of leading surgeon William Wilde, and grew up on Merrion Square in the heart of the city. Wilde excelled at studying languages and classics and was educated at Trinity College Dublin and Oxford University. By the early 1890s, he was writing society comedies and became hugely successful in London. Wilde and Douglas became infatuated with each other. Wilde indulged Douglas' every whim, whether material, artistic or sexual. Douglas initiated Wilde into London's underground world of rent boys. Wilde often met with these young boys, dined in private and went off together with them to a hotel room.

Queensbury fought regularly with his son and confronted Wilde and Douglas several times about the nature of their relationship. An infamously angry man, on one occasion, Queensbury accused Wilde of looking and acting homosexual and threatened to thrash Wilde if he was ever seen again in public with his son. Wilde was now ensnared in a family quarrel. Queensbury had already grieved for the death of his eldest son, Francis, Viscount Drumlanrig. Accused himself of having a homosexual relationship with the prime minister (the Earl of Rosebery), Drumlanrig took his own life once the rumours began to circulate. Queensbury was determined that his youngest son would not share a similar end.

It was fairly obvious to anyone who knew them that Wilde and Douglas were attracted both to each other and to people of the same sex. Acting against the sensible advice of his friends, but with Douglas's support, Wilde decided to sue the Marquess of Queensbury, who had publicly accused him of being a 'sodomite'. Queensbury, was arrested and charged with libel, which could carry a sentence of two years in prison. To escape this fate, Queensbury needed to prove that his accusation was valid and had some public benefit. Queensbury's lawyers hired private detectives to search for evidence. The lead barrister was Edward Carson (whom readers will meet again later as first signatory of the Ulster Covenant).

The trial opened at the Old Bailey on 3 April 1895. The judge was Richard Henn Collins, also from Dublin. The public galleries were packed. Journalists scribbled down details of the trial for their readers waiting in anticipation. Carson was from Dublin as well and, like Wilde, had attended Trinity College Dublin. He questioned Wilde on the immoral content of his writing, which Carson considered homoerotic. Wilde retorted by declaring that his writings were works of art. Carson dragged out a copy of Wilde's famous novel, *The Picture of Dorian Gray*, and read out scenes containing homosexual undertones. Wilde replied to all of Carson's questions with his characteristic wit, receiving many laughs from the audience, but Carson stood on firmer legal ground.

When quizzed about the rent boys, Wilde admitted that he had bought gifts for a few of them but insisted that nothing more untoward happened. Carson thought this unlikely. Wilde conceded that he platonically enjoyed the company of men. Carson then played his trump card. He revealed that several of the boys were willing to testify to having enjoyed sex with Wilde. The boys had been coerced into giving evidence with threats of legal action against themselves. Wilde finally saw sense and dropped the prosecution. Queensbury was found not guilty. The court costs bankrupted Wilde, who was then arrested for sodomy and gross indecency. He pleaded not guilty but begged Douglas to leave for Paris in case he was next to be arrested.

During this court case, Wilde was asked specifically about the meaning of 'the love that dare not speak its name'. Wilde explained eloquently that it is the great affection that can exist between an elder and younger man, a 'deep spiritual affection that is as pure as it is perfect'. The love being described was 'beautiful', 'fine' and the 'noblest form of affection'. 'There is nothing unnatural about it. It is intellectual and it repeatedly exists between an older and a young man, when the older man has intellect and the younger man has all the joy, hope and glamour of life before him,' explained Wilde. He added: 'The world does not understand. The world mocks at it and sometimes puts one in the pillory for it.' Although expressive and fluent, this statement hardly convinced beyond all doubt that Wilde had not had sexual relations with men. The jury was unable to reach a verdict. Even Carson was starting to think that it was time to ease up on this persecution of Wilde. Finally, Wilde was sentenced to two years hard labour at Reading Gaol. While imprisoned, he wrote a 50,000-word letter to Douglas, later published as *De Profundis*.

Released in 1897, Wilde spent the last three years of life impoverished and in exile. Douglas and Wilde reunited in August 1897 at Rouen. Families and friends of both men disapproved. Regardless, the couple lived together near Naples for a few months until both families threatened to cut off funds. Wilde refused to write anything new and slipped into poverty and alcoholism in Paris. After contracting meningitis, he died on 30 November 1900. Douglas served as chief mourner at the funeral.

In an unexpected turn of events, later in life, Douglas went on to have a strained marriage with a woman named Olive Custance. He adopted a staunchly Catholic lifestyle and spent his time trashing Wilde's reputation, in response to Wilde's searing *De Profundis*, which detailed their relationship. Only when Douglas himself was imprisoned for a while did his attitude towards Wilde soften. Later in life, Douglas gained a reputation as an unpleasant racist. Wilde's reputation much improved as society gradually accepted LGBTQ+ relations. In 2017, Wilde was among 50,000 men pardoned for homosexual acts that were no longer offences under new legislation known informally as the Alan Turing law.[28]

GIVING BIRTH

In Ireland today, the birth of a new child is usually cause for celebration but it's only recently that childbirth has stopped being a source of concern and anxiety. Until the twentieth century, both mother and child were at high risk of dying during birth. Effective anaesthetics were available only from the 1840s. Throughout most of Irish history, women gave birth without efficient pain relief.[29] Legal texts dating from 600–1200 reveal that pregnant married women were treated compassionately. Legal protections recommended that pregnant servants work less strenuously in the month leading up to a child's birth and the month afterwards. If a pregnant woman stole food, she was exempt from prosecution as mothers-to-be needed to eat. On a more poignant note, the content of these legal texts recognises childbirth as a time full of risks.[30]

We know only a little about childbirth in premodern Ireland. Aside from a few, the topic is almost absent from the historical sources. Even the rare accounts available tend to reveal the experiences of only wealthier families, particularly the settlers. Given childbirth's notoriously dangerous reputation, it might seem surprising that Irish women once gave birth to a seemingly endless supply of babies. Richard Boyle, the first Earl of Cork, established

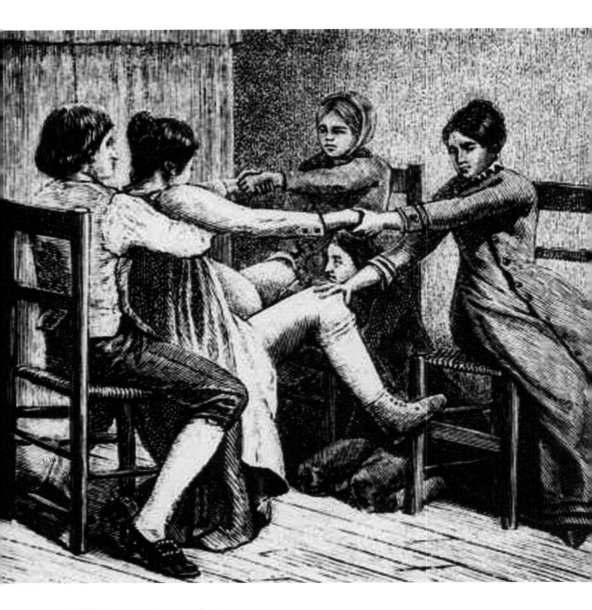

Childbirth was once a dangerous time for
both infant and mother. Maternal and infant
mortality rates remained high in Ireland
until well into the twentieth century.

numerous plantations (of English residents) in southern areas of Ireland in the early 1600s. When not busy taking land from the Irish, Boyle enjoyed procreating. His first wife, Joan Apsley, died in 1599 during childbirth along with her newborn son. Boyle's second wife, Catherine Fenton, fell dangerously ill in 1616 after delivering her eighth child. She survived and, undeterred, went on to have another seven children. After delivering Richard's fifteenth child in the space of 23 years, Catherine was understandably exhausted. Her health declined and she died relatively young, aged around 41. One of Boyle's many daughters, Sarah, died in 1633, five weeks after giving birth prematurely to a daughter, who also passed away, shortly after her christening.[31]

Births usually took place at home attended by other women. A straw bed was commonly used as this was easily disposed of, by either being burned or buried along with the afterbirth. (Beds were precious commodities, and women would have avoided ruining those used for sleeping at all costs.) Delivery in a kneeling position was preferred, although the ideal position was much debated. Warm drinks were administrated to help alleviate labour pains. Women considered childbirth to be a dangerous time when fairies might steal a newborn baby or swap it for one of their own.[32]

Women living in Dublin could attend the Rotunda Hospital, established in 1745 by Bartholomew Mosse, a surgeon and midwife appalled at the conditions in which pregnant Dublin women gave birth. The eye-catching building that now houses the hospital can be seen at the top of Dublin's famous O'Connell Street. As its name suggests, it has a distinctively round design. The Rotunda is the world's oldest continuously operating maternity hospital. Around 300,000 babies have been born there. However, the development of lying-in hospitals actually increased the number of patients dying of puerperal fever in the eighteenth century, as doctors with unwashed hands unknowingly cross-infected women as they attended them. Pregnant women who could afford the services of a doctor became more likely to die during childbirth than the poorer women who fortunately could not afford them.[33]

Following a successful birth, many mothers employed a wet nurse to breastfeed their child. Wet nursing had been common in ancient Ireland and the custom continued into more recent times. It gave middle-class mothers a break while allowing working-class women to return to work. Affluent families were more able to carefully choose a healthy, sober and respectable wet nurse. Robert Boyle paid his wet nurses handsomely and praised their services in helping to keep his many children in good health. Wet nursing also provided women with employment. In the nineteenth century, advertisements were still placed regularly in newspapers from recent mothers offering their services. These often specified whether the wet nurse was Protestant or Catholic (as if that really made much difference). Nineteenth-century doctors praised natural breastfeeding but criticised both recently invented artificial baby foods and drunken, unhygienic wet nurses.[34]

Handywomen helped with births. They lacked formal training but compensated with insurmountable practical experience. Eighteenth- and nineteenth-century male doctors criticised the handywomen, believing they could do a better job, and they unfairly held them largely responsible for the country's notoriously high infant mortality rates. In their place, doctors wanted formally trained midwives, nurses and doctors to attend births. Their propaganda depicted handywomen as dangerous, untrained and unsanitary.

In reality, handywomen were immensely respected figures in local communities. They commanded far more respect than male doctors, widely thought of as intrusive, moralistic, obsessed with experimenting on corpses, avid torturers of living animals and woefully unable to cure most illnesses. (This was a reasonably fair assessment of nineteenth-century doctors.) Hospitals were few and far between in remote rural areas, and the working classes distrusted them as places of death, disease and dissection (another fair assessment). The handywoman, regardless of one's opinion of her, was better trusted and readily available. However, her time was up. The 1918 Midwives (Ireland) Act made it illegal for children to be born without the assistance of a *qualified* practitioner. Families didn't welcome the strange new nurses with

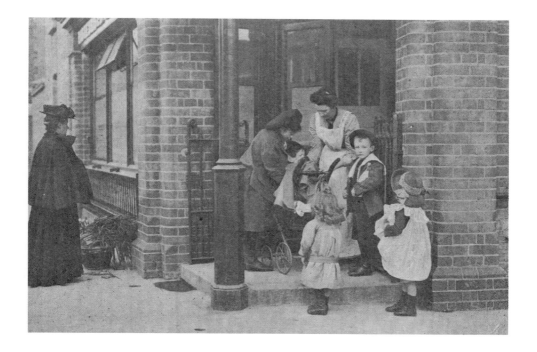

open arms, but gradually the medical profession and
hospitals assumed a greater role in childbirth. Over
the decades, the attendance of handywomen at births
petered out.[35]

From around 1900, mothers started
to receive improved advice on raising
babies, avoiding tuberculosis and
feeding them with healthy supplies
of milk.

The turn of the twentieth century was a time of
international obsession with motherhood, encouraged by eugenics, social
Darwinism and a determination to improve public health. In Ireland, these
campaigns intersected with the push for national independence. All health
promotion groups were aligned with political causes. The Ladies' School
Dinner Committee campaigned for a free school meals policy for poorer Irish
children. It was led by prominent republican Maud Gonne. A key tactic involved
accusing the British government of implementing deliberate genocide policies
by refusing to feed the Irish young, purposely invoking the Great Famine.
Strong words indeed, but they reveal how politics and public health were

deeply intertwined at the time. Another group, the United Irishwomen, ran practical schemes to improve infant welfare. Their name was derived from the United Irishmen, a group of rebels who had attempted a revolutionary approach to securing Irish freedom in the 1790s. The Women's National Health Association was led by Lady Aberdeen, wife of the lord lieutenant, and was viewed suspiciously because of its close state ties.[36]

These groups taught mothers the best ways to feed their children, protect infants from deadly diseases such as tuberculosis and ensure that youngsters grew up healthy. This undoubtedly benefitted Irish children, but it simultaneously narrowed women's social role to being little else but a mother. The Catholic Church, growing in influence, agreed that motherhood was a sacred role for Irish women. Mothers shouldered the responsibility of moulding future generations, and in the years immediately preceding independence, the Irish were looking towards an imagined future free from British influence. The new message was clear: producing healthy Irish children was women's primary role and *duty* to the nation.[37] And reproduce they certainly did. According to the 1911 census, the average Irish Catholic couple had seven children. Irish families became the largest in Europe. The lives of Irish women were dictated by endless cycles of pregnancy, birth and raising children.[38]

ÉAMON DE VALERA AND WOMEN

In 1937, Éamon de Valera enshrined Irish women's apparent function as mass producers of Irish babies in a new Irish constitution. Always a contentious public figure, de Valera had commanded the Irish Volunteers at Boland's Mill during the 1916 Easter Rising. Narrowly escaping execution at the hands of the British, he became a leading political figure during the War of Independence and opposed the treaty that established partition. After spending most of the 1920s refusing to take his Dáil Éireann seat (a strategy still used by Sinn Féin in the House of Commons), de Valera gradually warmed to the idea of constitutional participation in the Irish government, despite refusing to recognise that government as legitimate. He formed Fianna Fáil in March 1926, and the party won the general election in 1932. De Valera became taoiseach.

Fianna Fáil was intent on banishing British influence in Ireland once and for all. It refused to continue paying land annuities owed to Britain and implemented policies intended to allow Ireland to become economically self-sufficient from its problematic neighbouring island. An economic war ensued between 1932 and 1938.[39] Political and ecclesiastical leaders shared a belief that the revolutionary decade had encouraged many Irish women to vacate their homes and actively participate in fighting for Ireland. The conflict was now over, and it seemed essential that these women return to their supposed natural role as housewives.

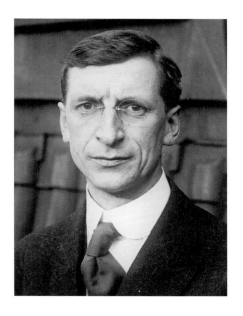

Taoiseach Éamon de Valera introduced a new constitution in 1937 that limited the role of women in Irish society to mother and housewife.

Partaking in public life distracted women from giving birth and attending to what were considered their domestic duties around the house. Women were simultaneously conferred a subordinate status while being landed with the onerous responsibilities of producing and raising a new Irish nation.[40]

Aside from its glaring sexism, de Valera's vision of an independent Ireland was romantic, nostalgic and anti-modern. Deliberately spared the misery and poverty of urbanisation and economic modernisation, Ireland would remain a traditional, rural country with a simple way of life. Its happy residents would speak Irish and dance only to traditional Irish music. Foreign (especially British) cultural material would be heavily censored to safeguard Irish moral standards. De Valera wanted to bring into fruition 'the Ireland that we dreamed of', populated by people 'satisfied with frugal comfort'. Drawing from the romantic myth of ancient Ireland as a land of 'saints and scholars', the new Ireland was to be a similarly spiritual place. The reality looked very different. Ireland in the 1930s was rife with poverty and misery. The country was poor, isolated and not particularly progressive. Nonetheless, this failed to deter de Valera from his national mission.[41]

The 1937 constitution promised to abolish the Oath of Allegiance, rename the state Éire, recognise the Catholic Church's 'special position' in guiding political policy, make divorce illegal (until this was revoked in 1995), claim the entire island as national territory (pointedly overlooking partition and the existence of Northern Ireland), replace references to the king of Ireland with the president and declare Irish the country's first language, with English as the second. On a warm summer's day at the start of July, men and women nationwide voted in a referendum to decide whether all of this was acceptable. They did and the new constitution came into force on 29 December 1937.

Article 41.2 of the constitution stated unambiguously that an Irish woman's duty to the state was to stay at home and attend to her domestic duties and many children. It discouraged women from taking on paid work, so as to ensure that they would not neglect their domestic and maternal tasks around the home. Not one single woman was consulted on the new constitution. Decades of suffrage and feminist campaigning might as well have never happened. The constitution discussed women's place in Ireland in relation only to their reproductive systems and household responsibilities. It had no aspirations for women beyond producing endless numbers of Irish children. The ideal Irish woman, constantly giving birth, was a bulwark against modernisation. Hardly known as an advocate of Irish women's rights, the Catholic Church described the constitution as a 'noble document'. Much to the annoyance of almost every woman living in Ireland, the offensive article remains part of the Irish constitution.

In 1937, suffragette Hanna Sheehy-Skeffington (and widow of an executed rebel) tried to remind politicians that Irish women had contributed immensely to the struggle for freedom, alongside campaigning for the female vote. Equal

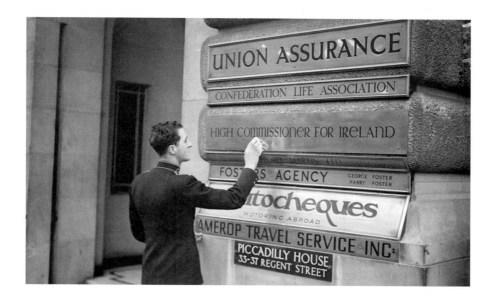

citizenship for both sexes had featured prominently in the 1916 Proclamation of the Irish Republic, but the reality of independent Ireland was a series of legislative measures that limited Irish women's role. The 1937 constitution proved to be the icing on the cake. Sheehy-Skeffington derided the constitution as being based on a 'Fascist model, in which women would be relegated to permanent inferiority, their avocations and choice of callings limited because of an implied invalidism as the weaker sex'.

The 1937 constitution changed the name of the country from the 'Irish Free State' to 'Ireland'. A new brass plate is fixed outside the office of the Irish High Commissioner in London to reflect the name change.

Many influences were at work, but Catholic social teaching was prominent among them. The 1937 constitution effectively enshrined Catholic principles into Irish law. Principles of 'Catholic womanhood' insisted that good Irish girls would acquire virtue by being steeped in a thorough moral education taught by nuns. The ideal Irish woman would not attend jazz dances, smoke, read 'evil literature', wear dresses cut less than four inches below the knee or attend to her sexual urges. Sheehy-Skeffington had raised an intriguing point. The cult of motherhood was indeed strong in fascist dictatorships in Italy and Nazi Germany, and it didn't look particularly different in Ireland.[42]

SEX AND IRISH TELEVISION

In the 1960s, many Irish political figures feared that the threat of the sexual revolution coming to Ireland would be spurred on by television. Indeed, the government had never been too keen on letting the Irish watch it. Britain had enjoyed a national television service since 1936 but the first glimpse of television in Ireland occurred only in 1949 when the BBC erected an 887-foot-high transmitter in Birmingham so powerful that the signal reached Ireland's east coast. From 1953, the BBC broadcasted from Northern Ireland. Southerners living close to the border were delighted to be able to pick up BBC1 and, later, ITV, and bought television sets in their droves. The Church and government were less impressed with British television signals spilling over the land and sea borders. Fears arose that the chaste, Christian Irish population would once again be exposed to immoral British cultural influence.

Ideas were floated that perhaps Ireland could have its own homegrown television station broadcasting material more suitable for the country, although the government insisted that the Irish did not want television. Despite this ungrounded presumption, a Television Committee was formed which excoriated British television as 'brazen', 'frank in sex matters' and driven by a desire to 'exalt the British royal family'. Only in 1961 did Ireland's own television station, Telefís Éireann (original spelling), start broadcasting. On its inaugural day, viewers endured a lengthy address by President Éamon de Valera warning of television's 'nuclear' power to destroy morals and cause decadence, followed by an even longer mass. The day after, the Catholic Truth Society described television as even more dangerous than the Antichrist.

The nation was rocked in 1962 when RTÉ screened an advert featuring sketches of women's underwear and again in 1966 when *The Late Late Show* presenter Gay Byrne asked Eileen Fox, a married female guest (whose husband was present), about the colour of the nightie which she had worn on her honeymoon. Eileen announced that she hadn't worn a nightie at all! Shocking stuff indeed. The next day, Thomas Ryan, bishop of Clonfert, Co.

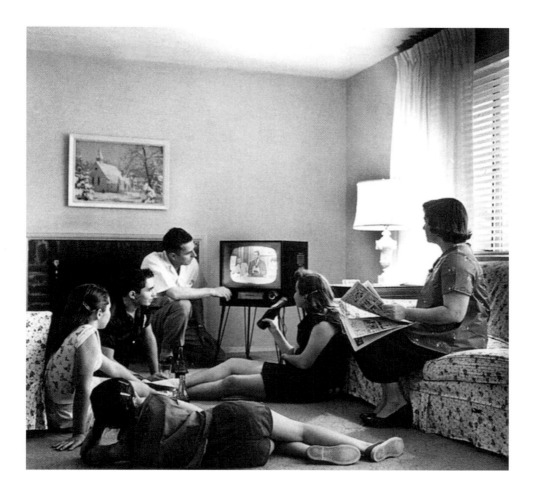

Galway, called on 'all decent Irish Catholics' to protest. Most people ignored him, not least the honeymooning couple, who found the bizarre situation rather amusing. It was against this backdrop that Flanagan launched his stinging attack on the immoral influences of television.[43]

Television came late to Ireland, but many viewers were able to pick up British television from Northern Ireland and across the Irish Sea.

PROBLEMATIC PREGNANCIES

Finding oneself pregnant outside of wedlock was the worst possible sexual crime, and the burden of this 'sin' naturally fell upon women. The father's culpability in the pregnancy was usually ignored. Unlike men, women exhibited the physical consequences of their sexual affairs for all to see as their pregnant bellies grew larger and larger. Women in these circumstances were regarded as a stain on good morals and their children a drain on national resources.

One solution was to murder the unwanted baby. It is an uncomfortable historical fact that, particularly during the nineteenth century, large numbers of unmarried Irish women killed their babies. If they could not face that gruesome task, unwanted children could be sold to baby farmers who, on the mother's behalf, would murder, neglect or underfeed them. Women discovered to have committed infanticide were condemned in the press as wicked, depraved murderesses. If a woman's primary role was to be a mother, those who murdered a child seemed all the more abhorrent. Between 1850 and 1929, 29 women were sentenced to death in Ireland for the murder of their infants, although their punishments were all reduced to imprisonment or transportation. Thousands more unapprehended women undoubtedly murdered their offspring (or attempted to).

Various means were employed to kill unwanted infants including suffocation, strangulation, drowning, leaving them outside exposed to harsh weather, poisoning, violent abuse, burning or neglecting to feed them. Ireland's bogs, fields, waterways, ditches and mountains offered ample space to hide the small corpses of dead babies. Sometimes infants, dead or alive, were found deposited outside church doors or railway stations. Occasionally, attempts were made to conceal a corpse at home underneath the floorboards. The problem of infanticide remained common until the twentieth century.[44]

Abortion was another option, but this was equally illegal and treated as akin to child murder. In Celtic Ireland, abortion was a relatively minor sin. Although religious leaders refute this, some historians believe that early

Christianity tolerated abortion. Four of Ireland's Sts were recorded as having performed abortions with God's blessing: Ciarán of Saigir, Áed mac Bricc, Cainnech of Aghaboe and Brigid of Kildare.[45] St Brigid, known for her work in fertility, is said to have met a young woman who had a crisis pregnancy. She prayed, blessed the woman, and laid her hands on the womb, and the fetus miraculously disappeared. By deliberately inducing abortion, Brigid restored the ailing pregnant woman to full health.[46]

Attitudes hardened in the nineteenth century. Abortion was prohibited under the Offences Against the Person Act (1861), regardless of circumstances such as rape, abuse or risk of death for the pregnant woman. Many beliefs circulated about the best way of inducing an abortion: drinking gin, eating washing soda, jumping off a chair. Drugs could be procured from chemists, although customers had to know the correct pills and powders to swallow without causing themselves harm, and chemists were liable for prosecution if implicated.

Despite usually wanting to be the same as Britain, the Unionist government of Northern Ireland refrained from allowing the 1967 Abortion Act to be passed there, even though it was legalised elsewhere across the United Kingdom. In the following decades, various female-led groups campaigned for legislative change, but Northern Irish women often struggled to unite in the 1970s given the Protestant–Catholic divide and the Troubles. In the South, after a 1983 referendum (with a low 54 per cent turnout), the law was amended slightly to give due regard to the lives of mothers facing life-threatening circumstances because of their pregnancy.[47]

Between 1967 and 2018, Irish women seeking to terminate a pregnancy typically travelled to Britain. An estimated 20,000 from across the island journeyed across the Irish Sea for this purpose. However, it seems likely that pregnant single Irish women travelled to England to escape the tyranny of Irish cultures of sexual shame and institutionalisation since the 1920s, if not before. In many ways, it was the tragic 2012 death of Savita Halappanavar in Galway that changed Irish public opinion once and for all. Halappanavar was 17 weeks

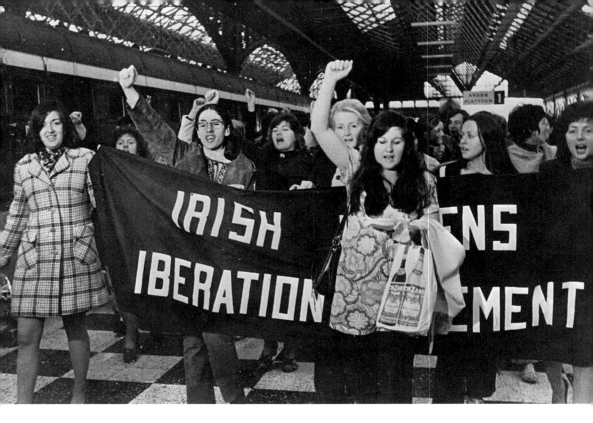

In 1971, a group of Irish feminists travelled to Northern Ireland to buy contraception (then illegal in Ireland), hoping to get themselves arrested.

pregnant when she arrived in hospital. She died of septicaemia a week later. Doctors had refused her request to have her pregnancy terminated until it was too late. Her death ignited a social movement across Ireland that led to the repeal of the Eighth Amendment.[48] Abortion was decriminalised in Northern Ireland in March 2020, although only because the British government passed new laws while the Democratic Unionist Party were refusing to take their seats in Stormont. No longer was there any need to travel to Britain. This was excellent timing. From March 2020, the COVID-19 pandemic closed down the island, making travel elsewhere extremely difficult, if not impossible.[49]

Perhaps the best way to avoid the situation altogether would have been to use birth control but this was banned too in the Republic of Ireland. In the nineteenth century, condoms were associated with prostitutes, harlots and courtesans. The reputation of contraception improved in the twentieth century when groups such as the Belfast Eugenics Society, formed in 1911, promoted birth control, although only in the hope of discouraging the working classes from having so many children. This approach to birth control was not simply about liberating women.[50]

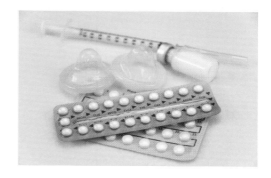

Contraception was illegal in Ireland between 1935 and 1979, and strong restrictions were imposed on its use even after legalisation. Throughout that time, contraception was legal in Northern Ireland but hardly embraced. South of the border, artificial contraception methods including condoms and the contraceptive pill (introduced elsewhere in 1961) were all outlawed. Owning contraceptives was not prohibited, but selling or importing

Between 1935 and 1979, contraception was illegal in the Republic of Ireland, including the contraceptive pill (which was introduced elsewhere in the 1960s).

them was. Loopholes were found, including 'gifting' rather than 'selling' contraceptives, but for much of the population contraception simply remained inaccessible or too much trouble to purchase. Family planning books and pamphlets were banned too on the grounds of indecency. Prohibiting this 'evil literature' denied Irish women full knowledge of their bodies and reproductive systems. Given the growing taboos around discussing sex, women were unlikely to learn about sex from their mothers. Sexual education was taught by nuns at schools, which was not particularly conducive to thoroughness. Sex was taught as something to be feared, not learned about, so it is ironic that improved education might well have helped stem the number of women becoming pregnant out of wedlock. Some women were so lacking in sexual knowledge that they believed babies came out of their belly button.

In 1971, forward-thinking Senator Mary Robinson (later president of Ireland) attempted to introduce a bill to liberalise the law but was not allowed a reading to discuss the matter. That same year, a group of 49 feminists from Ireland travelled to Belfast, risking the many bombs detonating there at the peak of the Troubles. While there, they bought lots of contraceptives, reboarded the 'Contraceptive

Train' (as they named it) and, upon returning to Dublin, provocatively waved their stash around in the hope of getting arrested. Thomas Ryan, the very same bishop of Clonfert who had disapproved of the honeymooning couple's television antics five years earlier, proclaimed that 'never before, and certainly not since penal times, was the Catholic heritage of Ireland subjected to so many insidious onslaughts on the pretext of conscience, civil rights and women's liberation'. Thankfully, the 1979 Family Planning Act allowed married couples to purchase contraceptives with a prescription (they had to wait until 1985 to buy them without a prescription). The AIDS crisis of the 1980s and 1990s brought successful campaigns for condom machines to be provided in public places.[51]

Clearly, aside from the misery of sexual abstinence, twentieth-century Irish women had few legal and reliable ways of avoiding becoming pregnant. When many of them inevitably did, social stigma tarnished their lives. Many single women mysteriously went missing after announcing a pregnancy. Their families never spoke of them again. Some ended up in the local asylum, their pregnancy seemingly a symptom of mental illness.[52] Between 1922 and 1996, over 10,000 girls and women considered to be 'fallen women' were sent to Magdalene Laundries. They endured forced labour and psychological and physical maltreatment.[53] Catholic Magdalen Laundries were found in various countries, but the Irish variety took on a distinctive character after independence. Well into the 1980s, many women entered these laundries involuntarily, sometimes remaining in these punitive, carceral institutions for the rest of their lives. In other countries, laundries had been closed down or reformed by then. Irish laundries were secretive and, as private institutions, actively dodged public scrutiny. All manner of Irish women ended up in the laundries, but most had been discovered being sexually active at a time when Irish women were expected to be morally pure. A large number had given birth to children deemed illegitimate or tried to conceal their pregnancy through abortion or infanticide. Others were unwilling victims of sexual abuse who ended up suffering further levels of psychological, physical and sometimes sexual abuse while detained in the laundries.[54]

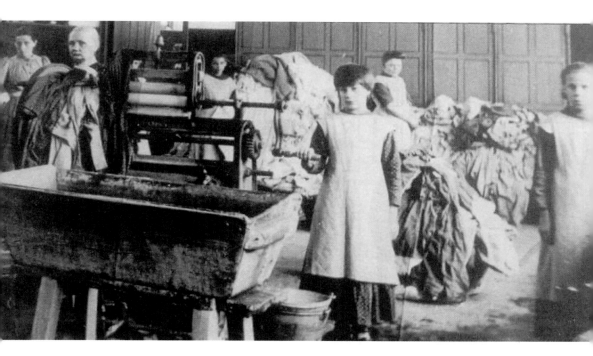

What of the children? The 1916 Proclamation had promised to 'cherish all the children of the nation equally' and provide them all with life's basic necessities. In practice, the needs of children born to unmarried mothers were disregarded. Like their mothers, many ended up institutionalised. Irish society did not want such children. Doctrines about the sanctity of a child's life bore no resemblance to the way Ireland treated them. Large numbers ended up in mother and baby homes, country homes and industrial schools. As with their stigmatised mothers, institutionalisation placed them at high risk of abuse, neglect and rejection, followed by a life of poverty, isolation, mental illness and further institutionalisation.[55]

'Fallen women' were shut away in Magdalene Laundries and Mother and Baby Homes right up to the 1990s, when the last home was closed.

Survivors insist that children born in mother and baby homes were neglected or starved. The public either didn't notice or didn't care, and the scandal has been depicted as Church and State collusion. Single motherhood was not a

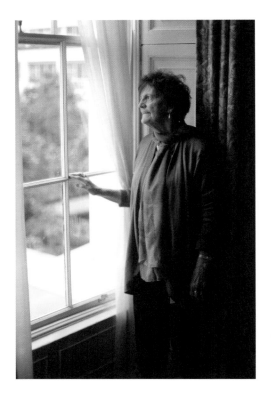

Philomena Lee was one of many women whose child was sent to America for adoption.

crime, but it might as well have been. Some of the more determined single mothers tried to raise their children and ignore the social stigma but risked having their children snatched away from them on the slightest pretext and dispatched to an institution.

One of the biggest scandals was the forced adoption scheme. Undoubtedly, the most famous adoptee is Philomena Lee, whose life was later chronicled in the 2009 book *The Lost Child of Philomena Lee* and a subsequent award-winning film starring Judi Dench. Philomena was born in 1933. Her mother died of tuberculosis when she was six. At age 18, Philomena became pregnant and was sent to the Sean Ross Abbey, Co. Tipperary, a place for unwed mothers. After giving birth, Philomena was forced to stay in the abbey for four more years. She was released only after the abbey had sold her three-year-old son to an American Catholic family. Philomena did not consent to this. She was forced to sign the adoption papers against her wishes, and the nuns refused to disclose details regarding her son's fate. Much later in life, Philomena tracked down her son's location with the help of journalist Martin Sixsmith. Tragically, it transpired that Michael had died of AIDS in 1995 after years of trying to find his birth mother. While anticipating his untimely death, Michael had arranged for his body to be buried at Sean Ross Abbey, hoping that his mother might someday find his grave, which she eventually did.[56]

Philomena's story illustrates the tragic circumstances that surrounded the life of women forced to give up their children for adoption. For a few decades, acquiring Irish babies was quite fashionable among Americans, and local newspapers happily announced their arrival while praising the wealthy benefactors engaged in rescuing Irish orphans from a life of poverty and misery. For the forgotten Irish mothers, these events were full of pathos, sadness and longing for their snatched children who weren't in fact orphans at all. The nuns organised the transatlantic export of babies stolen from the hands of mothers with the full support of archbishops such as John Charles McQuaid and the State, which quietly issued passports. Ironically, de Valera himself, president of Ireland between 1959 and 1973, and taoiseach for a total of 16 years before that, had been born in America to an unmarried mother.[57]

Thankfully, it's possible to end this chapter on a somewhat happier note. The controversies caused by the many institutional scandals caused a sea change in the amount of sexual repression that people in Ireland were willing to put up with. Particularly in the Republic, younger generations have rebelled against the historical activities of the Church. Several referendums in the 2010s ended restrictions on abortion and same-sex marriage but also symbolically announced a rejection of older repressive forces. Ireland could be said to have enjoyed its own sexual revolution, albeit one that occurred 50 years later than in most other Western countries.

Sheela-na-gig has returned too. In the twenty-first century, Project Sheela was launched by a group of feminists who sought to reclaim Sheela-na-gig and cast her in a more positive light. For them, Sheela-na-gig was a potentially empowering symbol for Irish women and should not be thought of as a clergy-led, male-designed warning about female sexuality. Members of Project Sheela placed the sexually provocative sculptures, with their wide-open vulvas, outside places where Irish women historically struggled. The former institutions where Irish women were housed have been prominent among these.

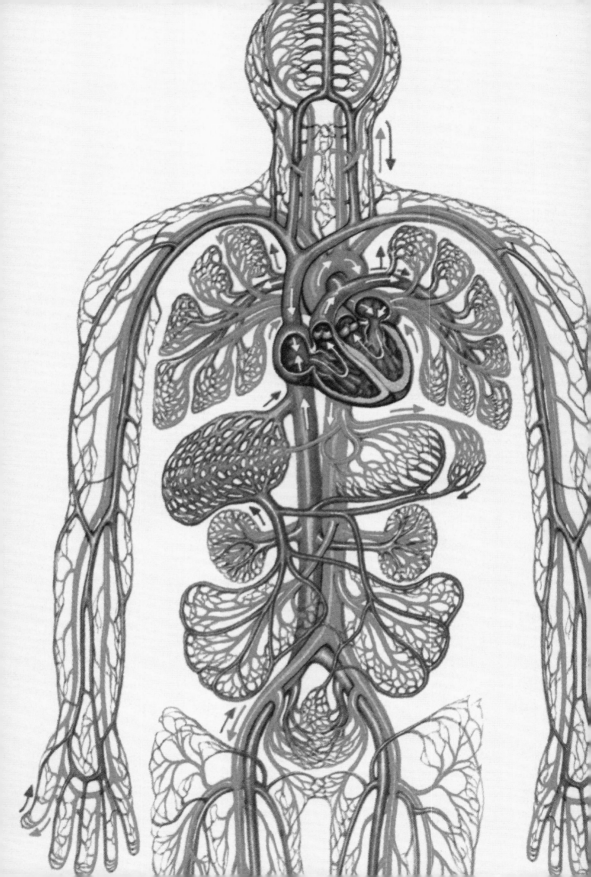

CHAPTER 6

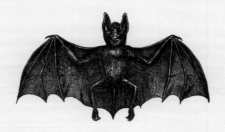

BLOOD

Blood carries oxygen and nutrients around our body, helpfully keeping our inner organs in good health, fighting infections and carrying out waste material through the kidneys and digestive organs. But, for humans, blood has held enormous symbolic importance beyond these basic physiological functions.[1] At the start of this book, we met Clonycavan Man, a mysterious ancient Irish man whose blood was offered to the gods as a gruesome human sacrifice. Many ancient cultures believed that the gods fed on sacrificed human blood, and perhaps the ancient Irish shared this belief.

In the millennia that followed, the course of Irish history remained interspersed with enthusiasm for all manner of blood sacrifices. Typically, these were associated with war. Given the sheer number of conflicts waged by Irish people, either among themselves or against the British, it is unsurprising that the idea of blood sacrifice retained such strong appeal through the ages. Various warring cultures, including those of ancient Greece and Rome, had glorified the honourable spilling of blood on battlefields. These ancient ideals surfaced once again in conflicts including the 1916 Easter Rising, alongside related principles such as 'blood brotherhood', 'blood vengeance' and 'blood baptism'. Ireland's revolutionary decade boasted other blood-related tales, including a bloody signature penned on the Ulster Covenant, an alternative to the more traditionally used ink. Important too is the matter of Irish bloodlines, the biological ties that bind together generations of Irish people.

IRISH BLOODLINES

In 2020, scientists performed a DNA test on the ancient remains of a man buried at the Newgrange monument, Co. Meath. This was a place of importance. Built around 3200 BC, the Newgrange monument is older even than Stonehenge and the Pyramids of Giza. The monument today is an impressively large circular mound, 4,500 square metres in area, which bulges from the ground. Surrounding it are 97 large stones decorated with megalithic art.

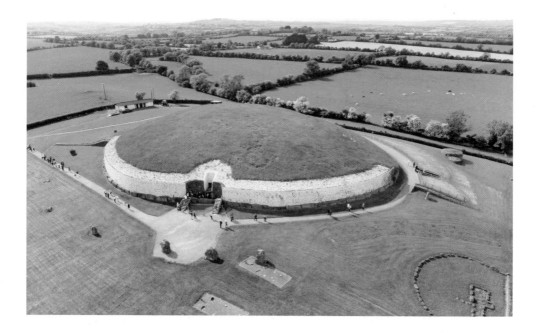

After walking around the circular ancient monument, visitors eventually come across a narrow entry carved into the side of the mound which leads them inside to tread unsteadily along a dark, narrow, rocky passage. At the end of this passage is a mysterious chamber that seems to serve no obvious purpose. Turning around, though, visitors' eyes may be drawn to a mysterious opening which lets in a small amount of light. The purpose becomes clear to visitors on the winter solstice, who are in for a truly amazing sight. Each year, as the sun rises, the beam entering the chamber widens. Sunlight floods in, beautifully illuminating the entire chamber. The monument perfectly captures the winter solstice. Understandably, access to the chamber on 21 December is in great demand; guests are randomly chosen in a lottery.

This was a technological feat indeed, especially for Neolithic times. No one knows why the prehistoric Irish bothered to build such a monument, although the scientist who set to work investigating the ancient man's DNA

Built around 3200 BC, the Newgrange monument is a large circular mound covering 4,500 square metres.

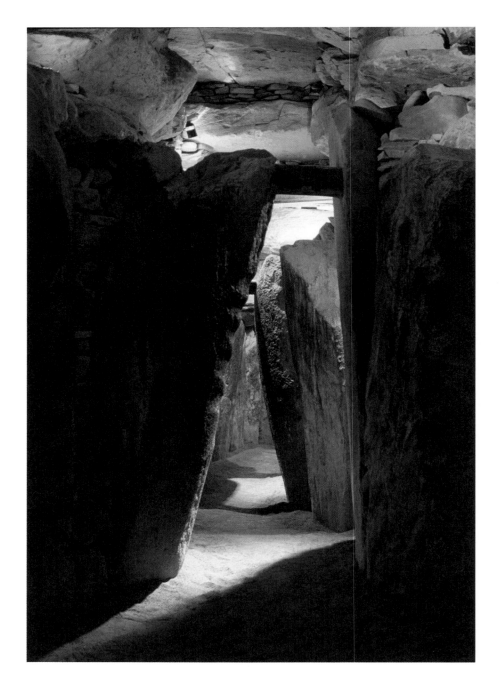

Sunlight pours through into an
inner chamber in the Newgrange
monument every winter solstice.

shed some light on the matter. DNA testing revealed that the man's parents were very close relatives. Far too close. Brother and sister, perhaps. His burial at such an elaborate monument indicates a family of immense social importance, probably royalty or Neolithic elite. For biological and cultural reasons, high-profile unions between family members of such closeness have always been rare and tended to take place only within royal dynasties.

Those familiar with Irish mythology pointed out something strange. The Newgrange monument has always been associated with myths and legends about sexual couplings between close family members. The Dindshenchas story of its sister site Dowth, also a giant hill built on the bend of the Boyne, tells of a king who wanted the help of every man living in Ireland to build a giant monument so that he could access heaven. Helpfully, the king's sister cast a spell on the sun to stop it moving across the sky, providing the builders with endless daylight. Then, somewhat unexpectedly in this so-far charming story, the king and his sister decided to have sex with each other, causing the spell to be undone. Darkness comes. The builders abandoned their task. The story has a clear moral message: don't have sex with your sister.

A variant of this tale dates from the eleventh century AD and tells of a builder-king who restarts the daily solar cycle also by copulating with his sister. In a different story altogether, Eochaid Airem, high king of Tara, is tricked into sleeping with his daughter. She becomes pregnant and the child is left outside to die, although a herdsman ends up raising her instead. With all this business going on in the area, it is unsurprising that the tomb also acquired the name Fertae Chuile ('Hill of Sin').[2]

Experts in DNA analysis have also broadened our understanding of Irish bloodlines since medieval times. Ireland is a small, quite insular country, meaning that gene pools are easily traced. In 2009, RTÉ broadcast a two-part documentary series which revealed the 'truth' about Irish genealogy. The programme claimed that one-fifth of men living in Ireland's north-westerly regions were directly descended from Niall of the Nine Hostages, the legendary high king of Ireland. Five Co. Donegal footballers were tested and found to

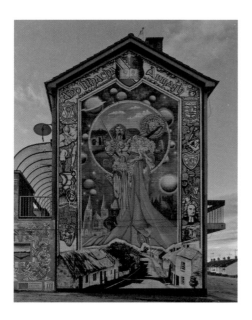

A fifth of Irish men living in the north-west are thought to descend from Niall of the Nine Hostages, a legendary high king of Ireland.

carry the relevant gene. Renowned Irish singer Daniel O'Donnell submitted his DNA for testing and also discovered that he was a descendant. Scientific research supported these claims and suggested that up to three million men worldwide are descended from Niall, who established a dynasty of powerful chieftains that dominated Ireland for six centuries.

Modern-day DNA techniques have revealed much about the historical bloodlines of the Irish. A shortened name for deoxyribonucleic acid, DNA is the genetic information contained in our body's cells. In simple terms, DNA contains the instructions (or codes) for how our bodies are made. When scientists look through a powerful microscope, they notice that DNA looks like a twisting ladder. Four different chemicals (or nucleotides) pair up to make the rungs of the ladder, and groups of these nucleotides make up our genes. Among many other functions, genes determine our physical appearance. DNA is stored in the chromosomes located in every cell. All of us inherit two sets of chromosomes, one from each parent.

In 2017, the Irish DNA Atlas was launched, a project which, as its name suggests, mapped the Irish gene pool over time. The project's curators collected DNA samples from 196 Irish people whose great-grandparents were born in Ireland within 50 kilometres of each other. The findings revealed 10 major genetic clusters that once existed in ancient Ireland, roughly aligned with the major ancient kingdoms. When investigating Ireland's genetic history, the scientists studied only the Y chromosome (passed down only through the male line) and found a hotspot in north-west Ireland where as many as 21.5 per cent of men carried Niall's genetic footprint. Appropriately, the surname Uí Néill translates as 'descendants of Niall'.[3]

Gene pools change over time as people move away from a region or new people arrive. Discernible in the Irish DNA Atlas was the genetic influence of Viking settlements, as well as the Ulster-Scot invaders of the 1600s.[4] There is genetic evidence of Irish ancestry in Norway due to the slave trade of Viking times. People were a valuable resource, and the Vikings eagerly took Irish men and women as slaves. Archaeological excavations in Dublin have unearthed large slave chains tied around the necks of captured Irish people who were presumably scheduled to be exported.[5] Apart from this anomaly, DNA analysis suggested relatively little population movement across Ireland until the nineteenth century. From this point onwards, the Irish travelled all over the world, interrupting the genetic make-up of other communities. Emigrating en masse, they mingled their DNA with others wherever they went. It is often said that people from Cork and Galway, two westerly port cities, tend to have darker hair than the rest of the population, due to mixing with Mediterranean bloodlines, although this claim about the so-called 'Black Irish' is largely unsubstantiated.

The DNA analysis also revealed that the Irish Traveller community were of Irish ancestral origin (and, despite presumptions, had no genetic ties with European Roma groups), but they did share a significantly different genetic make-up from other Irish communities. These differences arose due to hundreds of years of relative isolation. Travellers appear to have separated genetically from the rest of the Irish population around the seventeenth century, roughly twelve generations ago. Around 40,000 Travellers live in Ireland, less than 1 per cent of the population.[6]

Known in Irish as 'an lucht siúil' ('the walking people'), Irish Travellers speak both English and Shelta, a language of mixed English and Irish origin. Although their origins are vague, Irish Travellers seem to have diverged from the greater Irish population around the time of Cromwell's conquest. Traditionally, Traveller communities excelled in metalwork, which earned

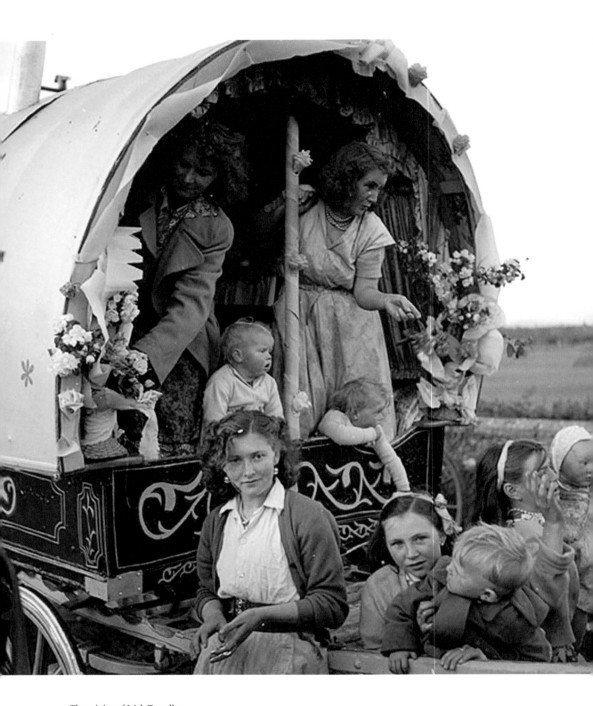

The origins of Irish Traveller
communities remain obscure.
Today, they are Ireland's only
designated ethnic minority group.

them the nickname 'tinker' (meaning 'tinsmith'), although this term was later used derogatorily. One theory about their origins is that the Travellers might be remnants of a people who lived in Ireland long before the Celts who enjoyed a lifestyle based on pastoralism rather than land tenure. Other theories suggest that this group were displaced during Cromwell's conquest in the 1650s or made homeless in the famines of the 1740s and 1840s. Historically, the Travellers were associated with vagrants (a Victorian word for homeless people), but since 2017 they have been officially recognised as Ireland's only indigenous ethnic minority who deserve specific rights.

Not everything passed down through the gene pool has proven beneficial. Known as the Celtic Curse, haemochromatosis is a genetic disorder which causes those affected to absorb excessive amounts of iron in the blood. If left untreated, this can cause organ damage or failure. One in 83 people in Ireland has the condition, which is also more common on Ireland's west coast. An alarming number of cases have been diagnosed on Inishbofin island.[7]

MAJOR CRAWFORD'S BLOODY SIGNATURE

On 28 September 1912 (known as Ulster Day), thousands of people travelled to Belfast City Hall to sign the Ulster Covenant. One Ulster man was not content with providing his signature the conventional way – with ink. Major Frederick H. Crawford took hold of his fountain pen, carved its sharp metal nib painfully through the surface of his skin and signed the covenant with his own blood. The signature still stands out today on the list of names and does indeed have a rich red colour. This bloody act was not entirely Crawford's idea. He had drawn inspiration from an ancestor in Scotland believed to have signed that country's National Covenant of 1638 in his blood.

Why did Crawford consider the Ulster Covenant so important that it was worth spilling his own blood over? Crawford was born in Belfast on 21 August 1861 into a Methodist family with an Ulster-Scots background. In his twenties,

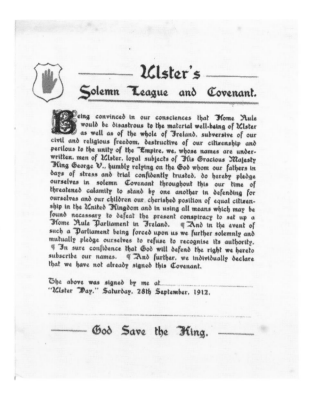

Ulster's
Solemn League and Covenant.

Being convinced in our consciences that Home Rule would be disastrous to the material well-being of Ulster as well as of the whole of Ireland, subversive of our civil and religious freedom, destructive of our citizenship and perilous to the unity of the Empire, we, whose names are underwritten, men of Ulster, loyal subjects of His Gracious Majesty King George V., humbly relying on the God whom our fathers in days of stress and trial confidently trusted, do hereby pledge ourselves in solemn Covenant throughout this our time of threatened calamity to stand by one another in defending for ourselves and our children our cherished position of equal citizenship in the United Kingdom and in using all means which may be found necessary to defeat the present conspiracy to set up a Home Rule Parliament in Ireland. ¶ And in the event of such a Parliament being forced upon us we further solemnly and mutually pledge ourselves to refuse to recognise its authority. ¶ In sure confidence that God will defend the right we hereto subscribe our names. ¶ And further, we individually declare that we have not already signed this Covenant.

The above was signed by me at _____
"Ulster Day," Saturday, 28th September, 1912.

——— God Save the King. ———

In September 1912, Major Frederick H. Crawford was so enthusiastic about the Ulster Covenant that he signed it using his blood.

Crawford worked as an engineer for White Star Line, and he returned to his beloved Ulster in 1892. During this time, Crawford would have read of the debates about Irish Home Rule that dragged on for decades. The Home Government Association was formed in 1870 by a small group of Irish Protestants who believed that a geographically distant, London-based government was failing to preserve their values and heritage. Unusually, membership consisted of both Catholics and Protestants. The group's leader, Isaac Butt, saw a place for both denominations in a new Ireland. A lawyer, he even defended Fenian prisoners.

In 1873, the Home Rule League was formed to call for limited Irish self-government and the re-establishment of a Dublin-based government. Once again, the group opened its arms to Catholics. In the 1874 general election, the league won an impressive 59 seats, including two in Ulster. Despite these successes, Butt was ousted from his leadership role by Charles Stewart Parnell, who was far more critical of British rule. During the 1880 election, he won seats in Cork. Parnell announced that he would not be content until he had destroyed the last links binding Ireland to England.

In December 1885, William Gladstone came around to the idea of Home Rule, irritating Queen Victoria so much that she remarked that her empire needed saving from 'Gladstone's reckless hands'. Two months later, Gladstone became prime minister for a third time leading the Liberal Party. In 1886, he put the first Home Rule Bill through parliament but was defeated by 30 votes. He took the country to the polls on the matter but lost. Lord Salisbury's Conservative Party held power until 1892 when Gladstone defeated him and reclaimed his role as prime minister. A second Home Rule Bill put forward in 1893 passed through the House of Commons but then needed the approval of the House of Lords, which voted against Home Rule by 419 to 41 votes. Gladstone retired in March 1894.

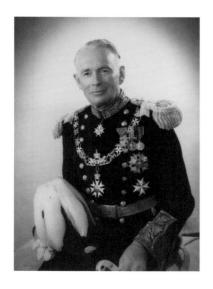

Frederick H. Crawford was considered too fanatical about Unionism even among his peers most dedicated to the cause.

In the meantime, Crawford had been serving in the Boer Wars with the Mid-Ulster Artillery Regiment of the British Army. In 1898, he was appointed governor of Campbell College, an exclusively rich school for Ulster's elite. The issue of Home Rule continued to bubble under the surface of British politics until the 1909 budget crisis, which led to the passing in 1911 of an act preventing the House of Lords from being able to veto policies already agreed in the Commons. Any bill that passed the Commons in three successive seasons would become law, regardless of what the House of Lords thought of it. Home Rule for Ireland was now a real possibility. In 1912, the third Home Rule Bill passed through parliament, meaning that Ireland was finally granted independence from Britain.

Crawford was enraged. Unionist and Protestant cultures were closely interlinked, but the influence of both was strong only in the north-east. Across the country as a whole, Protestants were in a minority. This raised fears that a Dublin-based government would be disinterested in Protestant needs, interests and culture. Unionists first complained in 1885 when Gladstone announced his support of Home Rule. In 1892, a major demonstration, the Ulster Unionist Convention, was staged when Gladstone returned to power. When the third Home Rule Bill passed, riots broke out across Belfast Notoriously, Catholic workers were expelled from the shipyards.

Horrified at the likelihood of Unionist culture being isolated if Ireland secured independence, in 1911 Crawford joined the Ulster Unionist Council. His heart rejoiced when the council first talked of organising physical force against Britain to resist Home Rule. Crawford was a pious, god-fearing man, but despite his godliness, he had an extraordinary knowledge of guns and openly suggested using them to murder Sinn Féin members. At Ulster Unionist Council meetings, he would ask attendees to step into another room where he had rifles, ammunition and bayonets laid out. However, even more militant Orange Order members looked at Crawford with puzzlement when offered rifles, finding him too bloodthirsty. Testifying further to his love of guns, Crawford started a secret society, Young Ulster. Members were required to own a Martini rifle, a Winchester rifle or a .455 revolver, plus 100 rounds of ammunition. His rifle clubs became hugely popular.

Crawford, who believed that God had personally chosen him to save Ulster, became a hero among Ulster Unionists. He played a major role in helping organise Ulster Day and thought that shedding a small quantity of blood would help secure Unionism's future. On Ulster Day, 471,414 people signed Ulster's Solemn League and Covenant. As leader of the Unionists, Edward Carson was the first person to sign it.

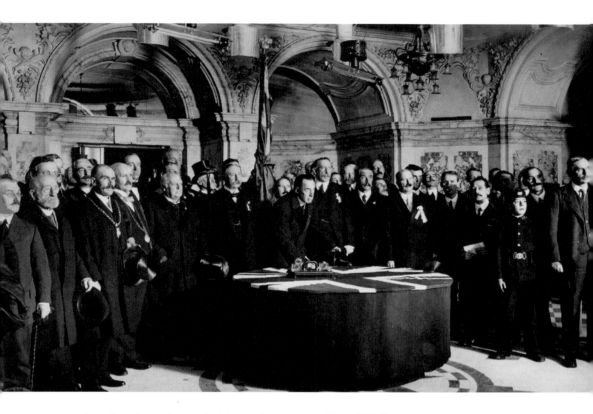

The Ulster Covenant was signed in Belfast City Hall on Ulster Day, 28 September 1912.

On that day, factories and shipyards across Belfast fell silent as Protestant workers made their way to City Hall to add their signatures. Church services ended early. Orangemen marshalled the crowds throughout the day. Carson left Belfast that evening on a steamer which made its way up Belfast Lough. Reportedly, a vast crowd stood at the edge of Belfast Lough singing 'Rule Britannia' and 'God Save the King'. The day's key message was that Unionists could, and were willing to, mobilise huge numbers if they wished. It was hoped that having signed a solemn, binding oath to resist Home Rule, the people of Ulster would act cohesively and collectively about the matter in the future. Ulster Day was also excellent propaganda. Crawford's bloody signature indicated Unionism's determination to fight Home Rule by all means necessary.[8]

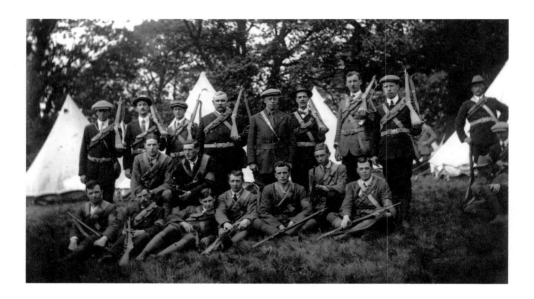

The UVF was formed in 1913 to protect Ulster from Irish nationalism.

After Ulster Day, Crawford kept up his enthusiasm for spilling blood, although this time not his own. The Ulster Volunteer Force (UVF), an armed military group, was formed in 1913 and Crawford was appointed as their Director of Ordnance. Much to his annoyance, customs officials were inclined to seize any arms which Crawford tried to smuggle into Ulster for the UVF. Crawford got smarter. He secured more than 25,000 rifles and millions of ammunition rounds from a German dealer. His daring plan involved switching ships halfway during the sea journey and sending a diversionary vessel into Belfast harbour. While the customs officials were distracted, Crawford smuggled the arms into Larne, Co. Antrim. By November 1913, the UVF had only imported only around 10,000 weapons (for context, the UVF had around 200,000 volunteers) but the gunrunning was symbolically significant. Murals of the UVF can still be found adorned on the sides of houses in staunchly Protestant areas of Northern Ireland.[9]

During the War of Independence and Civil War, Crawford continued to play an important organisational role in the UVF. Statements made in the early 1920s included 'I am ashamed to call myself an Irishman. Thank God I am not one. I am an Ulsterman, a very different breed' and a comment about 'killing a lot of the well-known Sinn Féin leaders and hanging half a dozen priests'. In 1921, he formed the Ulster Brotherhood, a group not afraid to use all means necessary to 'destroy and wipe out the Sinn Féin conspiracy of murder, assassination and outrage'. Even leading Unionists found his tactics somewhat extreme at this stage, and the Ulster Brotherhood lasted only a few months. Crawford died in 1952 and was buried at City Cemetery on the Falls Road, Belfast, a cemetery with a sunken wall that separated Protestants and Catholics.

Intriguingly, no one witnessed Crawford's blood signature. We know of the event only through a handwritten note on Crawford's personal copy of the Covenant Oath, which reads: 'I signed at 3.45 in City Hall in my own blood'. The story might well be yet another untruth in Irish history that has been passed down as historical fact. The sheer force of Crawford's beliefs perhaps meant that everyone simply believed him, given that he was just the type of person likely to consider shedding blood for beloved Ulster. More recently, scientists have investigated the signature and suggested that it doesn't contain blood after all. Nor has the signature darkened or discoloured over time as blood tends to do. Ulster Unionists still insist that the story is true, regardless of what the scientists claim.

BLOOD SACRIFICE

Four years after the third Home Rule Bill passed through parliament, Ireland was still being governed from Britain. The First World War led to Home Rule being temporarily placed on the backburner. It was to be dealt with when the war ended, but the conflict went on for years longer than anyone had expected. Some Irish people began to suspect that false promises had been made, or that the British government was secretly planning to renege because of the looming Ulster crisis. The shedding of blood for the sake of a signature had made clear

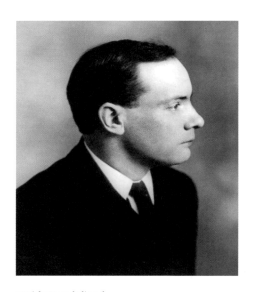

Patrick Pearse believed that blood sacrifice was necessary to free Ireland from British Rule.

the determinedness of Ulster Unionists, but some nationalists were willing to go further still. They planned to end their own lives in a glorious battle against the British to underscore their insistence that Ireland needed to leave the United Kingdom. If Ulster was worth fighting and dying for, so too was an independent Ireland. Blood sacrifice would prove this once and for all.

Patrick Pearse was prominent among Ireland's self-proclaimed saviours. Born in Dublin in 1879, as a child Pearse developed unusual fantasies of self-sacrifice for his country. His grandfather had been an active IRB member, and Pearse grew up listening to Irish rebel songs. On his mother's side of the family, the Irish language was spoken out of principle. Pearse's father was self-educated, and the house was filled with books. Pearse was exposed at a young age to eclectic readings, including ancient Irish mythology, writings of republicans such as Wolfe Tone and Robert Emmet, and the Bible. In 1900, Pearse was awarded a degree in modern languages (Irish, English and French) and actively contributed as a cultural nationalist to the literary outputs of the Gaelic revival.[10]

In 1913, Pearse was proudly sworn in to the IRB. His ideas of blood sacrifice fused Irish nationalism with Catholic teachings of Jesus Christ's blood sacrifice. By now, Pearse had developed an all-consuming yearning for martyrdom and dreamt of emulating Christ's sacrifice on the cross. Whereas Crawford thought he was God's messenger on earth for Unionists, Pearse imagined himself, like Jesus Christ, as a saviour of his persecuted people. He firmly believed that bloodshed in battle ('the red wine of the battlefield') cleansed and sanctified. Bloody battle was a regenerative force that cleansed the earth, a belief popular across Europe at the time. The rebels hoped to gain support across the nation by sacrificing themselves and regenerating the nationalist cause. How Pearse conjoined Christian doctrine and political violence remains controversial. Religious authors still consider Pearse's religious approach aggressively unorthodox and discordant with mainstream Christianity.[11]

Pearse was ecstatic when the IRB began to plan an armed insurrection, seeing this as Ireland's only hope of forever banishing the British. His dream of sacrificing himself for Ireland seemed to be coming to fruition. The IRB's last attempted rising in 1867 had been a fiasco. But the First World War reignited ideas about the value of insurrection, following the famous old republican saying: 'England's difficulty is Ireland's opportunity'. For republicans, the war was a rare moment when England was distracted and its soldiers were committed elsewhere. An opportune moment indeed for another uprising.

In 1915, the IRB Military Council was formed, with seven members: Éamonn Ceannt, Thomas Clarke, James Connolly, Seán Mac Diarmada, Thomas MacDonagh, Patrick Pearse and Joseph Plunkett. The IRB was aided by an Irish American group, Clan na Gael, which provided financial, logistical, and moral support. While Pearse romanticised about blood sacrifice, other council members aspired towards military success rather than martyrdom (or suicide, as sceptics called it). In 1915 the IRB was too small to stage a successful insurrection and teamed up with the Irish Volunteers.[12]

The Irish Volunteers had formed in November 1913 in direct response to the UVF's formation. The Volunteers were willing to defend Home Rule with as much physical force as the UVF would defend Ulster. When war broke out in autumn of 1914, the Volunteers boasted 180,000 members. The majority still favoured constitutional approaches, but a hardcore minority of 2,000–3,000 members resolutely opposed Irish men going off to war and thought a rebellion would be more effective. The IRB also joined forces with James Connolly, leader of the Irish Transport and General Workers' Union (ITGWU), who commanded the Irish Citizen Army and dreamt of an independent, 32-county, socialist republic in Ireland.

The IRB also allied with Britain's mortal enemy: Germany. It hoped that 12,000 German troops would land in submarines at Limerick, bringing thousands of rifles to arm the Volunteers. The Germans would sweep eastwards to support the Dublin insurrection. British troops would be massacred, and a victory march would take place along Sackville Street (now O'Connell Street). In return, Ireland would fight alongside Germany and help them win the war. The Germans were less enthusiastic about all of this and considered that sending over submarines would be too hazardous given Britain's naval strength. Perhaps hoping to placate their enthusiastic Irish friends, Germany sent over 20,000 captured Russian rifles and a million rounds of ammunition and explosives, dispatched on 9 April 1916 to Fenit Pier, Co. Kerry.

The Easter Rising was originally intended to take place on Good Friday, but this was shifted to Easter Monday, 24 April. Planning was done in top secret, and British intelligence failed to notice anything of interest. On the morning of Easter Monday, Dublin was unprotected and unprepared. Dublin Castle presumed that most people were happy enough waiting for Home Rule and did not expect an armed insurrection on its doorstep. Unbeknown to most people, a week before, on 17 April 1916, the seven leaders had signed the Proclamation of the Irish Republic, which announced a new provisional government for Ireland, initially composed of IRB Military Council members.

On the morning of Easter Monday, the rebels assembled at pre-arranged meeting points across Dublin. Just before noon, various units marched towards Dublin's key buildings and routes, occupying a number, including the General Post Office (GPO), the Four Courts, Jacob's Biscuit Factory, Boland's Bakery and South Dublin workhouse, as well as St Stephen's Green and, later, the Royal College of Surgeons. The rebels had the advantage of surprise. These premises were all occupied without opposition. The insurgents then defended them with sandbags and by seizing adjacent properties.

The GPO served as the rebellion headquarters and seat of the provisional government. Five of its members were based there: Clarke, Pearse, Connolly, Mac

The Proclamation of the Irish Republic was read out to passers-by at the start of the Easter Rising.

POBLACHT NA H EIREANN.

THE PROVISIONAL GOVERNMENT

OF THE

IRISH REPUBLIC

TO THE PEOPLE OF IRELAND.

IRISHMEN AND IRISHWOMEN : In the name of God and of the dead generations from which she receives her old tradition of nationhood, Ireland, through us, summons her children to her flag and strikes for her freedom.

Having organised and trained her manhood through her secret revolutionary organisation, the Irish Republican Brotherhood, and through her open military organisations, the Irish Volunteers and the Irish Citizen Army, having patiently perfected her discipline, having resolutely waited for the right moment to reveal itself, she now seizes that moment, and, supported by her exiled children in America and by gallant allies in Europe, but relying in the first on her own strength, she strikes in full confidence of victory.

We declare the right of the people of Ireland to the ownership of Ireland, and to the unfettered control of Irish destinies, to be sovereign and indefeasible. The long usurpation of that right by a foreign people and government has not extinguished the right, nor can it ever be extinguished except by the destruction of the Irish people. In every generation the Irish people have asserted their right to national freedom and sovereignty : six times during the past three hundred years they have asserted it in arms. Standing on that fundamental right and again asserting it in arms in the face of the world, we hereby proclaim the Irish Republic as a Sovereign Independent State, and we pledge our lives and the lives of our comrades-in-arms to the cause of its freedom, of its welfare, and of its exaltation among the nations.

The Irish Republic is entitled to, and hereby claims, the allegiance of every Irishman and Irishwoman. The Republic guarantees religious and civil liberty, equal rights and equal opportunities to all its citizens, and declares its resolve to pursue the happiness and prosperity of the whole nation and of all its parts, cherishing all the children of the nation equally, and oblivious of the differences carefully fostered by an alien government, which have divided a minority from the majority in the past.

Until our arms have brought the opportune moment for the establishment of a permanent National Government, representative of the whole people of Ireland and elected by the suffrages of all her men and women, the Provisional Government, hereby constituted, will administer the civil and military affairs of the Republic in trust for the people.

We place the cause of the Irish Republic under the protection of the Most High God, Whose blessing we invoke upon our arms, and we pray that no one who serves that cause will dishonour it by cowardice, inhumanity, or rapine. In this supreme hour the Irish nation must, by its valour and discipline and by the readiness of its children to sacrifice themselves for the common good, prove itself worthy of the august destiny to which it is called.

Signed on Behalf of the Provisional Government,

THOMAS J. CLARKE,
SEAN Mac DIARMADA,   THOMAS MacDONAGH,
P. H. PEARSE,   EAMONN CEANNT,
JAMES CONNOLLY.   JOSEPH PLUNKETT.

Diarmada and Plunkett. Pearse was designated president and commandant-general of the army. Connolly was vice president and commandant of the forces in Dublin. The task therefore fell to Pearse to read out the Proclamation of the Republic from the GPO's steps at 12.45 p.m. It was received with a mute response by bewildered onlookers. Hundreds of copies were then posted throughout the city.

Because telephone communication had been cut, the War Office only received news of the rising at 3.30 p.m. Once alerted, the military response was prompt and effective. Contact between Dublin and London was restored by early afternoon. By Monday evening, a large military force had gathered at Dublin Castle and begun assaulting the rebel-held buildings. The fighting lasted for the best part of a week. Soldiers were given official orders to shoot anyone suspected of being a rebel. In some areas, 'free fire zones' operated in which anyone visible on the streets was assumed to be an enemy and would be shot. Martial law was imposed.

As the week dragged on, conditions deteriorated in the GPO. Some men had not eaten for days. Lack of sleep, combined with hunger, caused debilitating exhaustion. Disorientated, traumatised Volunteers fell victim to paranoia and hysteria. Men deserted. At Boland's Bakery, one deranged volunteer was shot by his own men after killing one of the officers. The psychological pressure was intensified by the constant artillery bombardments. Liberty Hall, home of trade unionism in Ireland, was reduced to a shell. Sackville Street became a no-man's land. The rebels had underestimated the British Army's willingness to destroy the empire's second city. On Thursday, the bombardment intensified. The Rising was petering out and had clearly failed.

Pearse signed a general order of surrender on Saturday afternoon. Over the next few days, the rebels gradually surrendered. Some Volunteers had accepted that they would die for Ireland and planned accordingly, so they felt dispirited by this turn of events. Only when they left the buildings and witnessed the mass destruction around them did many Volunteers gain a less romantic perspective on the Rising.

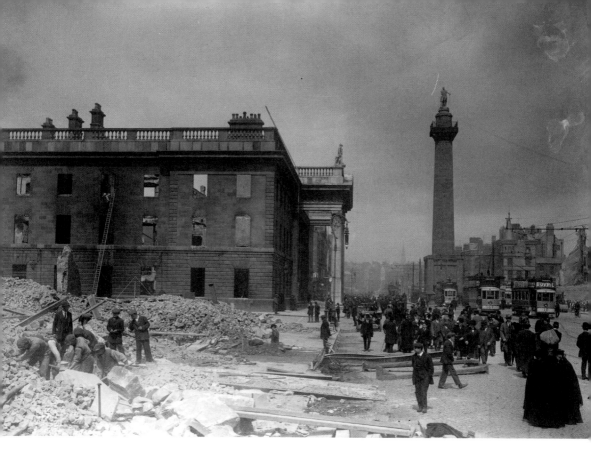

In terms of actual bloodshed, 450 people were killed during the 1916 Rising: 260 civilians, 143 British soldiers and 82 rebels. Pearse considered the behaviour of the rebels to be of utmost importance. Presenting themselves as a conventional army engaged in a legitimate form of warfare was a crucial strategy. For the most part, Volunteers avoided unnecessary bloodshed. Policemen and unarmed soldiers were not systematically targeted. Connolly's Citizen Army was more enthusiastic about shooting down policemen and was involved in several dubious killings around St Stephen's Green. Of all the leaders, Connolly was most opposed to shedding blood. In contrast with Pearse's grandiose military visions, Connolly insisted that war was not glorious, inspiring or regenerative. On the contrary, he thought, it was hateful, damnable and damning. Connolly added bluntly that 'any person, whether English, German or Irish, who sings the praises of war is, in our opinion, a blithering idiot'.[13]

Much of Dublin's city centre was destroyed during the Easter Rising of 1916.

Initially, Dubliners were infuriated by the deaths and extensive destruction. Around 16,000 Dublin families had family members enlisted in the British Army and at war. Home Rule was imminent anyway, they noted, so what was the point? For some, the idea of sacrificing oneself for Ireland simply felt silly. As the Volunteers surrendered and left their buildings, hostile, jeering crowds greeted them. Some rebels were surprisingly grateful for the presence of British troops, who protected them from the angry crowds. Although public opinion was generally negative, a few of Dublin's residents considered the rebels brave for holding out with relatively few arms for nearly a week against the military forces of an empire.

The Easter Rising might have gone down as a pointless episode in Irish history led by men with a grandiose vision of their own importance were it not for the events that followed. After the Rising, the Irish public mood changed. Acting against common-sense advice, the Cabinet introduced nationwide martial law on Wednesday 26 April. For several weeks after the rising, districts were cordoned off, ports kept under close surveillance and houses searched for rebels. The army swept up around 3,500 people. About 2,500 of these were interned in Britain, many of whom were not nationalists and not involved in the Rising. Although the rebellion had been largely confined to Dublin, the entire country was placed under martial law for six months. The indiscriminate punishment of so many people generated outrage, sympathy and protests from a wide circle of friends and family. The raids and arrests which extended throughout the country provoked resentment and support for the idea of the British as oppressors.

Major General Sir John Maxwell was appointed General Officer Commanding the British Army in Ireland. He was convinced that militant nationalism must be crushed and respect for law and order restored. Given the wartime context, he decided that the insurrection's leaders ought to be court-martialled and preferably executed. This was a foolhardy move. Eighty-seven civilians were tried by military court. Fifteen men were singled out for execution, including all seven signatories of the Proclamation. Éamon De Valera escaped

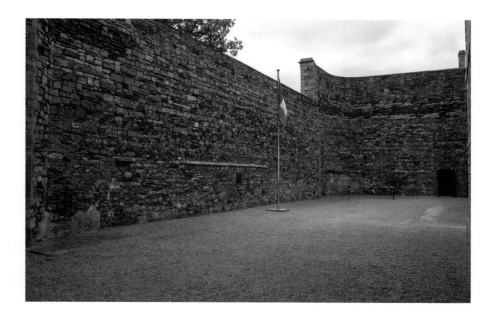

the death penalty despite being a commandant. The executions took place at Kilmainham Gaol, Dublin. Today, visitors can walk through the disused, renovated prison and follow guided tours to the fateful spot where the leaders were shot dead. The speed and secrecy of the executions were widely discussed. Some rebels had been tried and executed behind closed doors and with no access to lawyers.

The rebels were executed at Kilmainham Gaol, causing a huge public outcry.

The public saw the executions as draconian, and opinion shifted from hostility to sympathy towards the rebels. The rebels' willingness to die for their beliefs, and to commit blood sacrifice, started to evoke admiration. Perhaps the rebels had been right about the brutality of the British after all. Their embrace of death began to go down in Irish history as legendary, rather than foolish. Indeed, the blood spilt by the British during the Kilmainham Gaol executions began to form a powerful foundation myth for independent Ireland. Only one man was happy about the executions, and that was Patrick Pearse, whose dreams of martyrdom finally came true on 3 May 1916 when the British shot him dead. By all accounts, he whistled all the way to his execution.

Hec ē vndea
ma figura ano
thomie in qua a
mouetur os ca
pitis causa fnaē
di amotlpiā p
ipius ossis τ du
ar pelhaulax s̄ de
matsςt pie ma
ts ςt aerebu

CHAPTER 7

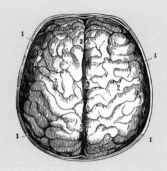

BRAINS

Human brains are intricately complex organs, located conveniently close to our sensory organs. Brains contain billions of tiny neurons which communicate to distant parts of the body. They control the processes that regulate our bodies: thought, memory, emotion, touch, vision, breathing, temperature, hunger. They also contain our mind which, of course, helps us to think and feel emotions. Considering the inherent complexity of our brains and mental processes, it may seem strange that Irish society long believed in the value of drilling or cutting holes into this organ, hoping to cure severe mental health issues. Such practices were performed by the ancient Irish to expel evil spirits thought to have taken over some people and, more recently, in Irish asylums when lobotomies became problematically fashionable.

It was only during the seventeenth century that Westerners started to believe that our minds and emotions reside in our brains. Before then, physicians and scientists thought that the processes of emotion, perception and imagination occurred in the digestive organs. (The stomach was said to be the seat of the soul.[1]) Since then, we have come to think of our brain as the site where we process our mental and emotional life.

The intensity of Irish emotions, particularly sadness, is reflected in the historical accounts of loss and misery felt during the Great Famine and the myth of the wailing banshee. In the decades that followed the famine, the Irish began to suffer staggeringly high levels of mental health problems leading to incarceration in the country's many lunatic asylums.

TREPANNING

Given the brain's neurological intricacy, the historical belief that drilling holes into the skull and brain was a good idea may come as a surprise. Twentieth-century psychiatrists, insisting that they were performing a complex neurological operation, called this lobotomy (or psychosurgery). Many people, including their patients, suspected that this smashing into skulls wasn't too dissimilar from

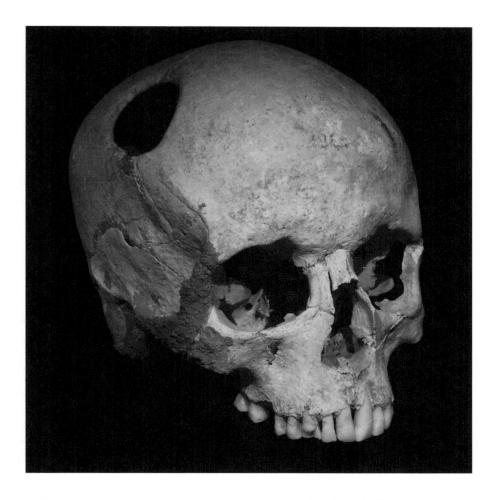

prehistoric trepanning (or trephining). Trepanning involved drilling or scraping a hole into the human skull. Ancient healers trepanned to help people who were behaving oddly let out the evil spirits thought to be afflicting them. (Presumably, many of these people would today be diagnosed with severe mental health issues.)

The practice of trepanning goes back to prehistoric times and appears to have been commonly used in ancient Ireland.

To date, archaeologists working in Ireland have discovered 18 trepanned skulls, more than enough to suggest that the procedure was once common on the island. All the holes were deliberately forged. Survival rates were surprisingly high, and new bone growth around the holes indicates that trepanned people went about their daily business despite having holes in their heads. Some people even wore the fragments of bone taken from their skulls as a charm to ward off evil spirits.[2]

When fighting in the Battle of Moyrath (Battle of Moira) of AD 637, Cennfaelad, a young Irish chief, was struck across the head with a sword. The pain was excruciating. He was carried to Tomregan Monastery to be healed. Like many people in Ireland, Cennfaelad was a direct descendant of Niall of the Nine Hostages. Even a year later, Cennfaelad still felt confused and disorientated, his memory no longer what it once had been. He sought help from a doctor at Tuaim Drecon, Co. Cavan – an ancient seat of learning similar in some ways to a university – who removed pieces of skull and brain, which cleared his intellect and brought back his memory. The 'brain of forgetfulness' had been removed. Not only that, but he went on to become one of Ireland's greatest scholars, earning him the name Cennfaelad the Learned. Cennfaelad wrote Primer of the Poets and founded the Derryloran school in Co. Tyrone. The fact that this story exists suggests the procedure was well known and recognised.[3] Even today, a significant number of people sign up for voluntary trepanning believing it will enhance their mental power or help them develop clairvoyance.

Brains also feature in another important tale in Irish mythology. According to lore, there once lived a king of Leinster named Mesgegra. Mesgegra was killed by an Ulster warrior named Conall Cernach. Delighted with his victory, and demonstrating his morbid sensibilities, Conall removed Mesgegra's brain, mixed it with lime and dried it in the sun, creating a trophy. Sometime later, the so-called 'brain ball' was stolen by the Connacht warrior Cet mac Mágach, who flung it in a sling shot at the Ulster king, Conchobar mac Nessa. The ball lodged in Conchobar's head, and his physicians were unable to remove it. They sewed up the wound and informed Conchobar that to survive he must not get overexcited. Seven years later, Conchobar was informed of the death of Christ and became so angry that the brain ball burst out of his head (the story most likely having been Christianised at some point). Conchobar died. There had

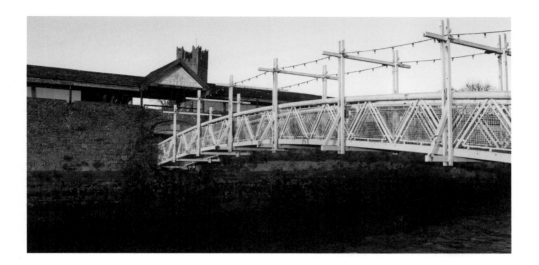

long existed a prophecy that Mesgegra would avenge his own death. That he certainly did. For seven weary years, Conchobar had ambled around with Mesgegra's brain poking out from the side of his head before revenge was enacted from beyond the grave by the bursting brain ball.[4]

A footbridge in Co. Limerick has been named after Dr Sylvester O'Halloran.

Over the centuries, Ireland produced an unusual preponderance of neurosurgeons and brain doctors. Limerick-born doctor Sylvester O'Halloran was among these. Writing in 1793, he believed that 'there is no part of the habitable globe that for half a century past has afforded such an ample field of observations on injuries of the head as Ireland in general [and] this province of Munster in particular'. O'Halloran blamed Irish people's fiery nature and love of whiskey for all the head injuries, noting that the Irish 'soon catch fire' to the 'slightest offence' leading to 'bloody conflicts'. He criticised the large amount of alcohol consumed at fairs and hurling matches and the violence, complaining that 'I have had no less than four fractured skulls to trepan on a May morning'. But O'Halloran considered himself fortunate to be working in this country and praised the 'superior advantages Irish surgeons have long possessed over those of the neighbouring nations'.[5]

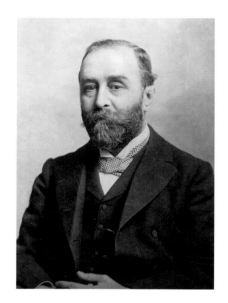

William Thornley Stoker was one
of Ireland's leading surgeons in
the nineteenth century and was
brother to Bram Stoker, famed
author of *Dracula*.

In the nineteenth century, following the advent of anaesthetics and aseptic techniques, surgeons performed increasingly complex and precise brain surgery. Everyone has heard of Dracula, the blood-obsessed vampire created by Irish author Bram Stoker. Less well known is that Bram had a famous brother, William Thornley Stoker, one of Ireland's leading doctors. When *Dracula* was first published in 1897, William was serving as president of the Royal Academy of Medicine in Ireland, the most prestigious position a physician could then secure. William became a brain surgery specialist and performed the first cerebral operations in Ireland while working at St Patrick's Hospital, Dublin. In the 1880s and 1890s, he saved the lives of numerous patients suffering from brain haemorrhages, tumours and abscesses. His success rates would seem low compared with today, but they were revolutionary by late-nineteenth-century standards.

These surgical feats were made possible by the new knowledge of the brain that had been recently accumulated. In 1802, Charles Bell, an accomplished English anatomist, published a radical new book: *The Anatomy of the Brain*. In this, Bell traced (for the first time) how the various nerve tracts connect to different parts of the brain which, in turn, control functions across the body. Bell found this all out by touching different parts of the spinal cords of living rabbits and observing the effects (e.g., muscle spasms) elsewhere in their bodies.

Bell beautifully embellished his book with engravings and drawings which revealed to readers the stunning anatomy of the brain and nervous system. Remarkable for their artistic skill and finish, they also granted surgeons and physicians access to a strikingly detailed map of the brain and its nervous

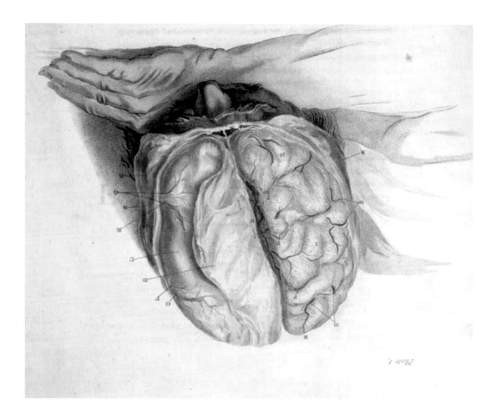

system connections.[6] Almost a century later, William Stoker would use David Ferrier's cortical maps, which visualised how certain areas of the brain were linked to specific body parts, discovered after electrically stimulating the exposed brains of unanaesthetised dogs

Charles Bell was an accomplished English anatomist who published striking images of the human brain for the first time in his 1802 book *The Anatomy of the Brain*.

and seeing which muscles contracted. Ferrier was a Scottish neurologist and psychologist who experimented on living monkeys in the name of science. He published two particularly notable books: *The Functions of the Brain* (1876) and *The Localisation of Cerebral Disease* (1878).[7]

As a staunch supporter of animal rights, William was at odds with both Bell and Ferrier. In the lead up to the 1876 Cruelty to Animals Act, which legalised

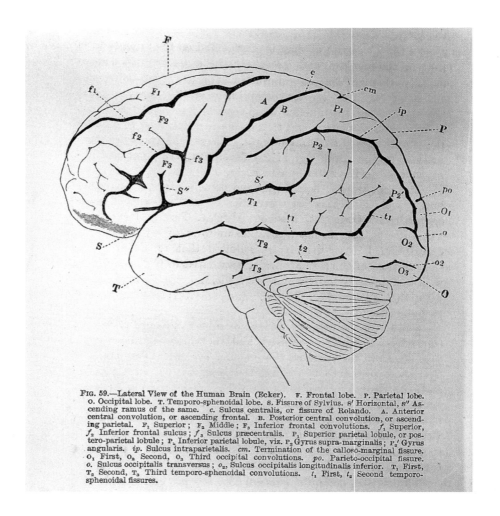

FIG. 59.—Lateral View of the Human Brain (Ecker). F. Frontal lobe. P. Parietal lobe. O. Occipital lobe. T. Temporo-sphenoidal lobe. s. Fissure of Sylvius. s′ Horizontal, s″ Ascending ramus of the same. c. Sulcus centralis, or fissure of Rolando. A. Anterior central convolution, or ascending frontal. B. Posterior central convolution, or ascending parietal. F_1 Superior ; F_2 Middle ; F_3 Inferior frontal convolutions. f_1 Superior, f_2 Inferior frontal sulcus ; f_3 Sulcus præcentralis. P_1 Superior parietal lobule, or postero-parietal lobule ; P_2 Inferior parietal lobule, viz. P_2 Gyrus supra-marginalis ; $P_2′$ Gyrus angularis. ip. Sulcus intraparietalis. cm. Termination of the calloso-marginal fissure. O_1 First, O_2 Second, O_3 Third occipital convolutions. po. Parieto-occipital fissure. o. Sulcus occipitalis transversus ; o_2, Sulcus occipitalis longitudinalis inferior. T_1 First, T_2 Second, T_3 Third temporo-sphenoidal convolutions. t_1 First, t_2 Second temporo-sphenoidal fissures.

In the 1870s, David Ferrier developed further knowledge of the workings of the human brain.

animal vivisection but only for scientists holding a licence, William gained first-hand knowledge of experimentation as an inspector for Ireland. William believed that animal experimentation was potentially ethical and valuable, but only in the right circumstances. Limitations needed to be imposed on experimental practices. He objected vehemently to experiments on dogs and monkeys as they seemed to feel more pain than rabbits and mice.

He also spoke out against experimenting on living animals for the sake of delivering a university lecture. In contrast, most doctors of the time ardently supported vivisection.

Bram consulted with his older brother on the scenes that fill the pages of *Dracula*, a book very much informed by the neuroscience of the 1890s. The novel's fictitious doctors, Abraham van Helsing and John Seward, both possess knowledge of cerebral localisation research. This is evident when they operate on Renfield, a madman who suffers a brain injury. Stoker describes Dracula as having a 'mighty brain', having acquired knowledge from animal and human experimental subjects. That scientists might start dissecting living humans before long was a genuinely felt fear at the time. Perhaps Dracula, as a character, stood in for the experimental scientist, a person who treated humans just as callously as laboratory-based scientists treated animals.[8]

One might presume, given all the scientific experimentation, that brain operations became ever more sophisticated. For the most part, they did. However, in 1941, Rosemary Kennedy, sister of future American President John F. Kennedy, had a lobotomy. The procedure became fashionable. Across Ireland, psychiatrists began operating on patients with an instrument similar to an ice pick. This would be smashed through the side of the eye socket to cut out part of the frontal lobe. An alternative procedure involved boring a hole in the skull. At Richmond Hospital, over 700 frontal lobotomies were carried out on patients between 1951 and 1960. Whether or not we had come far from the cruder ways of the ancient Irish was questionable.[9]

THE TEARS ON THE SHAMROCK

History is emotional, especially Irish history. Scientists haven't fully figured out how emotions work, but we know that the limbic system (a group of interconnected structures located deep within the brain), specifically the hypothalamus, plays a major role in controlling our emotions. Psychologists have identified six basic emotions: happiness, anger, sadness, fear, surprise and disgust. These correspond with Charles Darwin's idea about basic emotions. This interest in emotions was piqued by Charles Bell's 1824 book, *Anatomy and Philosophy of Expression*. In 1872, Darwin published *The Expression of the Emotions in Man and Animals*, an influential work ultimately overshadowed by his major works on evolution. Neuropsychologists now believe that emotions trigger parts of the brain and encourage us to respond in particular ways. Emotions are crucial to our existence. If we did not feel fear, we would not run from danger. Happiness is our preferred emotional state and allows us to feel sociable, energetic and fitter. From an evolutionary perspective, this makes us attractive to members of the opposite sex, with whom we then fall in love. Love is felt when the hypothalamus triggers the release of hormones including dopamine, oxytocin and vasopressin. Love is important and encourages us to reproduce with our loved one (or 'mate').[10]

Unfortunately, much of Irish history is desperately unhappy (largely thanks to the British, so the Irish would say), so it seems apt to focus on misery, agony, suffering and sadness. Perhaps the saddest song relating to Irish history is 'The Tears on the Shamrock', written in 1847 by British author and illustrator Alfred Crowquill:

> The sea moans with sadness around thy dark land
> And melts into tears as it touches the strand
> The cry from thy mountains comes wildly and low
> As the laden wind sighs with its burthen of woe
> And the notes that alone thy sweet harp strings can wake
> Are the dying laments that they give as they break
> Thy shamrock it glistens *Och hone! Wirrasthru!*
> With tears of dark sorrow, but not with the dew!
> With tears of dark sorrow but not with the dew!

The angel of Famine, with darkening wing,
Has thrown the cold shadow o'er each living thing,
Thy dwellings are fallen, thy children must mourn,
For the earth of its bounty is rifled and shorn,
And death claims thy champion, far from thy loved land,
But still must thou bow to the chastening hand
Thy shamrock it glistens, *Och hone! Wirrasthru!*
With tears of dark sorrow, but not with the dew,
With tears of dark sorrow, but not with the dew.

Poor Erin! Thy sister with fond love has flown
To dry up thy tears, and to hush thy deep moan
And with her, sweet Mercy and warm-hearted train
With bright feet have crowded across the dark main
So thy children shall smile, and thy heart bleed no more
For her succouring hands are spread out to thy shore
Then wall not, fair Erin, *Och hone! Wirrasthru!*
Thy shamrock shall glisten again with dew.
Thy shamrock shall glisten again with dew.

This was written in 1847, the most devastating year of the Great Famine (1845–52). The British still have a negative reputation, in Ireland, for their unsympathetic treatment of the famine-stricken Irish, but some British people felt genuine concern at the time about Irish suffering and resented their government for not doing enough. Crowquill was among these.[11]

During the famine, people from Co. Donegal said goodbye to their loved ones on the Bridge of Tears. Located between Dunfanaghy and Falcarragh, this attractive little stone bridge rests on the main road to Derry. Now a busy highway, a stagecoach would once have transported emigrants across it on their way to Derry, the region's largest port city. Visitors to the bridge today can read a small plaque written in Irish which translates as 'Family and friends

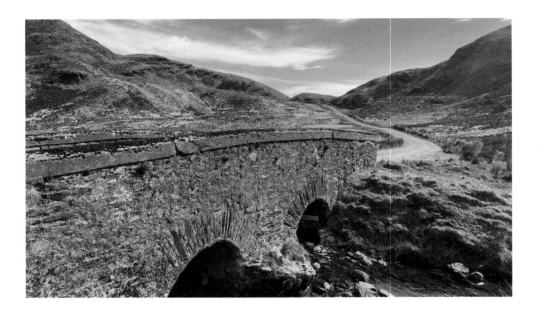

People used to say their goodbyes to emigrating relatives and friends at the Bridge of Tears in Co. Donegal.

of the person leaving for foreign lands would come this far. Here was the separation. This is the Bridge of Tears'. It was unlikely that the emigrants would ever return, so their departure was treated as a funeral by the living. Many tears were shed.

Tears also fell if a banshee arrived, for this heralded the death of a family member. It was impossible to ignore a visiting banshee, as she announced her arrival by loudly screaming, wailing and shrieking. Banshees are described in several ways. Usually, a banshee has long streaming hair and wears a grey cloak covering a green dress, her eyes reddened by constant weeping. She can appear as a beautiful, enchanting woman singing sorrowful songs only audible to the person for whom they are intended. Sometimes, she has a ghastly appearance: an old woman with rotten teeth and blood-red eyes whose mouth remains constantly open, emitting a piercing scream. Whether a good or bad banshee materialises can depend on how much the apparition liked the family they were visiting. On more than a few occasions, banshees seem to have been celebrating, rather than warning of, an upcoming death, if it involved someone they loathed. No one knows where the banshee gets her knowledge of the death.

Lady Wilde (mother of Oscar) neatly summarised the banshee's various forms in her *Ancient Legends, Mystic Charms and Superstitions of Ireland* (1887) as follows:

> Sometimes the banshee assumes the form of some sweet singing virgin of the family who died young and has been given the mission by the invisible powers to become the harbinger of coming doom to her mortal kindred. Or she may be said to appear at night as a shrouded woman, crouched beneath the trees, lamenting with veiled face, or flying past in the moonlight, crying bitterly; and the cry of this spirit is mournful beyond all other sounds on earth and betokens certain death to some member of the family whenever it is heard in the silence of the night.[12]

Banshees only appear to people of bona fide ancient Irish descent because they are remnants of Tuatha Dé Danann, who were defeated and driven underground by the invading Milesians. Each Tuatha Dé Danann member occupied a mound or hill (known as a sídhe) and turned into fairies. Banshee translates as 'woman of the fairy mound', or 'fairy woman'. In that sense, despite being dreaded, a visitation from a banshee could be a source of great pride and dignity as it signified a pure Irish-Celtic lineage untainted by foreign influences. Elizabeth Sheridan, a relative of Irish gothic writer Sheridan Le Fanu, claimed to have heard a banshee wailing in 1824, the night before Anglo-Irish novelist Frances Sheridan died in Blois, France. Elizabeth's niece greatly angered her by pointing out that the family were in fact of English descent. Being not pure Irish, she had no right to the guardianship of an Irish fairy.[13] For such families, even emigration failed to provide respite from the banshee's cries. Descendants of the O'Grady family, once one of Ireland's noblest families,

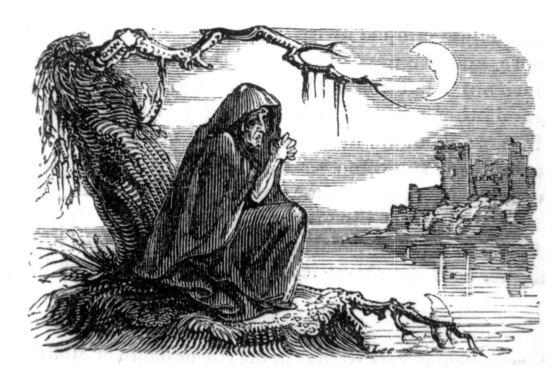

The arrival of a banshee, announced by her shrill screaming, was thought to signal an impending death.

moved all the way to Canada. One night, they heard a strange, mournful lamentation, a bitter cry of deepest agony and sorrow. The next day, the father and son of the household were found drowned.[14]

All noteworthy families fashionably claimed to have their own female spirit acting as a harbinger of death. The buildings once owned by these prominent families have also become associated with the wildly screaming fairies. Shane's Castle, set on the north-eastern shore of Lough Neagh, Co. Antrim, was built in 1345 by an O'Neill. Originally named Edenduffcarrick, its revised name came from Shane McBrien O'Neill, who ruled over it in the early seventeenth century. His many sons were all named Shane too. These O'Neills were also descended from Niall of the Nine Hostages. In 1816, the O'Neills threw a house party, and the spare bedroom was occupied.

A fire began in that room and burned down the main block of the castle.

This was no ordinary blaze. Some centuries before the fateful fire, one of the O'Neill lords had been out raiding and encountered a cow with its horns tangled in a hawthorn tree. The fairies regarded this tree as sacred, and no one would dare cut a branch to release the animal, apart from O'Neill. When he returned home, his daughter Kathleen had been carried off by the 'wee folk' to the bottom of Lough Neagh as punishment for the tree cutting. The fairies allowed Kathleen to return to let her father

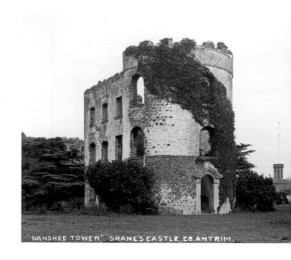

know she was safe in the fairy kingdom, but she had to promise to visit the family whenever misfortune was about to visit and loudly wail. The fairies also specified that a room had to be kept for her sole use in the castle.

The Banshee Tower at Shane's Castle in Co. Antrim.

Over the centuries, the family banshee paid regular visits. She became known as named Maeveen, the White Lady of Sorrow. In the room set aside for her, and where the fire started when it was temporarily occupied in 1816, chambermaids regularly reported seeing her impression on the bed. On the night of 15 May 1816, guests assembled on the lawn outside the blazing building saw a banshee hovering above the flames. Her cries were never heard around the estate again.[15]

In the 1890s, a furious debate erupted when the *Weekly Irish Times* published a letter dismissing belief in banshees as superstition and joyfully foreseeing the day when the Irish no longer believed in such nonsense. For years afterwards, letters poured in daily to the *Irish Times* offices from readers insisting that banshees were real. Many claimed to have personally witnessed their ominous presence and shrilling songs. How dare the anonymous letter writer dismiss such a cherished belief! Worse still, another sceptic claimed that those stupid enough to still believe in banshees lacked education and mistook the sounds of cats and birds in the night for banshees. Regardless of one's stance, the protracted debate reveals the persistence of traditional beliefs in the 1890s, a time when Irish society was becoming disenchanted and modernised.

One correspondent insisted that the banshee's cry sounded nothing like a wailing cat and described eerie sounds heard in Co. Down as follows:

> Its cadence, melancholy in the extreme, could not be mistaken for anything human; now shrill enough to be heard for miles, and sufficiently weird at the midnight hour to freeze the marrow in one's bones ... my first experience of the banshee was not a pleasant one, arousing me from a peaceful sleep to listen in fear and trembling to the death cry, which was felt by all in the household of which I formed a part to be the forerunner of dissolution for someone in the immediate neighbourhood.

Another correspondent wrote:

> I have heard her on three different occasions. The first time I did not even know that the banshee cried for the members of our family and was quietly sitting at a fire with a friend. Two large pointers were beside us. From outside the window came a wailing cry something like that of a child in great pain, but clearer and very sad ... [The dogs] lay stretched on the ground, the foam over their mouths and bodies, evidently too frightened to howl or move. A few days afterwards my sister, who seemed to be in perfect health, fell dead.
>
> Never did I again search for the banshee, as the cry once heard can never be mistaken. In our family, we always hear the cry a few days before a death. It is a curious circumstance that, as a rule, some one member, even though in the room with the others who hear it distinctly, cannot hear any cry.[16]

Belief in banshees persisted well into the twentieth century, although sometimes the wails of animals were mistaken for the banshee's cries. In 1931, a strange noise caused consternation and conjecture in Coolock and brought crowds flocking to the village. On this occasion, the banshee turned out to be a large barn owl. Its wings had been outstretched, its white breast was visible and its face appeared foggy and indefinite. If it was dark, it might well have looked just like a ghostly banshee. Residents described a 'piercing wail' 'so blood-curdling that it struck terror to the hearts of many who heard it, in one case causing the hearer to faint'. Locals presumed it was a troubled spirit, ghost or banshee.[17]

MENTAL HEALTH

Ireland has one of the highest rates of mental illness in the world. Currently, around 19 per cent of the Irish population is diagnosed with a serious condition such as bipolar, schizophrenia or depression. There is a long history to this curiosity. In the 1800s, asylum incarceration rates in Ireland rose rapidly. In the following century, Ireland shut away more people (proportionately) in psychiatric institutions than any other country in the world.[18]

At the start of the nineteenth century, Ireland had only a handful of asylums and 'madness' was not widely agreed upon as a medical problem that should be managed by trained doctors. Most people viewed it more as a social problem, not too dissimilar from crime. Over the decades, 'madness' became redefined as 'mental illness'. Professional psychiatrists (or 'alienists') emerged. As 'insanity' became a medical matter, it became less fashionable to treat the 'mad' as criminals or to chain them up in carceral institutions, as had previously been the case. People with mental health concerns were provided with their own institution: the asylum.

With the Irish Lunatic Asylums for the Poor Act of 1817, Ireland became the very first nation in the world to establish a publicly funded system of asylums.

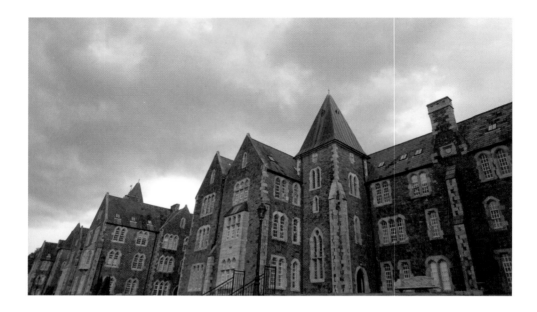

From the nineteenth century, thousands of Irish people with mental health difficulties were housed in asylums.

In the nineteenth century, social welfare was not a popular idea, so the creation of state-funded asylums across the country was a truly outstanding idea. The asylums were to be therapeutic, not punitive. By 1869, 22 public asylums had been built across the country, alongside many private ones. In some asylums, the number of incarcerated patients rose as high as 1,000. It was hoped that amassing the mentally ill in dedicated institutions would help psychiatrists develop more nuanced understandings of psychiatric problems, and perhaps even cure some of them. Asylums were meant to have a pleasing, cheerful environment, also seen as conducive to cure.

None of this happened. The asylums were expensive to build and operate. Costs were kept to a minimum and plans for an uplifting architecture were jettisoned. As anyone visiting an old Irish asylum today will testify, the buildings are difficult to distinguish from prisons, so grim was their construction. It was impossible for a small medical staff to pay much attention to patients, given how many people entered the asylums. Patients were no longer whipped and chained but still found themselves vulnerable to abuse, solitary confinement and milder restraints. Physical violence continued to be used to help discipline an unruly institutional population. Not one mental health condition was cured or much better understood. Asylums filled with chronic, incurable, hopeless cases. Some people with episodic mental illnesses came and went, but many patients never left, staying in the asylum until they died. Mental health conditions were stigmatised, and families often expressed no desire to see their tainted 'insane' relatives ever again.

By the twentieth century, the ageing asylums were dilapidated and falling into disrepair. Psychiatrists still couldn't cure anything. The number of patients entering through the doors rose and rose. Frustrated, some psychiatrists began to experiment on their patients' brains. From the 1920s, schizophrenics were treated with 'coma therapy'. Barbiturates made patients fall in and out of deep sleep but with a huge risk of overdose, irreversible coma and death. As an alternative, some psychiatrists used insulin instead, inducing around 50 insulin comas in each patient within a period of six to eight weeks.

An alternative was to shock brains back into functioning normally. From the 1930s, some psychiatrists came to believe that epileptic fits countered the symptoms of schizophrenia. It was an erroneous theory, but nonetheless psychiatrists used a substance called cardiazol to induce epileptic convulsions in schizophrenic patients. Patients hated and feared cardiazol. As the contractions started, patients lost consciousness. Between injection and seizure, a 10-second period of intense purgatory occurred during which patients felt as though they were dying. During the seizure which then followed, patients jerked and spasmed, their skin turned blue and their pupils widened; incontinence was common. After around 40 seconds, patients briefly fell into a comatose sleep. Extreme contractions caused joint dislocations and bone fractures, sometimes even lasting cognitive impairment. Patients rarely remembered the convulsions but never forgot the harrowing purgatory period. Nurses and attendants resorted to chasing terrified patients around the corridors who were trying to escape the treatment table. Psychiatrists named all this medical progress.

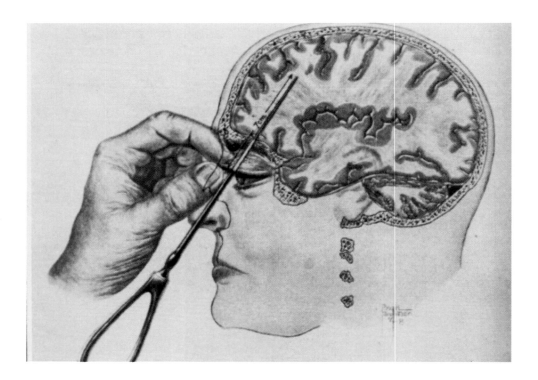

Lobotomies involve the surgical removal of part of the brain. The operation was widely used in twentieth-century Irish asylums.

Should their mental health still not have improved, patients found themselves wired up to the electrical mains and subjected to electroconvulsive therapy (ECT). Unlike with chemical injection, if something was going wrong during ECT, the plug could simply be pulled out of the socket. Electroshocks were given to severely depressed patients whose mental pain was not alleviated with other shock therapies. The maximum voltage used was usually 170 volts, producing an epileptic seizure lasting from 30 seconds to 1 minute. Despite its dubious reputation, ECT had some therapeutic benefits and remains in use today, although far less frequently.

Lobotomy was yet another option, which might leave readers questioning (again) how far Irish society had come from the ancient trepanning practices in its management of mental health issues. Patients were usually awake when their brains were drilled into. During the procedure, their utterances became more confused until they eventually fell silent. Most panicked at the beginning of the operation as they heard (and watched) the holes being drilled and the ominous accompanying grinding sound. Gradually, it became apparent that psychosurgery could cause irreparable brain damage. The behaviour of lobotomised patients improved in some regards, but they were now dull and subdued. Their 'mental amputation' had rid them of their symptoms, but also their personalities. They felt little anymore. Their emotional life had deadened. A heavy price to pay, indeed.

Fortunately for everyone involved, effective drug therapies were developed in the 1950s, with chlorpromazine being the most famous. Lithium was used to manage the symptoms of 'manic depression' (or bipolar disorder, as we know it today). Antidepressants became increasingly used later in the twentieth century. Tranquilisers became popular among people (especially women) with less severe mental health issues – those who felt nervous and anxious, for instance. By the late twentieth century, many people did not need to be institutionalised, as they could live a relatively 'normal' life thanks to the new drugs available to manage their symptoms. The asylums largely closed down or were reduced in size, and the various shock therapies which had terrified so many patients fell out of use along with their closure.[19]

However, even the curative drugs had a dark side. In the twenty-first century, Northern Ireland is thought to be in the grip of a deadly epidemic of addiction to prescription drugs, with nearly 200,000 prescriptions per year being handed out for tramadol (an opioid painkiller). Northern Ireland has one of the world's highest prescription rates for antidepressants in the entire world and proportionally higher mental health problems than all other regions that constitute the United Kingdom. Many people attribute this to the Troubles. Indeed, since the Troubles ended in 1998, many people have identified themselves as psychological victims of the conflict, with trauma being cited as an ongoing problem affecting their lives.[20]

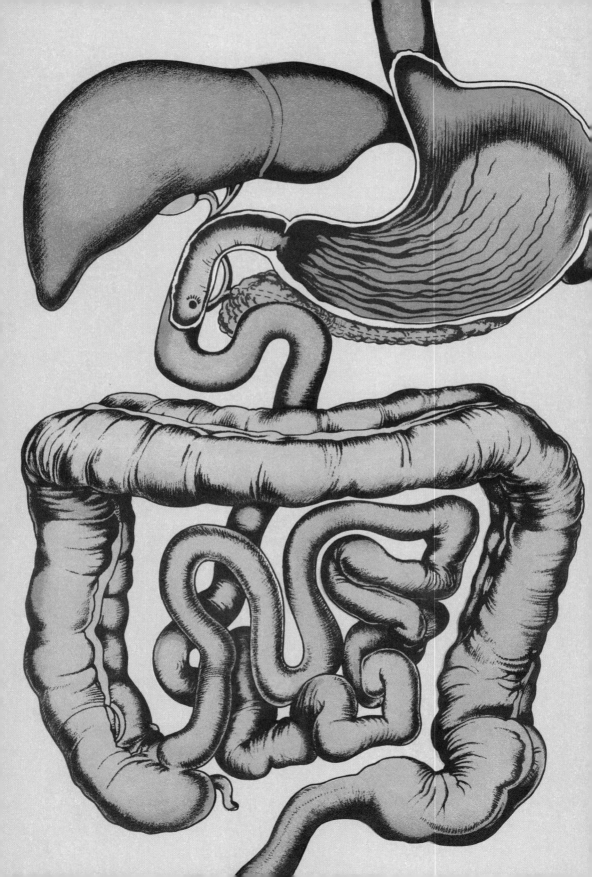

CHAPTER 8

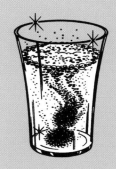

STOMACHS

An Irish fellow has been accustomed all his life to be what an
Englishman would consider half starved. Quantity or quality is
no great consideration with him. His stomach is like a corner
cupboard. You might throw anything into it.[1]

This harsh observation was made by former army lieutenant William
Grattan in 1847 in his reminiscences on his time with the Connaught Rangers,
a British Army infantry regiment, during the Napoleonic Wars (1803–15). It
puts forward a peculiar idea that Irish stomachs differed somehow from those
found in other countries. Irish people seemed willing to eat just about anything,
and extraordinarily large quantities too, caring little about quality, taste or
cuisine. But Grattan was wrong. At the time, Irish people weren't just throwing
anything into their stomachs. They ate large amounts of potatoes. Indeed, the
world once marvelled at the ability of the Irish to eat so many potatoes. Where
did they manage to put them all? Did they ever tire of such a repetitive diet? Did
potatoes keep the Irish in sound health?

The human stomach is a muscular hollow organ which takes in food from
the oesophagus, mixes it, breaks it down and then passes it downwards to the
small intestine. The entire digestive system is made up of one muscular tube
extending from the mouth to the anus, with the stomach being an enlarged
pouch-like section of this digestive tube. Its shape varies from person to person.
In the twenty-first century, scientists have become fascinated with the gut due
to the discovery of its microbiome, a collection of bacteria, fungi and viruses
that naturally live inside us. This inner microbiological realm contributes
immensely to human health and well-being. It protects against pathogens,
keeps our immune system healthy and helps us digest food properly. The gut
and brain are thought to be connected, with the health of the microbiome
having a major impact on our emotions and moods.

The Irish have long been ridiculed, and often condemned, for their dietary
habits, and also for the large quantities of alcohol which they enjoy consuming,
whether that's a hearty pint of Guinness or bottles of super-strong whiskey

(or poitín, as it's traditionally known in Ireland). Their dietary excesses were also believed to impact negatively upon their mental and moral state, but underlying the jovial stereotypes are sadder tales of poverty and famine that caused periods of distress, even in relatively modern times. Late in the nineteenth century, the Irish were accused of drinking tea to excess and even of getting themselves addicted to ether drinking. The public commentary that followed depicted the Irish as a reckless nation, a people with a lack of restraint over what they tipped into their stomachs. What people ate formed the basis of ideas about Irish national identity.

THE POTATO DIET

Walter Raleigh is thought to have first brought the potato over from South America to Europe in the late 1500s, during the reign of Queen Elizabeth I. During the Elizabethan plantation period, Raleigh owned 40,000 acres of land in Ireland, including the town of Youghal, Co. Cork, an acreage of such size that it attracted much criticism, given his close friendship at the time with the queen. He ran his colony of around 400 English people largely from London.[2] Raleigh is rumoured to have planted in Ireland (what later became known as) the 'hateful and pernicious potato', or the 'detestable root' (although the historical record is unclear on this).[3] Potato cultivation continued after the plantations and through the mid-seventeenth-century Cromwellian conquest of Ireland. The new settlers were enthusiastic about the crop, particularly in Munster and Leinster.

But potatoes became far too popular, a victim of their own success. The Irish poor became worryingly dependent upon them, using the potato almost exclusively as a dietary staple.[4] By the late 1700s, the poorest ate little else but potatoes, with a little milk, whiskey and the occasional fish. In the early 1840s, around 40 per cent of the Irish population lived chiefly on potatoes. At the time, Ireland's population was growing exponentially, meaning that many more mouths needed to be fed. Potatoes provided a simple solution, given how easy

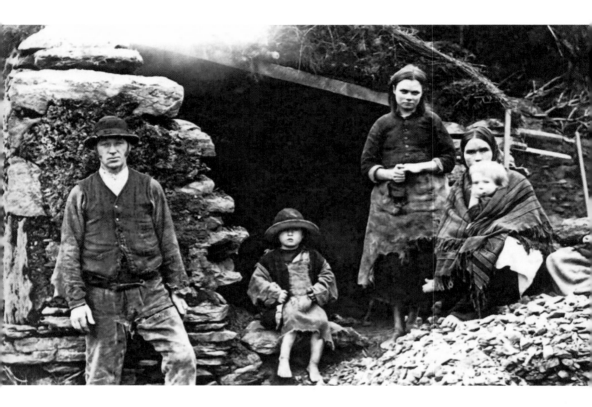

they were to grow. In contrast, the wealthier enjoyed a more varied diet of meat and vegetables and used potatoes to pad out their meals. Many of Ireland's famous potato-based dishes were developed around this time: champ (potatoes and spring onions), Irish stew (with meat, potato and vegetables) and boxty (fried potato cakes).[5]

This wasn't altogether bad. Most years, the potato crop was abundant, and it offered nutritious food for both people and pigs. Potatoes thrived in Ireland's damp, temperate climate and were adaptable enough to grow even in poor-quality, rocky soil. The 'lazy bed' in which peasants grew their potatoes was easily adjustable to suit different soil types, altitudes, slope conditions and rockiness, allowing steep, irregular or inaccessible slopes to be cultivated. Spade ploughing was hard

Until the Great Famine (1845–52), poorer Irish families lived almost entirely on potatoes, sometimes eaten with milk.

work but yielded excellent returns. Potatoes grow prolifically, and it is quite rare for the crop to fail for consecutive years. A single acre of poor soil can yield up to 6 tonnes of potatoes, an amount that proved necessary as Ireland's population boomed.

In 1842, the popular encyclopedia-style book, *Chambers's Information for the People*, commented that the Irish looked surprisingly healthy and robust, with the sheer quantity of potatoes being consumed compensating for a lack of meat and protein. Its authors, the Chambers brothers, surmised that Irish peasants ate up to 9 pounds of potatoes per day and explained that 'such a case is rather to be ranked amongst instances of extraordinary adaptations to a particular variety of food than as proof that an unmixed potato diet is healthy'.[6] In reality, average daily intake was close to 14 pounds (or 6 kilos). Potatoes were also gulped down by pigs and other farm animals, who then produced manure to grow even more potatoes.[7]

Nowadays, we know that potatoes are immensely healthy. Replete with protein, carbohydrates and minerals, they have a high energy value and low-fat content but are deficient in vitamins A, E and K. The Irish were unaware of these nutritional facts (knowledge of vitamins was developed only in the twentieth century) but sensed intuitively that a potato-heavy diet wasn't too bad for their health. That said, a lack of vitamin E could cause serious eye problems, and several Irish doctors linked potato consumption to scrofula, sore eyes and blindness.[8] Further negatives included the potato only being available for 9 or 10 months, meaning that other foods had to be sought out in July and August. Potatoes were difficult to transport, had little commercial value and were not a sound basis for economic development. This was the inherent contradiction of the potato diet. The Irish were generally healthy and robust, but contradictorily, the potato diet contributed greatly to their deep levels of poverty.[9]

For such reasons, critics aggressively scorned Ireland's over-reliance on potatoes. While many travel writers wrote with some astonishment of the Irish population's ability to eat so many potatoes, other visitors, particularly those from Britain, were less impressed. They were horrified at what they observed across Ireland: rows of tiny cottages, each with a potato patch and dung heap outside, and a pet pig living inside. Famously, English politician William Cobbett said that potatoes should be fed only to pigs, as among humans they encouraged 'slovenliness, filth, misery and slavery'.[10] These critics chose to ignore that the Irish peasantry were making efficient use of their land (boasting the highest potato yields in Europe) and that the offensive dung heap in fact indicated a proficiency in using manure effectively. Indeed, governments in other countries, including Italy, actively encouraged potato consumption, recognising its health benefits for the population.[11]

The British, and also the wealthier Irish, remained sceptical. In the 1840s, a lawyer named Thomas Campbell Foster visited Ireland regularly as *The Times* correspondent to report on 'The Condition of the People of Ireland'. Foster wrote often of his sheer despair and exasperation on constantly witnessing pounds and pounds of potatoes disappearing into so many Irish stomachs, Foster concluded that 'the Irish peasant, fed on potatoes, has a craving for a large quantity of food'. Potatoes contained little nourishment, thought Foster (wrongly), which explained why the Irish needed to endlessly consume such large quantities of them to remain in good health.

'By continually living on this large quantity of poor food', commented Foster, 'the stomach of the Irish peasant becomes enlarged, and craves for the quantity. It is a physiological fact, which dissection has established, that a potato-fed peasant has a stomach of nearly twice the ordinary size'.[12] A few years later, Robert Bentley Todd, a King's College Hospital physician, agreed that 'Pat' had a far larger stomach than 'John Bull', as the sheer quantity of potatoes caused the stomach to swell and dilate, simply to be able to fit so much bulk in.[13]

Also travelling around Ireland in the early 1840s was James Johnson, another famed doctor who, while compiling his travel book *A Tour in Ireland*, was revulsed by the sheer quantity of potatoes being consumed across Ireland, and also by how Irish people cooked them. Johnson revealed that Irish peasants half-boiled their potatoes, leaving a hard centre known colloquially as 'the bone of

In the late 1840s, blight killed much of the potato crop upon which the Irish depended, causing nationwide starvation, death and emigration.

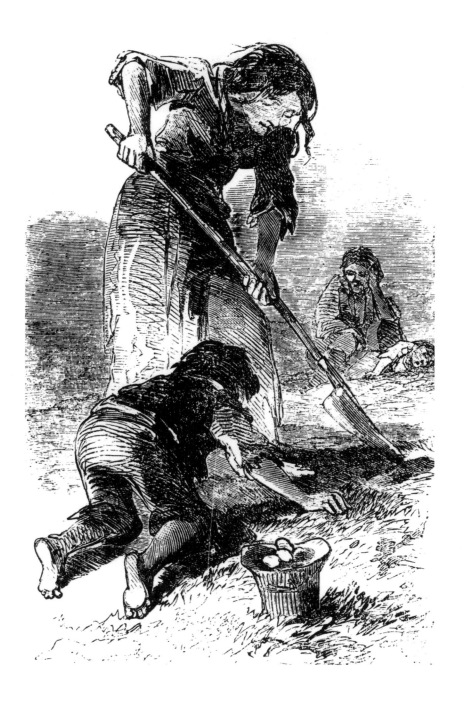

the potato'. (It was also known as the 'moon of the potato' due to the crescent-like shape of the hard bit.) Horrified, Johnson warned that 'there is scarcely a more indigestible substance taken into the human stomach than a half-boiled potato, and to a moderately dyspeptic Englishman, such a diet would be no less than poison'. When inquiring into why Irish people refrained from fully cooking their beloved potatoes, Johnson was told that under-cooking allayed the pangs of hunger for longer. Stomachs took longer to digest an undercooked potato, warding off feelings of hunger, for a while at least[14]

Johnson knew the Irish well. Born in Ballinderry, on the borders of Co. Tyrone, in 1792, he became an apprentice to a surgeon-apothecary in Antrim. After spending time in Belfast, he moved to London to complete his medical education. Subsequently, Johnson was appointed as a surgeon's mate on a naval vessel and worked in Newfoundland, Nova Scotia, Egypt and India. He gained public prominence when attending the Duke of Clarence (later King William IV) in 1814. So impressed was the future king with the quality of medical attention provided that he later appointed Johnson as physician extraordinary. In the meantime, Johnson settled in Portsmouth and, in 1816, founded the influential clinical journal *Medico-Chirurgical Review*, which was published until 1877. Better known for his publications on tropical diseases, Johnson also published books on a range of stomach-related matters: digestive ailments, gout, spas and mineral waters. Little surprise that he was so fascinated with the Irish stomach. He published *A Tour in Ireland* just a year before his death in 1845.

William Wilde was another esteemed doctor who despaired over the habit of leaving a hard lump of potato, around the size of a small walnut, to digest in the stomach throughout the day, although he conceded that this custom might serve a physiological purpose. Its remaining in the stomach for a few hours longer than the potato's more digestible parts meant that a second digestion started later in the day, staving off hunger for a few more hours. According to Wilde, 'every girl in an Irish cabin possessed instinctively what the most celebrated *chef de cuisine* never attained to: a power of knowing whether an egg or a potato was done by simply holding it for an instant in the closed hand'.[15]

Wilde was descended from a Dutchman, Colonel de Wilde, who served in the invading army of King William of Orange in 1690, and as noted earlier, was the father of famous playwright Oscar Wilde.

Critics also lambasted the type of potato being consumed monotonously throughout Ireland. In his 1837 book *Ireland: Picturesque and Romantic*, Scottish novelist and journalist Leith Ritchie wrote:

> Some misapprehension prevails in England with regard to the diet of the Irish peasant. By potatoes, we imagine is meant that dry, white, mealy vegetable we see at our tables – or used to see, for potatoes have grown vulgar! – and which we sometimes declare, as it breaks and crumbles under the fork, we could live upon ourselves, with the addition of a little milk or butter. This, however, is the potato which the peasant raises expressly for us. It is the true *pomme de terre*.[16]

In contrast, the Irish poor lived on a miserable-looking potato known as the lumper. The lumper flourishes on overly wet garden beds lacking in nutrients. Although quite suitable for Ireland's damp, rainy weather, it was regularly denigrated as a wet, nasty old potato, its appearance frowned upon as large, lumpy and knobbly. Its critics had a point. The lumper is not a pretty potato. Ritchie described it as 'moist and heavy, and said to be difficult of digestion, and therefore unwholesome', despite its being the main source of nourishment for millions of Irish people.[17] Other contemporaries described the lumper as a potato 'only cultivated in its most degenerate, unpalatable and least nutritive variety' and 'the vilest description of that vile root'.[18] Many doctors were convinced that the Irish peasantry suffered widely from a particular type of stomach affliction as a consequence of their enthusiasm for eating so many lumper potatoes. Its victims looked thin and fleshy, had a sallow complexion, complained constantly of crippling stomach ache, had a weak appetite and were prone to frequent vomiting. The treatment of the time for this chronic

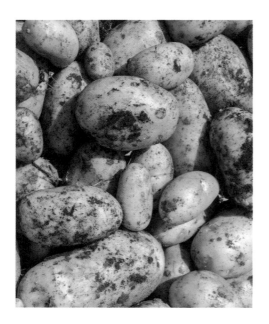

The lumper was a miserable-looking potato upon which the Irish poor relied heavily as a dietary staple.

dyspepsia (or indigestion) included leeching, blisters and cupping over the stomach.[19]

Other critics warned of the negative impacts of the potato diet on the Irish national character, believing that potato cultivation discouraged the poor from engaging in labour-intensive, and economically beneficial, forms of food production and cultivation. The potato was too easy to grow and cook and encouraged doing as little work as possible. This derogatory idea was also used to explain Ireland's relative lack of industrialisation, especially compared with Britain which had famously kick-started a global industrial revolution.

In 1848, Sandham Elly published a book with the intriguing title *Potatoes, Pigs, and Politics: The Curse of Ireland and the Cause of England's Embarrassments*. In this, he traced all of Ireland's socio-economic misfortunes back to potato cultivation and condemned peasants who felt perfectly content with their hand-to-mouth life of growing enough potatoes to feed their families and fatten their pigs. How was Irish industry to develop with such an unambitious mindset? Worse still, according to Elly, the peasants refused to eat their pigs. So enamoured were they with their pigs that families and pigs even lived together inside. In his words, 'nor does he enjoy any portion of the pork he fattens. No! He would scorn to eat the companion who shares his house, his food and his bed.'

In his diatribe, Elly concluded that eating the same food as their pigs reduced Irish people to the status of an animal. 'Man and swine feed alike on it [the potato]. Both meet on equal terms – not that the pig is elevated to the rank of man

– but that man has been sunk to the level of the brute', he opined. Elly longed for the day when 'industry and exertion' replaced 'idleness and crime', when 'tillage' replaced the 'lazy bed of potatoes', and when 'the indolent Irish potato growers' were 'transformed into farmers'.[20] Writing in the mid-1840s, little did Elly know that the potato diet was about to come to an abrupt, tragic end.

POITÍN

Stereotypes of Irish people often focus joyfully on their love of drink. The drunken Irish man, in particular, is a long-standing trope in literature and culture. In reality, Irish attitudes to drinking differed little from those of the Scottish, English or Welsh, but still, the caricature persists. Ireland is considered the birthplace of whiskey. Monks, on their long pilgrimages to the Mediterranean and Middle East regions, witnessed southern European techniques of distilling perfumes sometime between the eighth and eleventh centuries. Upon returning to Ireland, they modified these techniques to create a drinkable spirit. As the monks spoke Latin, the drink was originally called 'aqua vitae', meaning the 'water of life'. The Irish name was 'uisce beatha', from which the word whiskey is derived. This whiskey was flavoured with aromatic herbs, including mint, and more resembled a liqueur than the stronger spirit drunk today.[21]

The oldest known written record of Irish whiskey dates from 1405 and describes a clan member who died from drinking far too much.[22] Aside from this unfortunate incident, whiskey is largely missing from the Irish historical record until 1556, when an act was passed that restricted whiskey distillation to producers with a licence and that described whiskey as a drink 'drunken daily' and 'universally throughout this realm'.[23] Both Elizabeth I and Walter Raleigh are said to have preferred Irish whiskey even to their own English whiskey. The main difference today between Irish and Scotch whiskies is that Irish whiskey is distilled three times, whereas Scotch is usually distilled twice. Irish whiskey tends to be matured for longer than Scottish, usually somewhere between five

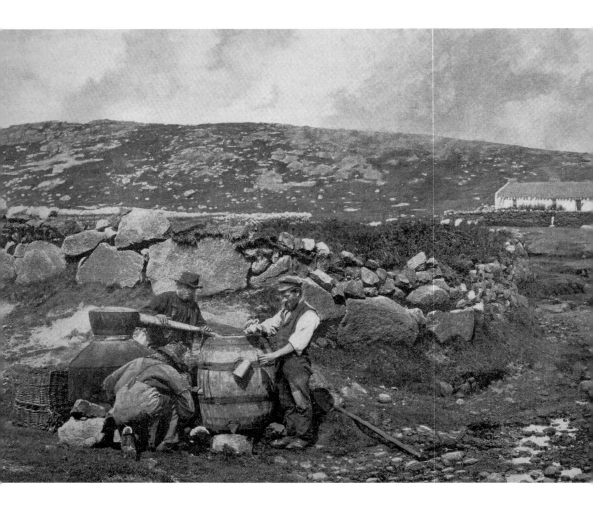

Poitín is an exceptionally strong
whiskey. Its distillation was
outlawed, or heavily regulated,
due to its potent strength.

and twelve years. This gives it a distinctive flavour that is more delicate than many Scotch whiskies, and with less of the mossy, peaty pungency.

Bushmills Distillery, in Co. Antrim, now a hugely popular tourist attraction, holds a whiskey production licence dating back to 1608 and claims to be the world's oldest distillery. Illicit distilling had thrived in the town long before 1608, and the licence essentially consolidated this ongoing activity. Bushmills' remote northern location meant that illegal whiskey distillation took place well out of sight of excise collectors. The nearby River Bush provided a constant supply of soft water, ideal for making whiskey, and local farms produced an abundance of high-quality barley. These were perfect conditions for making high-quality whiskey. However, Bushmills was not formally registered until 1784, which allows the Kilbeggan Distillery, Co. Westmeath, established in 1757, to also lay claim to being Ireland's oldest distillery.

On Christmas Day 1661, a tax of four pence was introduced on each gallon of whiskey produced. Initially, registration was voluntary; predictably, few whiskey producers signed up. From here on, whiskey produced by registered distillers was known as 'parliament whiskey', and illicitly produced whiskey as poitín, a Gaelic word meaning 'small pot', a reference to the still in which the whiskey was made. (The anglicised word is poteen or potcheen, and other names have included 'Irish moonshine' and 'mountain dew'.) The spirit duty was raised in 1775 and again in 1815, partly because Britain needed revenue for wars. However, this had a negative side effect. Whereas poitín had usually been made for personal consumption, the extra taxes placed on parliament whiskey meant it was out of the financial reach of many Irish people. Those who knew how to produce and sell cheap, although illegal, whiskey now had many potentially lucrative options ahead of them. Another change made in 1775 meant that distilleries had to manufacture a minimum number of gallons per week to hold a licence. Whiskey makers had to work faster and faster to meet this quota, and the quality of their parliament whiskey soon dropped. In contrast, illicit poitín makers still had time on their hands to work at a steady pace and produce a better-tasting product.[24]

Meanwhile, the notorious Distilling Act of 1779 imposed a steep levy on pot stills based on their capacity. It aimed to stop widespread undeclared distilling by legitimate distillers. The logic ran that if such producers habitually produced extra whiskey on the sly, then the still itself should be taxed and not its output. Distillers could then produce as much or as little whiskey as they wanted, and the government would still receive its duties on the still. Numerous legal distilleries closed down. Many legitimate distillers became moonshiners.[25]

In the eighteenth century, whiskey's popularity grew significantly. By 1790, whiskey accounted for 66 per cent of the total duty on spirits received by the exchequer.[26] Regardless, by the early 1800s, Ireland was the largest spirit market in the British Isles, the whiskey capital of the world. Due to the various laws, the number of registered distilleries across Ireland dropped rapidly from 1,228 in 1779 to 246 in 1790 and 32 in 1821. While this might suggest a rapid decline, in fact smaller distilleries went underground while larger ones became increasingly profitable, creating a monopoly. Dublin's distilleries, including Jameson, became the largest in the world. Only in 1823 were the restrictions on legal distilleries lifted, although illicit poitín production remained hugely popular until the 1840s.[27]

Throughout much of the nineteenth century, Dublin was the whiskey powerhouse of the world. It boasted half a dozen distilleries which between them produced nearly 10 million gallons of whiskey each year. The 'Big Four' companies were those of John Jameson, William Jameson, John Power and George Roe, and their products were considered among the finest whiskies in the entire world. The Irish whiskey industry was at its zenith between around 1870 and 1890. Its popularity continues today. Jameson whiskey was first produced in 1780. Its unique taste came from using less malt, which was then subject to tax. The public soon acquired a taste for it. Nowadays, Jameson is among the best-selling Irish whiskeys in the world.[28]

Until the late nineteenth century, people drank alcohol out of necessity as well as for revelry, socialising and pleasure. Water supplies were often polluted or contaminated. Tea and coffee remained relatively expensive until

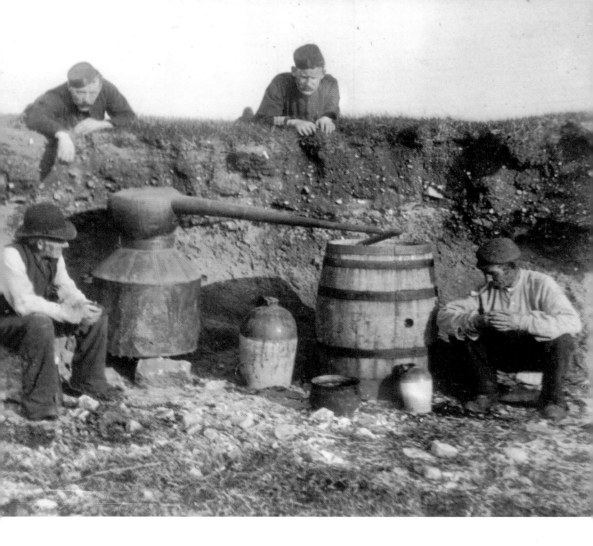

the late nineteenth century and were more popular among the affluent. Doctors and the public alike saw many health benefits in consuming alcohol. Alcohol was processed and (although

this was not known at the time) free from germs.[29] Little beer was produced in Ireland, but parliament whiskey was too expensive for much of the populace to drink regularly, and so the illicit poitín industry filled a market gap for a cheap, palatable alcoholic drink.[30] In the cottages of the Irish poor, the whiskey jug under the bed became as common as the potato pot on the hearth.[31] A travelling doctor wrote in 1889 that 'you can scarcely enter a country house by a road side that has not its crock of contraband whiskey'.[32]

Poitín was usually strong; its alcohol content could be as high as 90 per cent. It could be made from cereals, grain, whey, sugar beet, molasses or even potatoes. The Irish word for a hangover is póit. For poorer families, poitín production provided a supplemental source of income. Landlords overlooked these illegal goings-on, as extra income increased the chances of their tenants being able to pay their rent. Many excisemen turned a blind eye too and were open to bribery. Illicit production was concentrated mostly in the northern and western parts of Ireland, where mountainous regions concealed the whiskey-making from the prying eyes of excise officers.[33]

One popular song about poitín went like this:

> Oh, poteen
> The nice poteen,
> The mellow, mild and rich poteen
> The chosen toast
> Round Erin's coast,
> That darling drink, the poteen.
> Unfathomed by the Exciseman's rule,
> Our native shines in bottle green
> And where's the drink so mild and cool
> As barley juice, our smoked poteen?
> Let Britons boast their ale and beer,
> For whiskey good they've never seen,
> Or else another tune we'd hear
> In praise of thee, our prime poteen.[34]

In 1846, the *Irish National Magazine* published a poem about poitín, although with the rejoinder that 'we only regret that the writer's powers have not been employed on a worthier subject'. The opening lines read as follows:

Oh! A dainty drink is the pure poteen,
That comes from the secret still,
By a lonely stream is he found I ween,
On the side of a heathy hill.
Oh! The heart must be heavy that he can't cheer,
And he brightens the eye that is dim,
And the head of the peasant, the prince, the peer,
Has each been a home for him.[35]

There were three stages in poitín production: malting, brewing and distilling. Malting involved steeping a sack, partly filled with grain, in a bog or stream. When the grain had swollen, it was spread out to sprout, perhaps in an empty house or underground cave. It needed to be turned by hand once or twice per day to ensure it sprouted evenly. After 10 days, the malt was usually ready for drying or grinding, after which it was placed in a vessel. A vat of boiling water was poured over the malt, and the liquid was left to ferment. This mixture of water and malt was known as wort. Boiled hops and yeast were then added to the wort, and the mixture then had to be shielded from contact with the air. The fermentation process took around three or four weeks, although illicit distillers, fearing detection, were prone to working more quickly. The poitín would then be distilled using a still, which could hold between 10 and 80 gallons, depending on its size.[36]

William Richard Le Fanu was an Irish railway engineer and Commissioner of Public Works, born into a literary family of Huguenot, Irish and English descent. A year before his death in 1894, Le Fanu published his reminiscences of Irish life. In this, he recalled going on a fishing exhibition in a village near Glen Lough. Le Fanu had never seen poitín being made before and told his friend, Dolty, that he would like to see an illicit still. Dolty guided him through a remote lane, sheltered by thorn bushes, where, by a stream, three young men were working at a still. The men wore stockings, rather than shoes, so that they could run more quickly over rocks and rough ground if detected.

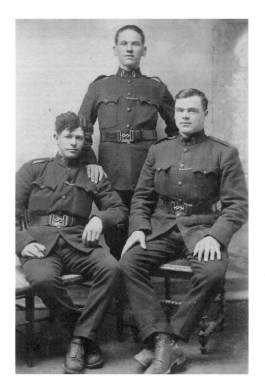

The RIC reportedly disliked the arduous task of locating and chasing poitín makers in the mountains.

Enjoying a drink of poitín together, Le Fanu asked Dolty and the men if the smoke ever attracted police attention but was told that distilling made little smoke. It was the malt drying that created a great deal of smoke, so they always performed this task in early July when the police were busy in Derry putting down the annual twelfth-of-July riots there. Le Fanu also recalled watching five policemen carrying a still through the village one morning. Dolty was in fits of laughter. The still was old and worn out. Dolty explained that the police had been deliberately tipped off, probably by a poitín maker, in the hope of receiving a pound reward for a now useless still.[37] (It was not uncommon for 'real' informers to be chased out of the district, with neighbours shunning their presence.)[38]

The Irish constabulary hated the task of hunting down illicit poitín producers. David Russell McAnally recorded in his 1888 book, *Irish Wonders*, the 'days and nights of toilsome climbing, watching, waiting and spying, often without result', only for an alarm to be raised and the whiskey makers flee, leaving nothing but the 'pot and the smell'. The job was dangerous. In the mountains of Donegal, Mayo, Galway, Clare and Kerry, the distillers owned firearms and felt 'no more compunction for shooting a policeman than for killing a dog'. Residents in the local neighbourhood, very fond of drinking the poitín, resented constabulary efforts to halt illicit production. They were more than happy to be 'on the lookout for the enemy', and 'there are always friends to give the alarm'. As

McAnally elaborated:

> To hide the still in the ground or in a convenient cave is the work
> of very few minutes, after which the distillers are quite at leisure
> and turn their attention to shooting at the police, a job attended
> with so little risk to themselves and so much discomfort to the
> constables that the latter frequently give up the chase on very
> slight provocation.[39]

Ferocious armed battles took place between gangs of up to 80 distillers
and revenue officers, the constabulary or soldiers.[40] In 1808, six distillers
were prosecuted in Co. Louth for murder when a sergeant, David Forbes, was
shot dead after helping seize a quantity of malt in the Ardee area. Men were
prepared to put their lives in danger by participating in the illicit spirit trade,
and constabulary members sometimes paid with their lives in defending
government policies on spirit taxation which many people considered
excessive.[41] If the constabulary entered a house to break up a poitín party, the
drinkers would smash the bottles, an attempt at destroying the evidence. It
was known for the constabulary to try to pick up a few drops with a spoon
from the floor and later provide a jury with these sparse drops of evidence to
smell.[42] Efforts to break up poitín drinking in pubs and bars led to vicious fights
between constabulary and customers, which the latter often won.[43]

But what was to be done with any poitín confiscated? In 1872, a distiller
named James Crimmins was caught outside Ennis District Lunatic Asylum
with 70 gallons (5 kegs) of poitín and sentenced to pay a £6 fine. The poitín
itself was sentenced to be destroyed but had a market value of around £90.
Some people suggested that the poitín might as well be sold, now that it had
been made, and proceeds given to a local charity. Or perhaps it could be sent to
the hospital wards and used medicinally or as a disinfectant? The *Irish Times*
quipped: 'Why the innocent poteen should be destroyed to punish the guilt of
the still-owners by the mountain side we cannot understand'.[44]

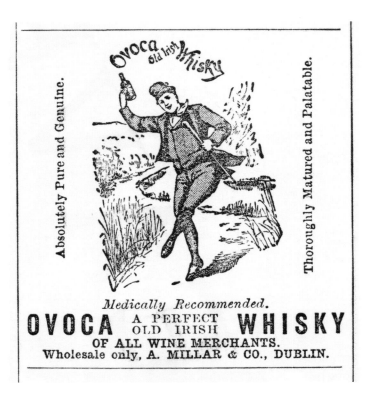

Whiskey is one of Ireland's biggest exports.

By the century, many people were fed up with the drunken ways of the Irish. In 1829, even Mr Fearon, famous for opening London's first gin palace, felt 'grieved' by the number of whiskey shops at Edgeworthstown, Co. Longford, and declared that one shop out of every four across Ireland seemed to be a whiskey shop.[45] When Poor Law Commissioner George Nicholls travelled to Ireland in the 1830s to plan his widely hated workhouse system, he was similarly astonished by the number of spirit shops in every town and village, noting that almost every type of shop sold cheap whiskey. In his words, 'a man can get beastly drunk for 2d., and I understand their potato diet renders the Irish people more easily affected by the spirit than others – it may possibly increase their love for it.' Nicholls added that: 'many of the acts of violence and disorder which occur in Ireland are planned in some obscure whiskey shop and executed under the influence of the poison there imbibed'.[46]

One line of thought insisted that Irish people were naturally kind and cheerful, but that their demeanour changed quickly when overexcited by a mixture of strong whiskey and politics. Whiskey corrupted the very spirit of the Irish, so some thought, an idea eagerly picked up on by temperance advocates, who actively sought to remove the joys and temptations of the whiskey bottle from the Irish peasantry.[47] 'In the Irish stomach,' one critic opined, 'a refuse of diseased potatoes and decayed vegetables have ruled there supreme, with here and there a bit of meat as a treat on Sundays'. Commenting on the collective effects, this author added: 'No wonder that beastly drinking, so stupefying everywhere else, should have produced such fatal effects upon poor Ireland, and that this deplorable craving should have extinguished in many Irish minds the last redeeming link with humanity'.[48]

Well over a century later, John McGuffin – a Northern Ireland anarchist who actively campaigned against the British Army presence there during the 1970s – wrote several books on political topics such as internment. Then, in 1978, he wrote *In Praise of Poteen*, which lauded the anti-authoritarian spirit of the poitín makers. McGuffin insisted that illegal poitín had received an unduly harsh press, encouraged by groups and individuals with a vested interest in slamming the drink, including licensed distillers, revenue departments, temperance groups and even famed Irish writer Brendan Behan, who publicly declared himself more partial to a drop of the parliament whiskey.[49]

Such critics included James Johnson, who believed that poitín and lumper potatoes were a dangerous combination. Perturbed by this, he wrote:

> A glass of poteen would be useful to the labourer as a digester to his potatoes with the bones in them. But alas! The finest theory is not always the most practicable. Among a people so excitable and social as the Irish, there is no safe resting place between total abstinence from whiskey and actual ebriety. There is no middle

point or neutral ground in the shape of temperance. The moment
that a single glass of whiskey is swallowed, you throw a blazing
faggot among dry wood which will almost certainly cause the
whole to ferment.[50]

Evidently, Johnson didn't trust the Irish peasantry to stay sober for very
long and portrayed poitín as a drink that dangerously excited their passions
and emotions. To help resolve the problem, Johnson proposed placing higher
duties on strong spirits, to persuade, or perhaps force, the peasantry to instead
enjoy lower-strength alcoholic drinks such as beer, 'a far safer manufacture of
stimulants for the Irish stomach than fiery poteen,' thought Johnson.[51]

Intriguingly, Johnson also blamed Irish supernatural beliefs in fairies,
goblins and demons on poitín drinking, blaming it for causing alcohol-induced
hallucinations. Johnson thought that the stomach and mind were intimately
connected via the nervous system. In fact, Johnson had written an influential
clinical book on indigestion which outlined his theories on this matter, first
published in 1827 and then regularly reprinted in subsequent decades. In this,
Johnson hypothesised that indigestion, including alcohol-induced varieties,
spread its evils throughout the body via the nerves, infiltrating the brain and
causing mental distress. Like many contemporary physicians of the time,
Johnson was obsessed with indigestion (or dyspepsia), considering it the starting
point of all manner of physical and mental disorders. Chronic dyspepsia also
signalled a lack of restraint when it came to eating and drinking, an idea that
mapped easily onto derogatory perceptions of the bodies of the Irish poor.[52]

Johnson's clinical writings contained numerous warnings about the hazards
of overeating. 'The body is tortured for years, and the mind ultimately wrecked'
if chronic dyspepsia set in, he warned.[53] Stomachs were as sensitive to bad food
as eyes to blinding lights and noses to pungent smells.[54] Johnson thought that
the Irish needed to be calmed and that a more suitable national diet would be
moderate and plain, unlike the current one consisting of excessive amounts of
poitín and potatoes that overexcited and over-exhilarated.[55]

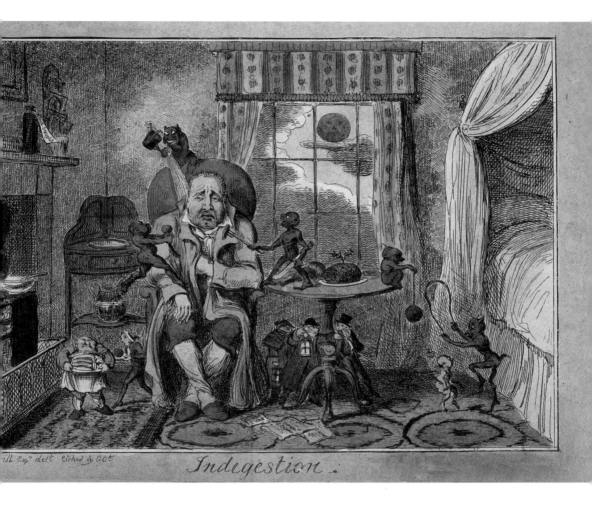

Indigestion.

Johnson believed that indigestion led to a poor night's sleep. During slumber, the stomach's irritated nerves set to work. Seeping into the brain, 'the stifled groans of the nightmare' became audible, while a hangover developed due to the digestive disruption at play. 'The head aches. The intellect is not clear or energetic. The eyes are muddy. The nerves are unstrung. The tongue is furred. There is more inclination for

In 1825, George Cruikshank published his image of the 'Demons of Dyspepsia'. Chronic indigestion was thought to trouble the Irish due to their heavy intake of potatoes, poitín and strong tea.

drink than food', as he described it.[56] Johnson referred to the poitín-fuelled nightmare as an 'incubus' (a male demon in folklore thought to have sexual intercourse with sleeping women, who had a female form, the succubus). In his words:

> Indigestion is the key by which Incubus unlocks our closet door, pounces on his prostrate and sleeping victim, presses on him with the weight of an elephant, whirls him over rocks and mountains, chains him in dungeons, plunges him into the lake or strangles him with a giant's grasp! These, and many others, are the feats of the nightmare.

Johnson was convinced that the Irish (and the Scottish, too) were more vulnerable to 'these forays of the tyrant nightmare than their neighbours of England'. His reasons? Poitín and the half-boiled potato. Stomachs were forced to continue their digestive work at night, due to Irish peasants having gulped down undercooked, indigestible food. Worse still, these undercooked potatoes had been washed down with excessive quantities of poitín. The hallucinations and nightmares caused by the disturbed sleep – goblins, fairies and the like – were remembered the following morning as very real indeed, so vivid had the mental impressions been.[57] Reading between the lines, Johnson's writing here betrays his views that Ireland needed to modernise, become disenchanted and abandon non-science-based beliefs. Abandoning a reliance upon potatoes and poitín might provide a sounder socio-economic basis for future development. But then a national disaster occurred.

THE GREAT FAMINE

There was an obvious problem with living on one food alone: what would happen should the crop fail? In the 1720s, grain failures caused food shortages across Ireland. Facing starvation and disease, around 15,000 Irish people departed for the American colonies in that decade. In this instance, potatoes saved many people from starvation and cushioned against famine. Then, on 27 December 1739, temperatures across Ireland dropped far below freezing. A harsh frost set in, made even less bearable by a week of strong easterly gales. The cold weather lasted without remission for seven weeks and was followed by a long period of unusual weather that lasted until September 1741.

On that bitterly cold December night, most of Ireland's potatoes froze, making them inedible – the very first potato-related crisis in Irish history. Food shortages were worsened by cattle, sheep and horses all freezing to death. No potato seeds were left for the next growing season, but in the autumn of 1740, the cold returned anyway. This was a European-wide crisis, meaning that food couldn't be readily imported from elsewhere. Tens of thousands of people were reduced to wandering the roads and begging for food. In 1740, Ireland had a population of 2.4 million people. The 1740–41 famine killed off between 13 per cent and 20 per cent of them (proportionately, the deadliest famine in Irish history).[58]

Around a century later, in 1845, the potato crop looked likely to be abundant. Irish farmers had sown a much greater acreage than usual, and the plentiful supply appeared likely to last well into 1846. Then the potato blight arrived.[59] By November, over a third of the crop was destroyed; by December, around half. In Britain, Robert Peel's government purchased £100,000 worth of Indian corn (maize) and meal from America and dispatched £46,000 of its own maize and oatmeal from Britain. Through 1845 and 1846, hundreds of relief committees distributed this food and helped conserve limited supplies for the summer months ahead.

However, the starving Irish didn't take kindly to Indian meal and contemptuously nicknamed it 'Peel's brimstone' because of its bright-yellow

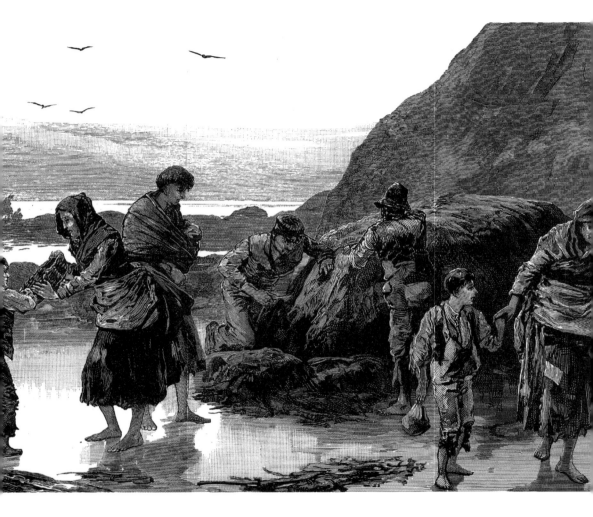

Debates on British responsibility for the Great Famine (1845–52) still rage today.

colour. Much of the meal was imported unmilled and was not sufficiently ground by private millers when it arrived in Ireland. When sold and eaten without being boiled for long enough, as was often the case, it was coarse, lumpy and unappetising and caused severe and crippling bowel complaints. Many people chose to starve rather than eat it, and the British in turn interpreted this as Irish ingratitude.

There existed a general expectation that healthy potatoes would resume growing from August 1846, but this was not to be. That year, blight attacked the potato crop earlier in the year, and far more destructively. For the potato to fail in two consecutive years was highly unusual. However, sowing new potatoes on the same land previously occupied by diseased potatoes reinfected the crop. Heavy rain and thunderstorms spread the blight across the island from east to west, expanding its geographical spread. (Although it was not known at the time, the blight was fungal.) By October, around three-quarters of the crop had been destroyed.

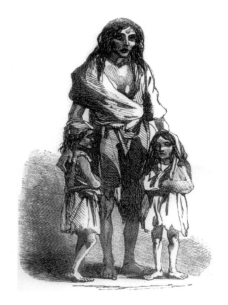

The Great Famine accelerated trends of emigration to countries including America, Australia and Britain.

Now that their potato patch was defunct, people needed hard cash to buy food, but landlords refused to make cash payments. There were massive rent defaults, followed by cruel forced evictions and land clearances, causing lasting controversy and resentment. These evictions reduced even further the number of labourers available to work the land for the next potato season. In autumn 1847, the potato crop acreage was a mere one-seventh of what it had been a year earlier. Here was a cruel irony. The quality of the 1847 potato crop was excellent. Blight was largely absent, but due to minimal planting, the crop yield was smaller than ever. 'Black '47' was the worst year for starvation and suffering. The situation improved in subsequent years, but the effects of the blight were still felt in some parts of the country well into the early 1850s.

Debates about British culpability for the Great Famine have raged since the 1840s. During the famine years, relief decisions were made by an ideologically driven political ruling elite who shared preconceived notions of the Irish (and we have seen above the amount of scorn poured onto the Irish). From their perspective, the famine was a good thing, or at least a necessary evil, as it might

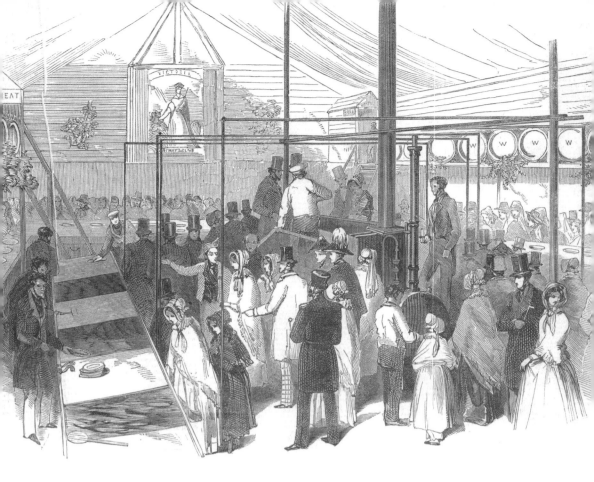

In 1847, famed French chef Alexis Soyer opened soup kitchens across Ireland.

finally encourage the peasantry to abandon their lifestyles of potatoes and poitín, having now seen the folly of their ways, improve their moral character and partake in rejuvenating Ireland's socio-economic life. Perhaps so, but such perspectives were devoid of empathy and compassion. The government's laissez-faire economic approaches, which involved 'letting things be', worsened conditions considerably in Ireland. Most shamefully, principles of not interfering with trade meant that food continued to be exported from Ireland to Britain while the Irish starved.

Rather than directly feeding people, between 1846 and 1847 the government implemented public works schemes, forcing starving people to work for a wage, which would then allow them to buy food. The work was largely pointless; roads were built that led nowhere. People were so weak (physically and mentally) that they were unable to perform much hard labour without collapsing. The workforce soon became malnourished and debilitated. Frequent delays in wage payments occurred. Food prices rose while supplies dwindled. Wages were unpaid if work was called off due to sickness or bad weather (a common problem in rainy Ireland). Labourers had to work a 12-hour shift, 6 days a week. The winter of 1846–7 was particularly harsh, and snow was still falling as late as April. Destitute workers had inadequate clothing to offer the protection needed for outdoor work.

During Black '47, many Irish people resorted to eating birds, frogs, rats, dogs, cats, snails, nettles, weeds, seaweed and grass; the latter two contributed to the folk memory of people dying with their mouths stained green. A lack of investment in fisheries meant that eating seafood wasn't an option for most people, despite Ireland being surrounded by the sea. Throughout the summer of 1847, another relief system was introduced which, this time, provided food directly to starving people via soup kitchens.[60] The government called upon famed French chef Alexis Soyer to fill the empty stomachs of the Irish peasantry. Soyer was dispatched to Dublin, where he set to work co-ordinating his nationwide network of soup kitchens.

Soyer's recipes angered a number of prominent medical men. Prestigious Edinburgh physician James Simpson wrote to the chief secretary of Ireland criticising Soyer's soups for not containing health-sustaining meat.[61] The Lancet, a medical journal, derided Soyer's recipes as 'soup quackery' and as 'soups of pretence … taken by the rich as a salve for their consciences' as part of 'a spasmodic feeling of benevolence'. The Lancet then undertook a thorough chemical analysis of the content of each soup, dismissing some of its contents – turnip parings, celery tops and salt – as items not even describable as food.[62] Even Queen Victoria's doctor, Henry Marsh, argued in a widely distributed pamphlet that soup was an unhealthy, even dangerous, form of relief. Labourers needed solid food, he insisted, as liquid food digested far too quickly, causing further hunger and debility. Marsh noted that, unlike soup, the eating of the 'bone of the potato' had long served this useful purpose.[63]

The soup kitchens were intended as temporary, and after they closed in 1847, the starving Irish were deposited in overcrowded, disease-ridden workhouses, or they decided to emigrate instead. Workhouses struggled to keep up with increased demand, but disease was rife on the 'coffin ships' that transported people, in most cases permanently, to England, America and Australia. Some compassionate landlords paid for their tenants to emigrate, but these were few and far between. It is estimated that between 1841 and 1851 Ireland's population fell by around 20 per cent, a drop from 8.2 million to 6.5 million. Ireland never recovered its 'lost' population. Today, the country still has a population of only 5 million and a deeply entrenched tradition, which accelerated during the famine, of emigrating. Between 1845 and 1855, around 2.1 million Irish people left the country rather than risk starvation and the lethal diseases which accompanied it.

EXCESSIVE TEA DRINKING

The potato diet ended abruptly, but what was to replace it? After the Great Famine, the potato remained important in the Irish diet, particularly in impoverished rural areas, but no longer did the Irish rely almost entirely upon it as a dietary staple. Instead, they ate potatoes with a variety of vegetables, meats, fish and bread. The opening up of grocery shops across Ireland helped end over-reliance upon the potato patch. However, the potato diet had at least been nutritious, whereas post-famine diets were typically of poorer nutritional quality. By the 1890s, Irish people seemed shorter, thinner and frailer than they had before the famine. Their mental health also seemed to be rapidly declining. A more diverse diet did not necessarily improve national health.[64]

The discussion moved swiftly away from potatoes to another vice: 'excessive tea drinking'. Nowadays, the Irish are renowned across the world for their love of tea. The fictional character Mrs Doyle (from the TV show *Father Ted*) famously and comically insists that

After the Great Famine, tea became hugely popular across Ireland. Doctors thought that excessive tea drinking caused chronic indigestion and severe mental health issues.

TODD'S
INDIGESTION
_{AND} LIVER
MIXTURE

IS A CERTAIN CURE FOR
**INDIGESTION, FLATULENCY, PAIN IN
STOMACH, FULNESS AFTER EATING,
HEARTBURN, PILES, CONSTIPATION,
LIVER AND KIDNEY COMPLAINTS,**
and all Disorders arising from a Sluggish
Liver or Deranged Stomach.

DOSE. Half to one tea-spoonful after each meal
in a wine-glassful of water; a smaller or larger dose
may be taken if required.

PREPARED BY

HORATIO TODD, M.P.S., F.C.S. Pharmaceutical
Chemist,
72, HOLYWOOD ROAD, BELFAST.

her house guests consume endless cups of tea. The average Irish person is thought to drink anywhere between four and seven cups a day, making Ireland one of the leading nations in the world for tea consumption. However, nineteenth-century doctors genuinely feared that too much tea drinking was literally driving the Irish mad. In 1872, an alarmed lady wrote to the *Freeman's Journal*:

> Taking shelter in a cottage, near Banbridge, Co. Down, some time ago, during a shower of rain, and noticing the teapot on the hob, I observed that tea stewed in that way did a great deal of harm. The woman who lived in the cottage at once admitted that the parish doctor had said 'the folks were killing themselves with tea', and that it caused him more trouble than anything else.
>
> A few days ago a gentleman, just come up to town, was mentioning that the poor people in his neighbourhood suffered dreadfully from 'tic'. I replied that this was a disease often caused, I believed, by excessive tea-drinking. 'Indeed', he answered, 'well I must say, they do take immense quantities of tea'.[65]

While the exchange initially appears humorous, especially given what we know today of the Irish love of tea drinking, it reveals various problems inherent in the move away from the potato diet. Irish cookery skills were woefully poor and remained so until the twentieth century. Most families knew how to cook nothing but potatoes, which had at least kept them in relatively good health. As early as the 1870s, doctors were complaining of a national health decline seemingly linked to the new Irish diet which, for the poorest, was sparse and consisted of only tea and white bread – though, tea had once been a luxury item enjoyed mainly by the middle and upper classes. The situation worsened from that decade when a deep economic depression set in, causing widespread poverty.

Once again, the 'demon of dyspepsia' was called up. Nineteenth-century psychiatrists believed that women were delicate, emotional and prone to 'insanity', especially those who didn't eat properly. Excessive tea drinking was thought to cause chronic dyspepsia by over-exciting the stomach, with this 'nervous excitement' then affecting mental functioning, paving the way for psychiatric issues. In the 1890s, psychiatrists were using terms such as 'tea drunkards' and 'tea mania', a condition with the following symptoms: headache, vertigo, insomnia, heart palpitations, mental confusion, nightmares, nausea, hallucinations, morbid depression of spirits and suicidal feelings.[66]

Concern peaked in the 1890s when Dublin Castle initiated an official investigation into rising asylum admissions. At the time, emigration was causing a population decline in Ireland. This made the problem of rising asylum admissions seem even more curious, as surely asylum populations should also have been declining proportionately. When asked what they thought might be causing the situation, almost every asylum superintendent across the island blamed excessive tea drinking (and its related dyspepsia and mental health problems).[67] Prominent psychiatrist Thomas Drapes wrote, 'We see [tea's] effects in the number of pale-faced children, who are brought up on it instead of the old time-honoured, but now nearly abandoned, porridge and milk.'[68]

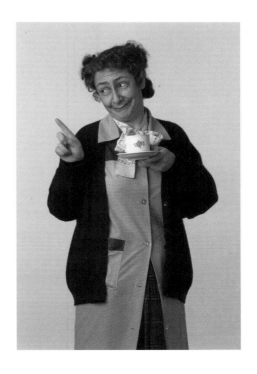

Tea was once consumed strong and dark after being stewed on the stove all day.

As with the potato diet, doctors discussed excessive tea drinking as a problem of both health and morals. By this time, the temperance movement had campaigned successfully against the consumption of alcoholic spirits, but now some doctors were claiming that tea, long lauded as a suitable alternative to alcohol, might be just as pernicious and addictive. It was a nervous stimulant, they claimed, which, when consumed excessively, caused mental excitability and overstimulation. Doctors criticised poor women for using tea like a drug, prioritising mental exhilaration above nutrition. They accused working-class women of lacking the knowledge for correct tea preparation, stewing tea on the stove all day long and, in consequence, recklessly succumbing to a life of stomach problems, addiction and psychiatric issues.[69]

'Tea and coffee,' warned the Belfast News-letter in 1887, 'offer the opportunity for abuse – an opportunity quite often availed of. Their devotees drink for the mere love of them, more than they ought.' The article continued by melodramatically describing hospital waiting rooms filled with dyspeptics suffering the consequences of their tea addiction. It then outlined a cycle of events whereby the tea-obsessed housewife gradually lost her appetite, started to loathe food due to her dyspepsia and eventually found solace for her woes in the teacup. Once hooked, she adopted tea preparation methods that allowed her to secure as much tannin as possible, such as stewing tea on the stove all day long, to quell her ever-intensifying cravings.[70]

These perspectives failed to acknowledge that milk was often adulterated, watered down, infected with tuberculosis or simply too costly. In reality, over-reliance on tea was often a necessity, not a choice. Doctors failed to grasp bleak working-class realities. In times of need, working-class mothers made hard decisions to go without and economise by serving nutritious food to other household members. Fathers needed strength for the workplace and the young needed to ensure healthy physical growth. Mothers sacrificed their own health, using tea to suppress appetite and quell hunger pangs. They were not recklessly seeking hedonistic pleasure but instead navigating 'food poverty'. However, as with the pre-famine Irish, they were widely regarded as reckless, immoral and responsible for their own conditions of abject poverty.

ETHER DRINKING

In 1891, *The Times* wrote of an epidemic sweeping through northern parts of Ireland. The infected area was very large indeed, covering around 600,000 acres. The outbreak was worsening daily, and no one of any class, age or gender was safe from its contaminating influences. However, the problem in question was not a disease or infection. It was ether drinking.[71]

Ether was an anaesthetic first introduced into surgical practice in the 1840s, although it had been used medicinally since the previous century. In eighteenth-century London, a quack physician named James Graham first came up with the idea of inhaling ether to get high. In the nineteenth century, 'outbreaks' of so-called 'etheromania' took hold among the rural peasant populations of Lithuania, Germany, Russia, Galicia and Norway.[72] Ether was usually smuggled into Ireland from England to avoid additional carriage rates imposed due to its being an explosive substance. It was then carried illicitly into the main towns by railway or cart, and the police had problems tracing it. It has been estimated that up to 4 tonnes of ether entered the north of Ireland illegally each year in the late nineteenth century.[73]

Ether drinking became popular in the north partly because of the success of the temperance movement in discouraging the Irish poor from drinking so much poitín and whiskey. A Catholic priest named Father Mathew had waged a dramatic campaign against ardent spirits and had reportedly discouraged thousands of Irish people from heavy drinking by the time of his death in 1856.[74] In the following decades, the temperance movement continued to be effective in the north, where a substantial Protestant population resided who were often willing to forsake alcohol.[75]

Between the 1840s and 1860s, the consumption of spirits plummeted. Despite having once boasted of being the world's whiskey capital, Irish consumption dropped below that of Scotland and America. Around the same time, land reforms and scarce barley supplies led to the decline of illicit poitín making.[76] Instead, the brewing industry took off. Many Irish people still drank

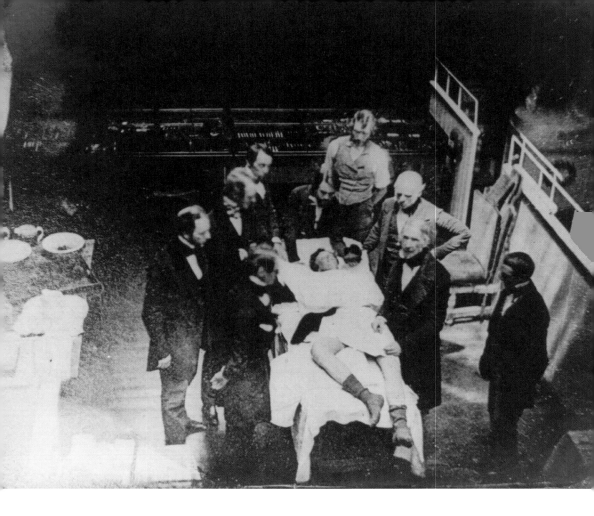

Ether had first been developed as a surgical anaesthesia but many people in Ireland used it for recreational purposes.

alcohol, but usually lighter beers and stouts.[77] From the late nineteenth century, pubs came to be a major feature across Ireland and new centres of social life.[78]

Ether's introduction was often blamed on a mysterious, unqualified Draperstown physician, Dr Kelly, who came up with the idea of dispensing small bottles of ether mixed with water in the 1840s to people seeking non-alcoholic intoxication. By all accounts, Kelly himself used to drink far more whiskey than was good for him, and when he gave it up, he found ether to be a suitable alternative.[79] Those new to ether drinking endured watery eyes, a burning stomach and considerable vomiting, but with perseverance, they became more accustomed to it. Pleasure and fun then awaited. Ether caused a sharp, sudden and intense drunkenness and a 'trip' that lasted for 20 minutes, followed by a rapid return to sobriety, all without a hangover and few side effects once the user had sobered up. This could be repeated half a dozen times a day, and cheaply too.[80] Ether had similar effects to alcohol when consumed but contained no alcohol. It was a substance 'on which a man might get drunk without violating his conscience'.[81] Hence its appeal in areas of temperance success. The ether drinker could get intoxicated and sober up again around six times per day if they wished and suffer less of a hangover than someone who had been drinking strong spirits the previous night. Ether was cheap, and it was possible to get drunk on a small glass of ether three times each day for as little as sixpence.[82]

In Maghera, in Co. Derry, a parish priest in the 1870s cursed ether in the hope that Catholics would no longer sell or consume it.[83] In 1888, and again in 1889, the Catholic Synod contacted the British Parliament in the hope of convincing politicians that ether drinking was a great social evil in the north and that 'great moral and material injuries' had befallen the lower classes as a result of the 'epidemic'.[84] These concerns truly began to be raised at government level after Ernest Hart, editor of the *British Medical Journal*, delivered a talk to the Society for the Study of Inebriety in October 1890, which received considerable public attention.[85]

The apparent prevalence of ether drinking, seemingly unnoticed until 1890, led to much hyperbole. In 1890, the *Irish Times* reported:

> Enter the humblest cabin and you will see decrepit, white-haired men, tottering and feeble, inane as far as brain power is concerned, who have become the miserable wrecks they are – helpless to themselves and loathsome and disgusting to others – through long-continued use of ether. How can we expect children born of parents whose lives consist of one long-continued series of ether debauches to be other than impaired, if not irretrievably and hopelessly ruined?[86]

In 1889, rumours spread that in the small town of Cookstown alone, ether sales in a single shop averaged 20 gallons per year.[87] In 1891, Thomas Mackenzie Ledlie calculated that 17,000 gallons of the 'vilest forms of impure ether' were consumed around counties Derry and Tyrone, an area containing 100,000 people.[88] Even children were seasoned ether drinkers. Many shopkeepers gave the substance to youngsters in their shops to bribe them to keep returning.[89] Grocers encouraged children to run errands for them in return for a small bottle of ether.[90] One 14-year-old boy was discussed in the national press due to his ability to drink 5 ounces each night; he belonged to a family celebrated locally for their ether drinking abilities.[91]

However, doctors struggled to decisively link ether drinking with a specific medical complaint. A few people blamed the rising asylum admissions of the 1890s on ether drinking, but excessive tea drinking was still considered the most likely culprit.[92] If anything, ether drinking seemed to have medicinally beneficial properties. It was popular among elderly women as it produced immense quantities of wind that could be belched from the stomach. One 'ether hawker', interviewed by T.J. Stafford, a doctor dispatched by the government to investigate, claimed to drink up to four draughts of ether each day as it 'warmed' her and helped her sleep well. She recalled that she and two friends had once consumed a wine glass of ether. All three of them had quickly swollen up to such an extent that they feared their clothes were about to burst Apart from this potentially unfortunate problem, she had seen no indications that ether drinking might be bad for her health and praised it as a very useful medicine for shortness of breath and flatulent dyspepsia. There were all sorts of reasons why ether was taken, among them 'wind on the stomach,' 'stuffing on the chest' and 'smothering of wind on the heart'. [93]

The key danger with ether drinking seemed to be misadventure. In 1877, a publican explained to one investigator that he knew a man who always drank ether and who, after one particularly strong dose, had lit his pipe. The flames caught his breath, which was set alight. Fortunately, another man came to his rescue and poured water down his throat.[94] Subsequent decades saw numerous reports of people accidentally setting their breath, mouth or face alight by smoking while drinking ether.[95]

Aside from misadventure, and the potential to set oneself alight, the main complaint was antisocial behaviour. When asked in the House of Commons about the effects of the substance in March 1891 Reverend Dr Carter, rector of Cookstown, complained that 'it produces combustive instincts, high state of exhilaration, shouting and singing, and has been found provocative of words, strife and outrages.'[96] An *Irish Times* report complained similarly about violent excitement, stupor, quarrelsomeness, loss of self-control, violent crime and dishonesty.[97] In 1890, ether was scheduled under the Poisons Act of 1870 and legal sales dropped dramatically overnight. Black market ether became quite expensive but reports of its consumption lingered on into the 1920s.[98]

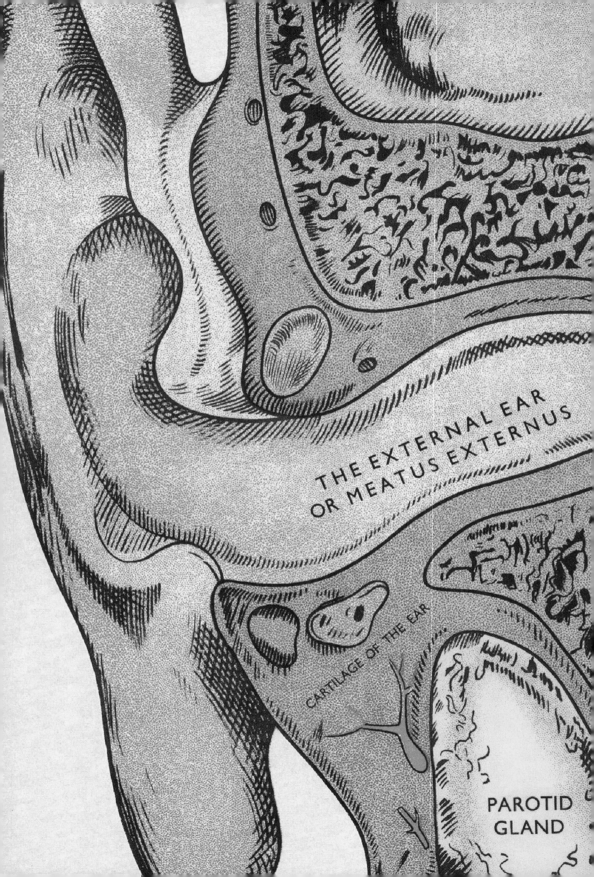

THE EXTERNAL EAR
OR MEATUS EXTERNUS

CARTILAGE OF THE EAR

PAROTID
GLAND

CHAPTER 9

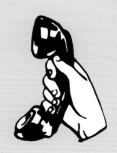

EARS

Humans have five basic senses: hearing, touch, sight, smell and taste. Our sensory organs transmit information to our brains, helping us to perceive and understand the world around us. Until relatively recently, information was transmitted orally. Most people could not read or write and saw few reasons for learning to do so. Listening (and remembering information) was crucially important.

Being able to hear one another allows humans to communicate verbally, rather than simply gesturing. Over time, humans developed a multitude of languages which constantly change and evolve. Which languages are used (and where and when) has proved to be a hugely contentious sociopolitical matter. This is particularly the case in Ireland, where the right to communicate in Irish, rather than English, took on huge cultural significance.

Given the emphasis on oral communication, political campaigners have relied heavily upon prowess at public speaking. In the early 1800s, Daniel O'Connell gained an international reputation as Ireland's 'Great Orator' and agitated successfully for Catholic emancipation – the granting of equal rights. His oratory strategies formed part of a culture still based largely upon oralism and finding people willing to listen to radical political messages.

Of course, many people in Ireland have been unable to listen due to being born deaf or acquiring hearing-related problems later in life. How to educate deaf children, and in what language, was a controversial and much-debated matter. Many nineteenth and twentieth-century educators insisted that deaf children should learn to speak conventionally, and in English, viewing sign language as a primitive, unsuitable form of communication.

SPEAKING IRISH

The earliest known forms of the Irish language are (somewhat dismissively) referred to as 'Primitive Irish'. We know of this language only through a few fragments inscribed on stone between the fourth and sixth centuries AD. It looks broadly similar to Latin, Classical Greek and Sanskrit. Around 300 of these Ogham inscriptions have been found in Ireland: 121 are from Co. Kerry and 81 from Co. Cork. For the most part, these are mostly memorials containing the name of a deceased person (and sometimes those of their father and grandfather).[1]

From the sixth century, Old Irish, a more complex language, evolved unusually quickly. The reasons for this speedy linguistic transition are uncertain but it was probably related to the arrival of Christianity and the introduction of Latin learning. Examples of Old Irish writing are rare, although scholars have been able to reconstruct the language reasonably well.[2] Middle Irish was spoken between around 900 and 1200, and its written form is thought to be close to the actual language spoken in everyday life. English-speaking voices began to be heard after the Anglo-Normans arrived in 1169, especially in larger port towns and around the Pale. Surprisingly, though, the Normans developed a love of speaking Irish. This annoyed King Edward III so much that he issued the Statutes of Kilkenny in 1367, after starting to believe that his settlers were becoming more Irish than the Irish themselves. To encourage Anglo-Normans to resume their native linguistic customs, speaking English was made compulsory under threat of having their property confiscated. However, Irish speaking withstood the threat.[3]

At the very start of the 1600s, the traditional Gaelic aristocracy was defeated. In September 1607 members of some of Ireland's leading families fled Ireland for Europe – the Flight of the Earls – opening the way for an intense period of plantation of English settlers. The Irish language became associated with Catholicism and disloyalty; English with loyalty to the Crown.[4] The Elizabethan conquest of Ireland is often depicted as a linguistic turning point in which the

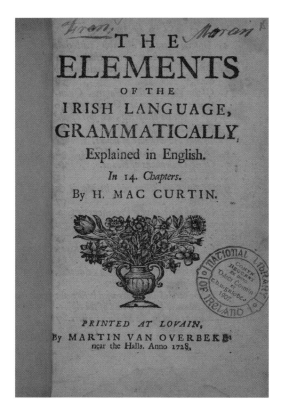

THE ELEMENTS
OF THE
IRISH LANGUAGE,
GRAMMATICALLY,
Explained in English.

In 14. Chapters.

By H. MAC CURTIN.

PRINTED AT LOVAIN,
By MARTIN VAN OVERBEKE
near the Halls. Anno 1728.

Speaking in Irish was historically looked upon with suspicion by the British authorities in Ireland.

national language shifted decisively from Irish to English.[5] In practice, various languages co-existed for the time being. Latin was the language of learning, Irish that of the bards and peasantry. Middle English remained the preferred form of communication among the 'Old English' (descendants of the Anglo-Normans), while planters spoke 'Early Modern' or 'New' English.[6]

It is often said that by the nineteenth century, Irish was a dying language. This wasn't entirely the case. In 1851, up to 30 per cent of the population still spoke Irish. Nor was Irish confined to rural western regions. It could be heard being spoken in Ulster and all of Ireland's major towns and cities. In Dublin, Irish was widely spoken in the Liberties area. People from across the social classes, and not just the poorest, communicated in Irish. Priests continued to address their flocks in Irish from the pulpits well into the late nineteenth century, and numerous religious-themed books were published in Irish that same century.[7]

However, the English language now undoubtedly dominated formal settings such as the courts. The Irish language was under siege from the growth of a bureaucratic state which preferred to operate in English. In 1831, when National Schools were introduced, Irish was omitted from curricula and pupils were told not to speak their language on school premises. Pupils overheard speaking Irish would have to wear a wooden stick around their neck, which teachers would mark whenever they spoke in Irish. At the end of the school day, the ticks would be counted, and pupils punished accordingly. Even when Irish learning was reinstated later in the century, it remained secondary to English, Latin, Greek and French. Nonetheless, more than 1 million people still spoke Irish in 1861.

Despite the relative vibrancy of the language, the Great Famine undoubtedly reduced the number of Irish speakers, through either death or emigration. Irish was far from being on its deathbed, but some people feared that it was at risk of disappearing altogether. In founding the Gaelic League (Conradh na Gaeilge) in 1893, Douglas Hyde was determined to salvage the language. The league ran classes all over the country, teaching native speakers how to read and write in Irish. One popular book, *Simple Lessons in Irish*, was written by priest, scholar and league member Eugene O'Growney. Learning Irish was a symbolic rejection of British rule (de-anglicisation) intended to bolster campaigns for Home Rule and national independence. Nationalists eagerly learned Irish (with varying degrees of success) largely to make a point. Patrick Pearse became editor of an Irish-language newspaper and opened an Irish-speaking school for boys in his own house in Rathfarnham. Speaking Irish was a political statement, despite being seen by some as a 'badge of a beaten race'.[8]

Contradictorily, the independent Irish state formed in 1922 retained English as its administrative language. Irish was the Republic's official language, but English usually proved more practical. It was hoped that over time proficiency in Irish speaking would spread from the Irish-speaking regions, including the Gaeltacht areas, but English would suffice for the time being. A qualification in Irish was required to hold state jobs, although little fluency was required. Irish was made a compulsory subject in schools in 1928.

Ironically, the number of people who spoke Irish as a first language sharply declined after independence. Even many Irish people were unenthusiastic about having to learn Irish. Many pupils, parents and teachers insisted that emphasising Irish learning diluted the overall quality of education: more valuable subjects were neglected. In a globally connected world, whether or not proficiency in Irish would open up many opportunities beyond Ireland seemed questionable. Ireland joined the European Union in 1973, and the government removed the requirement of passing Irish to obtain the Leaving Certificate (the final secondary school exam) that same year. From 1975, Irish was no longer needed to secure a job in the civil service. Irish-language advocates pushed back. All-Irish schools (gaelscoileanna) opened across the country, and state-funded television (TG4) and radio stations were created. Since 2003, everyone has had a right to avail of any public service in Irish if they wish. Irish become an option, although one fiercely defended.[9]

The Northern Irish state expressed little enthusiasm for formally recognising Irish as an official language. Associating Irish with Catholicism, it conveniently forgot that Protestants also spoke Irish. The Ulster Gaelic Society was founded in 1830, and an Ulster Branch of the Gaelic League was even formed in 1895. Alice Milligan was a key northern advocate. (The league is regularly commented upon favourably for opening up prominent positions to women, including Milligan, Lady Gregory, Lady Esmonde, Mary Spring Rice, Máire Ní Shúilleabháin and Norma Borthwick.) Even after partition, many people in Northern Ireland remained interested in learning Irish and would often hop over the border to Co. Donegal to practise their language skills. Unlike in the Republic, the Northern government had no vested interest in preserving or protecting this particular linguistic tradition. While it would be going too far to expect to hear many dedicated Northern loyalists asking 'Cad é mar atá tú?' (How are you?) anytime soon, the issue of Irish speaking is more complicated than it initially appears, given its appeal to quite a number of Protestants.[10]

Recognition of the Irish language was enshrined in the 1998 Good Friday Agreement. In practice, the Irish language has since regained popularity mainly in Catholic areas. Belfast even has its own hip-hop trio, Kneecap, who rap in Irish. Their first release recounted the night when Móglai Bap was arrested for spray-painting and refused to respond to the police in English. The PSNI had to find a translator. In reality, Irish speaking is more symbolic than practical in Northern Ireland.[11] This powerful symbolism explains why Unionists were

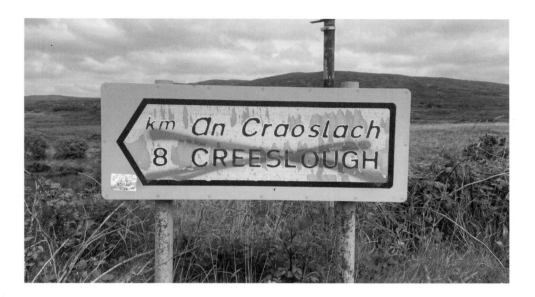

adamant that an Irish Language Act would never be enacted in the North. Where's the need for having road and street signs in both Irish and English? Why bother to speak Irish in Stormont? Who would fund all this unnecessary expense? These sorts of questions were asked regularly by Unionists, which critics interpreted as part of an ongoing effort to marginalise Irish culture. With some irony, though, the British government intervened while the Northern Irish government was not sitting in Stormont and the Identity and Language (Northern Ireland) Act of 2022 conferred official recognition on the Irish language in Northern Ireland.[12]

The Irish language remains a contentious political issue, particularly in Northern Ireland, which until recently did not accord it any legal status. In parts of Ireland such as Co. Donegal, it is common to paint over English translations of Irish place names on road signs.

Northern Protestants more readily identify with the Ulster-Scots language, and provision was also made for this in 2022. Scots used to be the national language of Scotland and arrived in Ireland during the seventeenth century when Scottish people settled en masse in Ulster. Scots was then the language of Scotland's lowlands and also its courts. Bad harvests in Scotland and religious persecution encouraged an ever-increasing number of Scots to settle in Ulster. In 1688, the 'Glorious Revolution' saw the Catholic King James II deposed by

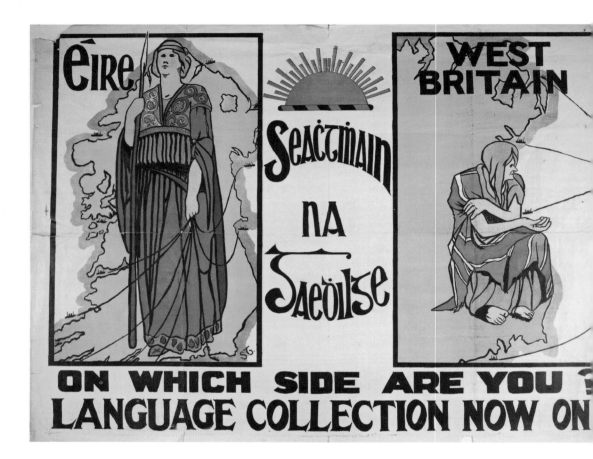

In the Irish revolutionary period, groups such as the Gaelic League actively promoted the Irish language and urged that English be spoken less often.

the Protestant prince of Orange, who was crowned King William III. James fled to France but then took up his struggle in Ireland with the support of its Catholic population (the Jacobites). Conflict ensued between the native Irish Catholics and the settlers of English or Scottish descent. For five long months, Derry was under siege and effectively starved into submission. The 1690 Battle of the Boyne saw William victorious, ensuring the continuation of the Protestant Ascendancy in Ireland. This encouraged further Scots speakers to move to Ireland.[13] Ulster-Scots remains spoken today, mainly in the north-east. Many Ulster-Scots speakers see their language, heritage and culture as under threat and campaign just as vigorously for its preservation as do Irish-language enthusiasts.[14] Language, after all, can be a deeply contested matter.

DANIEL O'CONNELL –
THE GREAT ORATOR

In the early nineteenth century, through his powerful mastery of words, a great orator transformed conditions for Catholics across Ireland. Since 1695, when the first Penal Law was decreed, Catholics have faced endless barriers and restrictions. Enacted by the Irish Parliament, the Penal Laws secured the Protestant Ascendency's monopolisation of property, power and public office, acknowledged the British monarch as supreme governor and rejected 'foreign jurisdictions and powers', a thinly veiled reference to the Pope.

The Penal Laws purposefully weakened Catholic power, brazenly attacked Catholic culture and actively anglicised (or, as the Protestants termed it, 'civilised') Ireland. Catholics were no longer permitted to bear arms, serve in the army or navy, work as a weaponsmith, own horses worth more than £5, bequeath their entire estate to one child, take time off work for unauthorised holy days, hold public office, marry Protestants, work in legal professions, inherit Protestant land, build lasting churches made of stone, construct churches close to a main road, teach in schools and so on. A lengthy list indeed. Catholics probably wondered what they were still actually allowed to do.[15]

Eighteenth-century Ireland was a separate but dependent kingdom, united to Britain through the monarchy. It enjoyed its own separate executive parliament, headed by a lord lieutenant based at Dublin Castle. Nonetheless, the British Parliament at Westminster could veto Irish legislation and the highest appointments were always of British appointees. The Penal Laws were gradually dismantled later in the century, but Catholics remained second-class citizens. From the 1780s, some liberal Protestants, led by Henry Grattan, campaigned for parliamentary reform, less British influence and improved rights for Catholics and Presbyterians. However, the typical Irish peasant had little interest in the concerns of middle-class reformers, such as exclusion from public office, a problem that they would never personally encounter. Leaders failed to communicate meaningfully with potential grassroots supporters.[16]

Across Europe, the 1780s and 1790s were a time of revolution and political unrest. Set against this turbulent backdrop, the United Irishmen formed in Belfast during 1791 with barrister Theobald Wolfe Tone as its secretary. The group initially worked constitutionally but was increasingly swayed by ideas of staging an uprising. It transformed into an oath-based secret society with cells across the country. In 1796, Wolfe Tone attempted to arrange a French invasion of Ireland, but this was thwarted by storms. On 23 May 1798, a rebellion took place, but the French reneged on their promised support by not bothering to show up. The Dublin rising was soon quelled, and the rebellion continued, largely unsuccessfully, locally across Ireland. Mass atrocities were committed on both sides, and that summer, 30,000 died. Despite this failure, romanticised ideas of a violent rising took hold in Ireland.[17]

Two years on, and not coincidently, the Act of Union received the royal signature. Prime Minister William Pitt thought that the union would work better if Catholics were granted rights. Given its large size, it was best if the Catholic population could be persuaded to become more loyal to Britain. Pitt crossed paths with ardent opponents (including the mad King George III) and the union passed into law without a Catholic settlement. Protestants still monopolised positions of power, but the post-union period also saw the rise of middle-class Catholicism, a revitalised Catholic Church and a renewed impetus for full emancipation of Catholics to secure them equal rights.

This is where our 'great orator' enters the story. Daniel O'Connell was born on 6 August 1775 in Co. Kerry into a Catholic gentry family who had survived the punitive eighteenth century. In the 1790s, O'Connell became fascinated by radical politics. He sympathised

The Penal Laws were a series of draconian laws that severely restricted the rights of Irish Catholics.

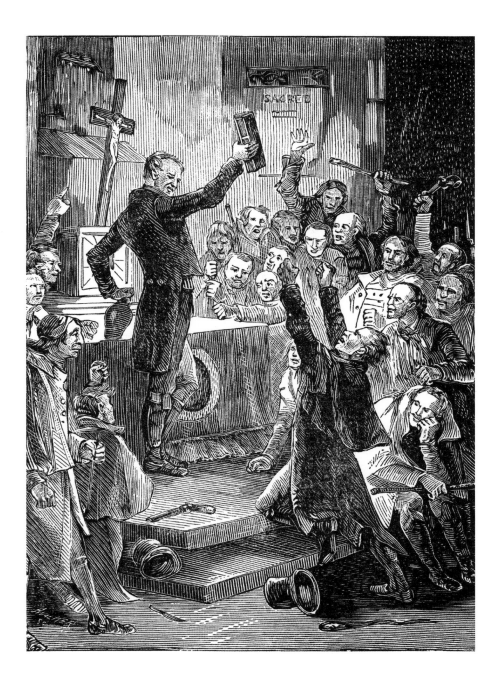

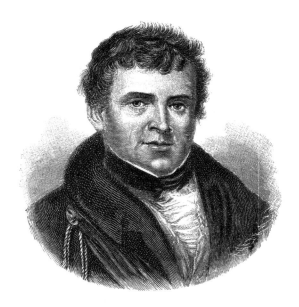

Daniel O'Connell is remembered in Ireland for successfully campaigning for Catholic emancipation in the early nineteenth century.

with the United Irishmen's aims but was horrified by the bloodshed of 1798. From then on, O'Connell remained steadfastly opposed to using violence to effect political change and wondered if other means were possible.

In 1823, O'Connell founded the Catholic Association, a group which used constitutional, not revolutionary, approaches to emancipation. O'Connell wanted to reform 'the system' from within rather than radically overthrow it. Unlike those before him, O'Connell actively engaged with the Catholic masses by offering cheap membership. Local branches, set up across Ireland, collated local grievances and forwarded them to headquarters in Dublin, allowing direct lines of communication between leaders and peasants. The association soon attracted significant publicity. Membership applications spiralled. By 1824, the demand for emancipation had undergone a whirlwind transformation. Catholic emancipation became the leading Irish question of British politics.

O'Connell's oratorical adeptness was crucial to this success. O'Connell has many biographers, all of whom consistently struggle to extract a particularly eloquent quote or sentence from his speeches. O'Connell had no 'I have a dream' moment. Rather, it was the way O'Connell articulated and delivered his poignant words that moved his listeners. As he spoke, 'the passions of mighty multitudes rose and swayed and sunk again beneath his hand, as tides heave beneath the moon'.[18] Contemporary accounts confirm that O'Connell's speeches were neither ambitious, ornate nor well-prepared. Their language was not especially elegant. Nonetheless, those speeches delivered at the hugely attended 'monster meetings' were forceful, powerful and skilfully improvised. Believing the Catholic masses to be broken in spirit, O'Connell gained popularity by appealing directly to their concerns.

As one biographer later wrote:

> His appearance, his personality, his record of services, his variety and grace of elocution, the inflexions of his voice, his command of gesture, his expressive countenance and the mobility of his features, his power of evoking sympathy – all these must have affected his audiences as much as what he said. He had in his youth frequently heard [William] Pitt speak and imitated that statesman in the management of his voice. It is with some surprise that one learns that he was a rapid speaker, and that the newspapers complained of the difficulty of reporting a man who could utter two hundred words a minute for three or four hours together.

O'Connell's powers as a speaker were also enhanced greatly by the day-to-day knowledge which he accumulated of his audience's lives, worries and tribulations. As another biographer elaborated:

He played on the national prejudices and weaknesses of the Irish as on a musical instrument. He could indulge in pathos or jest, fiery denunciation, or subtle argument, as it suited his purpose, with consummate skill. Many testimonies to his power of swaying vast audiences have been given by those who heard them.[19]

Frederick Douglass, himself an impressive public speaker, and who shared O'Connell's anti-slavery perspectives, wrote:

Until I heard this man, I had thought that the story of his oratory and power were greatly exaggerated. I did not see how a man could speak to 20 or 30,000 people at one time and be heard by any considerable portion of them, but the mystery was solved when I saw his ample person and heard his musical voice. His eloquence came down upon the vast assembly like a summer thunder shower upon a dusty road. He could at will stir the multitude to a tempest of wrath or reduce it to the silence with which a mother leaves the cradle side of her sleeping babe.

Such tenderness, such pathos, such world-embracing love and, on the other hand, such indignation, such fiery and thunderous denunciation, such wit and humour, I never heard surpassed, if equalled, at home or abroad. He held Ireland within the grasp of his strong hand, and could lead it whithersoever he would, for Ireland believed in him and loved him as she has loved and believed in no leader since.[20]

In yet another example of the glowing praise showered on O'Connell, Arthur Houston later wrote:

Marvellous voice, powerful ... sonorous, melodious, penetrating, capable of expressing every shade of human feeling. But a voice is nothing without a command of words, and words are nothing where ideas are lacking. O'Connell had an abundance of both ... Nor was it the masses alone that fell under the spell of his eloquence. Judges and juries bowed to his influence, and this wonder at his eloquence was affirmed later by those who heard him in the House of Commons.[21]

Strong testimonials, but what did O'Connell's grand speeches actually achieve? In the 1820s, several bills for Catholic emancipation passed through the House of Commons, but the House of Lords rejected them all. Undeterred, O'Connell placed additional pressure on the government by putting forward Catholic Association members for election. In 1826, George Thomas Beresford, brother of the archbishop of Armagh and son of the marquis of Waterford, also one of the most powerful proprietors in Ireland, lost his Waterford seat to a Catholic emancipationist. Henry Villiers-Stuart's victory signalled a firm rejection of political and social deference to the Protestant Ascendency. In many other constituencies, the victory was repeated, signalling the death knell for Protestant political supremacism.

In 1828, O'Connell himself stood for election, winning the Clare county by-election. With an elected leader of a mass movement on its hands, Irish Protestants bowed to the inevitable. After the Catholic Emancipation Act was passed in 1829, Catholics could hold offices of state (apart from regent, lord chancellor or lord lieutenant of Ireland) and sit in parliament. But initially the act was more symbolic than anything else, and social change for Catholics was a far more gradual process. It rejected centuries of discrimination and withholding of social rights. Through his powerful oratory, O'Connell had finally given Irish Catholics control over their own future.[22]

But anyone attending one of O'Connell's famous monster meetings would have been hard pressed to hear their grievances being discussed in Irish. Despite being a native Irish speaker, O'Connell considered the language primitive and backwards. In 1833, he expressed indifference to the gradual abandonment of

Irish speaking, commenting that linguistic diversity was a curse inherited from the building of the biblical tower of Babel, adding that the 'English tongue' was 'superior'. O'Connell never actively tried to stamp out Irish, but his indifference to the fate of the language remains a bone of contention to this date.[23]

DEAFNESS

Not all Irish citizens have been fortunate enough to have been born with fully operating senses. Like all other countries, Ireland has a significant population of people living with disabilities that present barriers to their lives. Today, around 8 per cent of the population suffers from deafness or severe hearing loss.

While recovering from an illness in 1815, an Irish physician named Charles Orpen became determined to find ways of teaching language to deaf people. He practised on a deaf boy named Thomas Collins. Just four months later, Orpen was convinced that he had managed to teach Thomas an extensive vocabulary, improved pronunciation and even some basic arithmetic. He announced his success in a series of lectures delivered at Dublin's famous Rotunda Hospital and then printed 1,000 copies of a book outlining his findings, which he distributed to missionary societies.

Donations began flooding in to fund Orpen's new idea: a School for the Deaf and Dumb. Orpen visited a number of similar institutions in Europe and was particularly impressed by what he saw at the Institution for the Deaf and Dumb in Paris, led by Abbé Sicard, a French educator who excelled in developing methods of teaching the deaf. Opened in 1816, Orpen's institution was Ireland's first school for the deaf. Three years later, the school moved to Claremont in Glasnevin, a site boasting 18 acres of garden and meadow. Over 100 pupils enrolled each year until 1931, when a new school opened in Belfast: The Ulster Society for Promoting the Education of the Deaf and the Blind.[24]

In 1845, the Catholic Institution for the Deaf and Dumb sent two nuns and two deaf girls to a deaf school in Caen, France, to learn the most up-to-date

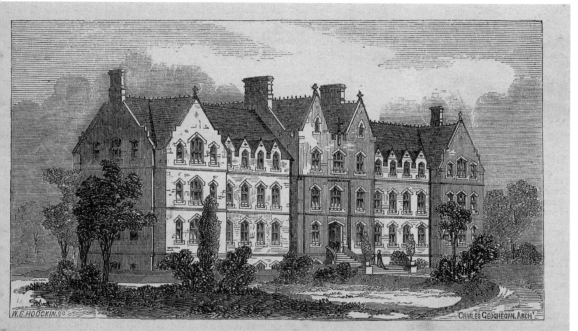

STITUTION FOR THE DEAF AND DUMB, CABRA, IRELAND.——Mr. C. Geoghegan, Architect.

methods of deaf education. A year later, it opened a specialist school – St Mary's – for the deaf in Cabra, Dublin. The first student was Agnes Beedem, an eight-year-old girl from Capel Street. The school was residential, meaning that boys and girls were separated. Some residents were moved to the school from workhouses. The establishment of these various schools for the deaf helped forge a sense of community among deaf people.

In the nineteenth and twentieth centuries, many children with deafness were taught in the Institution for the Deaf and Dumb, Cabra.

Between 1846 and 1849, Irish sign language (ISL) was developed. ISL is its own unique language and bears no resemblance to any spoken or written languages. Peculiarly, it has different signing for men and women. However, serious tensions were soon to erupt about the nature and purpose of deaf education.[25]

On 21 April 1861, Francis Maginn was born in Castletownroche, Co. Cork. He was the sixth of 12 children, the son of a Church of Ireland rector and a relative, through his mother, Mary, of the Elizabethan poet Edmund Spenser. At age five, Francis caught scarlet fever. Tragically, the infection caused him to lose his hearing, much of his memory and his power of speech. Disabilities were stigmatised in nineteenth-century Ireland. Some saw them as a punishment from God. Francis' parents struggled to cope and reserved a place for him in the Asylum for Deaf and Dumb Children in Bermondsey, London, where sign language was taught.

In 1880, the institution's headmaster, Richard Elliot, travelled to Milan to attend a notoriously controversial meeting: the second International Congress for the Education of the Deaf. Attendees passed resolutions that caused a storm in the world of deaf education worldwide: two essentially banned the teaching of sign language in schools. Some educators in attendance insisted that spoken language was far superior to sign language. Sign language, they insisted, was little more than gesture, pantomime and mimicry. No one thought to ask the deaf what they thought about this. Spoken language had many advocates, including Alexander Graham Bell, inventor of the telephone, who agreed that sign language should be banned and deaf people barred from marrying each other. This approach was known as 'oralism'. Despite his views, Bell was selected to provide evidence for the Royal Commission on Deaf Education, whose report was published in 1889 and proved highly influential across Ireland and Britain.

Upon returning from Milan, Elliot told Maginn of the harsh restrictions being placed on sign language. Thoroughly disgusted, Maginn decided to campaign for its retention. He returned to Ireland in 1883 but then received an offer to attend Gallaudet University in Washington, DC, the world's only higher education institution for deaf students. Sadly, due to his father's illness, Francis returned to Ireland in 1887 without completing his studies. Between 1888 and 1918, he was active in a mission that provided hostel accommodation for 30 deaf people. He travelled around the country and once helped deaf people secure employment in Belfast's shipping industries.

ISL is the sign language of Ireland, used primarily in the Republic of Ireland, and also in Northern Ireland alongside British Sign Language.

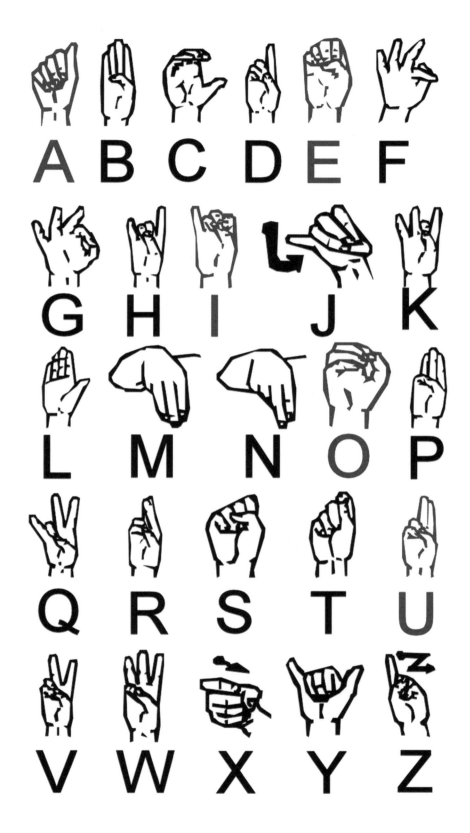

Maginn founded the British Deaf and Dumb Association in January 1890, although he became disillusioned after people who could hear assumed the leadership roles. Instead, Maginn began to focus his attention on his work with the Ulster Institute for the Deaf and Dumb and Blind, Belfast. In 1918, he attended a gala evening at which two deaf men became involved in an altercation. While attempting to intervene, Maginn was accidentally punched in the chest. He later died of his injuries aged 57.[26]

For decades after Maginn's death, debates about deaf education rumbled on. Advocates of oralism largely ignored the successful integration of deaf people into the workforce, including those who communicated via sign language. Claremont, now a Protestant institution, proudly switched to oralism in the 1880s. During the 1940s and 1950s, Catholic schools implemented oralism: St Mary's moved to an oral approach in 1946.[27] This was heralded as a panacea to cure all the problems of the deaf and help them integrate more fully into 'normal' society. Oral schools opened in Dublin, Cork and Limerick. In 1946, a group of Irish nuns toured 12 oral schools in England and Scotland with a view to upgrading deaf education back home in Ireland. They influenced the introduction of oralism at Cabra in 1946. In turn, eminent visitors arrived from England to promote the apparent benefits of oralism.

However, much of the work being done in these schools was guided by a sense that the Catholic Church had a divine task of caring for the weaker elements of society. Irish institutions concentrated primarily on religious instruction, speech training and a watered-down version of the standard school curriculum. At Cabra, nuns tended to view deafness as a medical infirmity that could be cured if the deaf learned to speak like everyone else.[28]

Traditionally, children had learned speech and lip-reading in the classroom and then reverted to sign language on their breaks and mealtimes, or when the teachers were not looking. However, from the 1940s, a stronger anti-signing ideology developed which essentially prevented deaf people from communicating in their own language. It did not help that the hearing people in charge who considered this a good idea had not asked any deaf people for their views. Deaf people needed to assimilate into society, not have their own language and culture, so critics insisted. The use of sign language was suppressed, further stigmatising the language. Even compared to other countries, the Irish regime was regarded as harsh. Oralist approaches formed part of a broader punitive institutional environment in which vulnerable Irish children faced various types of abuse. In 1972, an oral approach to education became official state policy.[29] ISL was only formally recognised again in 2017. However, activists still insist that deaf children are being denied a full and adequate education due to the ongoing stigma attached to sign language, even if it is now finally recognised as one of Ireland's official languages.

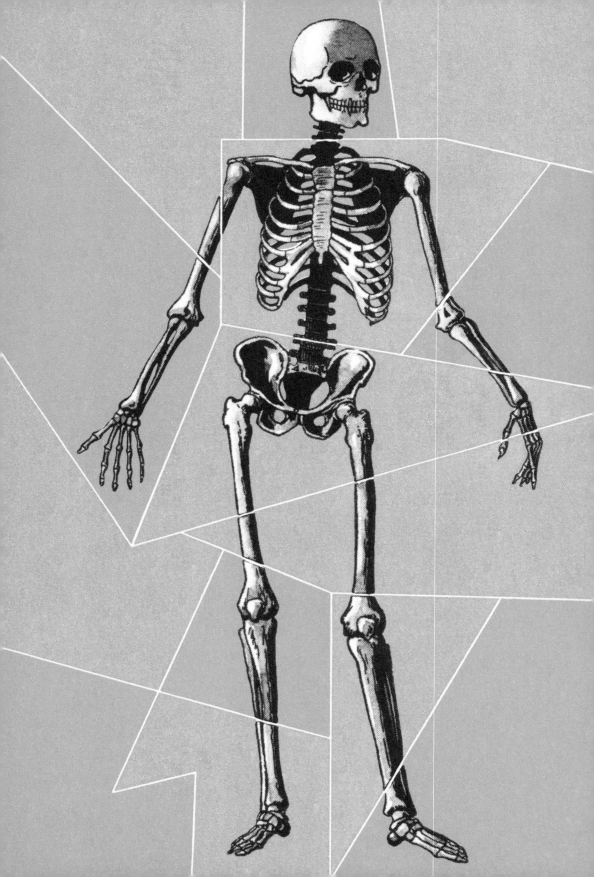

CHAPTER 10

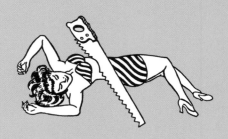

CORPSES

The end is nearly upon us. Death, our finale, comes to us all. When it arrives, our hearts stop beating, depriving cells of oxygen. Our bodies self-digest as enzymes consume cell membranes, a process that commences in our softer organs: livers and brains, for example. (Some scientists believe that our brains still work for 10 minutes or so after death, meaning that we might have some awareness that we are dying.) Our muscles relax, pupils dilate, and jaws fall open. Our bodies pale and whiten as blood drains from our veins. Damaged blood cells settle in the capillaries and veins, discolouring our skin. Body temperature cools, bringing on the 'death chill'. As the hours pass after our final breath, rigor mortis – the 'stiffness of death' – sets in. Beginning with the eyelids, jaws and neck, our muscles become rigid. Joints lock together. Not altogether dead, our decomposing corpses start to teem with new life, transforming into a vast, complex ecosystem which flourishes as we decompose.

The basic biological experience of dying has stayed more or less the same throughout human history, but the customs and concerns surrounding dead bodies have taken on peculiarities in different societies and cultures. Today, the Irish retain long-standing traditions, once a loved one has sadly passed away, of holding a wake, essentially a party at which even the deceased is present, providing an opportunity for relatives and friends to say one final farewell. In many other western countries, it became more common in the twentieth century for death to occur in a hospital and for professional undertakers to care for the corpse, but not so in Ireland. Broadly similar traditions are seen among both Catholic and Protestant mourners. However, some funerary practices have fallen out of fashion, including keening. A keener was a woman (usually unknown to the grieving family) who would attend funerals and perform the task of crying and wailing on behalf of the family. Also of interest is the rise of a world-famous Irish medical profession in Dublin early in the nineteenth century that broke traditional customs relating to corpses through unpopular activities such as bodysnatching and anatomy. Dead bodies and funerals also took on special significance in cases of Irish martyrdom, including the famous deaths of hunger strikers, prisoners who deliberately starved themselves to death to help secure Irish freedom from Britain.

CARING FOR CORPSES

Historically, the Irish developed customs for caring for corpses designed to ensure that they maintained a pleasing, respectful and almost still-alive appearance. Until the 1950s, most people died at home, not in hospitals. Families, not morticians, looked after bodies, a custom known as laying-out. Home was widely considered the best place to die, surrounded by relatives and friends in our final moments. When death came, mirrors were covered to ensure that the deceased was not trapped inside the house. Windows and doors were opened to let the soul depart. Around the house, clocks were stopped at the time of death, restarted only after burial. Neighbours brought food and drink, sometimes even mortuary clothes and a coffin. The time had now come to prepare the corpse for its public viewing.

Between death and burial, corpses shared domestic space with the living. Clergymen, doctors and public health workers looked on aghast, warning that putrefying bodies, no matter how diligently laid out on the kitchen table, were virulent sources of disease and contagion. Their pleas fell on deaf ears. For close relatives, the act of washing and laying-out a corpse represented a final gesture of intimacy and affection. Critics weren't entirely wrong. Weather and indoor fires hastened the decomposition of soft organs, causing corpses to fester and emit pungent odours. In the warmer summer months, a corpse smelled rancid within hours.

Preparing a corpse for burial was not an easy job. Physical strength was required to lift and roll a heavy body. Squeamishness and fear needed to be assuaged. The task of laying-out a corpse usually fell upon female family members, handywomen or female neighbours. Preparing the corpse for burial was carried out silently. Bodies were laid out facing south east, pointing to holy places, due to a common belief that evil spirits came from the north. Washing the corpse was the first task; a baptism for the afterlife and a purifying ritual that helped secure the soul a place in heaven. Washing commenced at the head and moved down the body, eventually reaching the feet. Water and other used

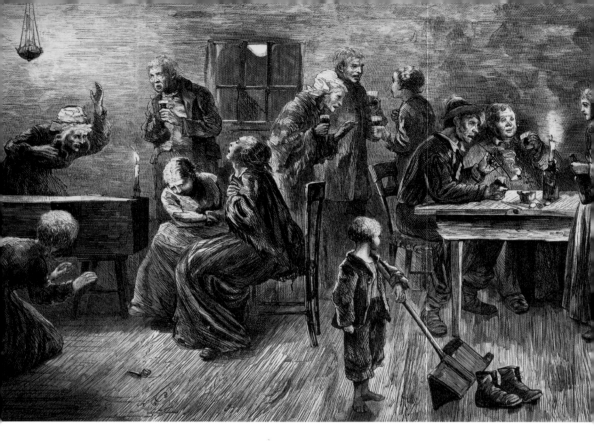

Irish funerals could be surprisingly jovial occasions and it remains common to hold a wake with the deceased person present.

items were carefully disposed of afterwards, committed to the earth just like the body was about to be.

After the body was cleansed, it was made presentable for burial. Eyelids are the first part of the body affected by rigor mortis, and so pennies were placed on them, to hold them shut. The mouth was closed. A band or shroud cap held the chin up. Limbs were straightened and held together with string, arms placed crosswise over the breast or stomach, orifices plugged with herbs to prevent undesirable bodily fluids leaking out. Faces were shaved, hair brushed and fingernails scrubbed. Finally, the corpse was dressed in a nightgown or simple shroud.[1]

There were many other customs. As Christ died on Friday, 'a Friday death, a Saturday prayer and a Sunday funeral' was considered ideal. If an illness started to look quite serious, Catholics called in a priest to hear the sick person's confession and help them arrange their affairs. Should death seem imminent, the priest issued the last sacraments. Blessed candles, consecrated in his church, would be lit around the room.² In Connemara, it was customary to hang unsalted butter from the rafters in a piece of a cloth and let the sick person die alone if they were dying of tuberculosis. Family members returned to the house only when convinced that the person was 'well dead'. Rather than passing on to other household members, the tuberculosis seeds were inhaled by the butter, it was believed, warding off consumption for the next seven years.³

After the laying-out had finished, watching and waking took place – a continuous watch kept on the deceased until burial. Relatives gathered around the spruced-up corpse to express their grief and solemnly acknowledge the passing. Irish wakes could be surprisingly jovial, a drinking orgy, even. To outsiders, this revelry and boisterousness jarred with the occasion's sombreness. For centuries, the clergy objected to boisterous wakes. In 1888, American ethnographer James Mooney described a typical Irish wake:

> As soon as the news of the death gets abroad, the friends begin to arrive to pay their respects to the deceased. They never enter the house singly, but should one come alone, he waits on the outside until joined by one or two others, when they open the door a little way, take off their hats and recite in an undertone the prayers for the dead. Then entering the room, they salute those present, take seats and join in the conversation ... The friends arrive all through the day, some coming from long distances, and by nightfall there are as many present as the house can well accommodate.
>
> When the family and the caoiners [keeners] sit or stand about the corpse, the others pass the time in smoking, gossiping, telling stories, singing songs and playing games, all of which seems strangely out of place in the presence of death. At intervals, one of the company will say 'let us repeat a Pater and Ave for the soul of the dead', when all rise and say a short prayer in silence, after which the talk and merriment go on as before.⁴

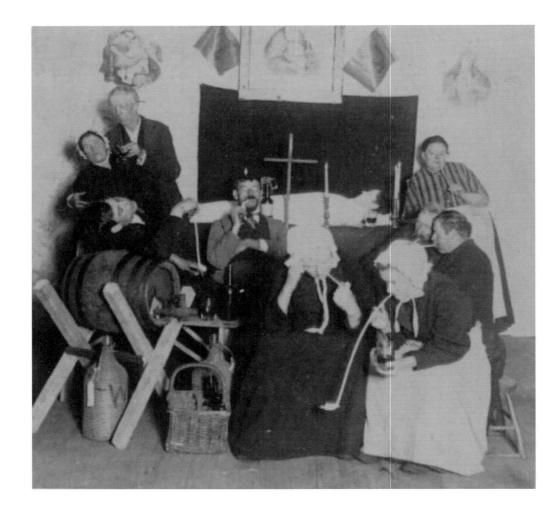

Wakes provide opportunities for relatives, friends and neighbours to say their final goodbyes to the deceased.

This sociability, and the sheer number of people assembled around a rotting human body, shocked and disgusted public health officials and caused consternation whenever the Irish emigrated to new places. In 1840s England, public health reformer Edwin Chadwick regretted that 'the body is never absent from their [the Irish's] sight. Eating, drinking, sleeping, it is still by their side'. Relatives remained over-familiar with the deceased and even desecrated corpses. According to Chadwick's description, 'the body, stretched out upon two chairs, is pulled about by the children, made to serve as a resting place for any article that is in the way, and is not seldom the hiding place for the beer bottle or gin if any visitor arrives inopportunely'.[5]

In the 1960s, folklorist Seán Ó Súilleabháin published a book entitled *Irish Wake Amusements*, which similarly confirmed the joviality that once characterised Irish wakes, which he described as 'far merrier than weddings'. Tales were told, songs were sung and games were even played. The most common games were card-playing, riddles, tongue twisters, versifying and repeating jingles. Strength contests had also been common, with tests of endurance including lifting the corpse (not the actual corpse, thankfully, but a stout man pretending to be dead), wrestling and various other competitions in agility and dexterity. In some districts, athletic contests would continue all night. Games still familiar to us, such as blind man's bluff and hide and seek, were commonly played.[6]

Critics of the Irish (and there were many) failed to appreciate the importance attached in Ireland to a good send-off and a proper funeral, particularly among less affluent communities. Of particular importance was avoiding a farewell that resembled a pauper's funeral. To better grasp the significance of a good funeral, the writings of Cork-born antiquary Thomas Crofton Croker are helpful. In 1824, he wrote:

'An easy death and a fine funeral' is a proverbial benediction amongst the lower orders in Ireland. Throughout life, the peasant is accustomed to regard the manner and place of his interment as matters of the greatest importance. 'To be decently put in the earth, along with his own people' is the wish most frequently and fervently expressed by him. When advanced in life, it is usual, particularly with those who are destitute and friendless, to deny themselves the common necessities of life and to hoard up every trifle they can collect for the expenses of their wake and funeral.

> Looking forward to their death as to a gala given by them to their acquaintances, every possible preparation is made for rendering it, as they consider, 'creditable'. Their shroud and burial dress are often provided many years before they are wanted. Nor will the owners use these garments whilst living, though existing in the most abject state of wretchedness and rags. It is not unusual to see even the tombstone in readiness.[7]

Avoiding a pauper's funeral mattered more than ever when the British government introduced the Poor Relief (Ireland) Act in 1838. Rather than offer financial support to the poor, this law punished unemployment with a spell in the workhouse, which remained Ireland's most feared institution for almost a century. The basic idea was that if conditions inside workhouses were made unrepentantly grim, 'welfare scroungers' would choose to work instead. (Work wasn't always available in Ireland even for those actively seeking it, but this practical matter evaded the Poor Law Commissioners' attention.) Over time, workhouses became less punitive and even a social security net for vulnerable groups such as the elderly. Still, the stigma persisted.

When walking through graveyards in Ireland today, our eyes can be drawn to curious grassy spaces, usually rectangular in shape. In this expansive area rests no gravestones, pathways or ornamental features. These mysterious spaces stand out all the more because Victorian graveyards are always packed and overbrimming with crumbling tombs and plots. Buried six feet under the surface are hundreds of unknown, nameless bodies. The many victims of the workhouses, these bodies once belonged to individuals so excluded and exiled from society that the Poor Law Guardians deemed them unworthy of a decent burial. Everyone knew about pauper burials. That was their intention, for they provided a deliberate reminder that everyone needed to work, or else.

The poor had no say about how they were to be buried. Nor did their relatives or friends. Parish coffins were cheap, unmarked and unsentimental. Even the ringing of bells was banned at pauper funerals. Worst of all, pauper graves

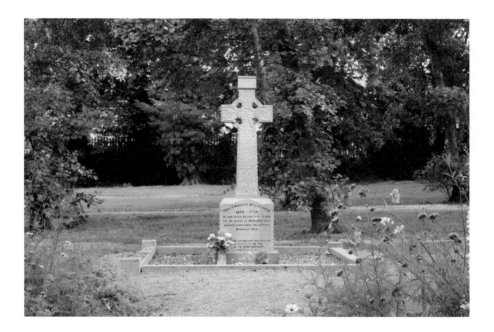

had no headstones. Only those in the know would be aware that a mass grave existed. Remaining relatives were given no clues about where they might visit the deceased. (Even today, pauper graves are still unexpectedly found when major building works commence, and the bodies are respectfully moved to a proper burial site).[8]

Between the nineteenth and twentieth centuries, the bodies of workhouse paupers were thrown into unmarked mass graves as a punishment for living in poverty.

In light of all of this, a proper send-off began to matter greatly, especially among the least affluent in Irish society. In 1888, Mooney wrote:

> The poorest old woman will hoard up year after year from her slender means in order that she may be buried respectably when life's struggle is over, and above all that she may not have a pauper's funeral, while the most poverty-stricken family will strain every nerve to perform the same office for the departed father, mother, brother or sister.[9]

DUBLIN'S SCHOOL OF MEDICINE

In the early nineteenth century, Dublin was one of the world's leading medical centres. Its heyday didn't last long. After the Great Famine, medical graduates emigrated to England and elsewhere due to a dearth of professional medical jobs in Ireland.[10] But for a brief period the Dublin School of Medicine was truly world-leading. To advance medicine, and their own careers, doctors relied upon stealing working-class corpses, a gross indignity to families who believed wholeheartedly in the good send-off. Modern medicine had developed in late-eighteenth-century France, overlapping with the tumultuous revolution of 1789. Until then, physicians had relied upon the ancient Greek humoral theory and attempted to cure illness with bloodletting, applying lots of leeches and similar practices. Medicine hadn't really moved on since ancient times. The modernising influence of the French Revolution encouraged doctors to look more closely at specific body parts and accumulate knowledge scientifically, rather than continue to depend upon ungrounded theories.

Hearts, stomachs, lungs. All the major body organs came under the scrutiny of the modern physician. New technologies such as the stethoscope were designed in the modern spirit to examine specific organs (e.g., by listening to hearts beating). Medicine became organ-centric. (Knowledge of cells, DNA and smaller bodily constituents followed later on.) To advance their scientific knowledge, French medical scientists depended heavily upon anatomy, and dissecting dead bodies, hoping to match symptoms displayed while alive with any bumps, lumps, ulcers or anomalies discovered in the corpse's body organs. So, if a patient had experienced severe stomach pain while alive, the anatomist would know to explore their gut after death, and the same with all other organs. The overarching goal was to build a strong corpus of scientific knowledge to improve diagnosis and save more lives.

Clinging to the old ways, the upper-class physicians who dominated medical teaching at Trinity College and the Royal College of Physicians of Ireland initially refused to teach modern, scientific medicine. As an alternative,

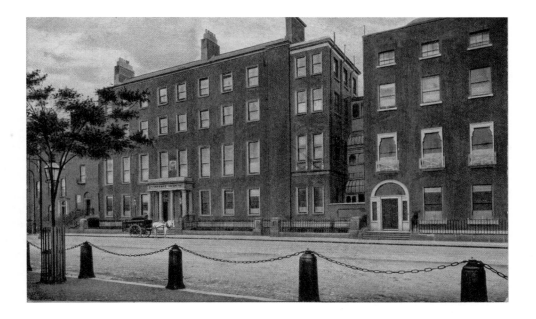

the new breed of French-trained doctors opened private teaching schools across Dublin. Many made an impressive international name for themselves. From the 1840s, William Wilde, Oscar's medical father, became a major international specialist in eye and ear problems and also established a

In the nineteenth century, Dublin transformed into one of the world's leading medical centres. It remains home to numerous hospitals.

new professional journal, the *Dublin Journal of Medical Science*. William Stokes published the first treatise in the English language on the use of René Laënnac's stethoscope. Robert Graves played a huge role in improving fever treatment by feeding rather than bleeding and purging. The Rotunda Hospital became one of Europe's best maternity hospitals. Unusually for the time, the government financially supported the building of a network of hospitals, infirmaries, asylums, dispensaries and workhouses, all of which housed healthcare facilities accessible to the entire population.[11]

Presumably, the Irish would have been delighted. That was not quite the case. Doctors remained deeply distrusted, and many people preferred

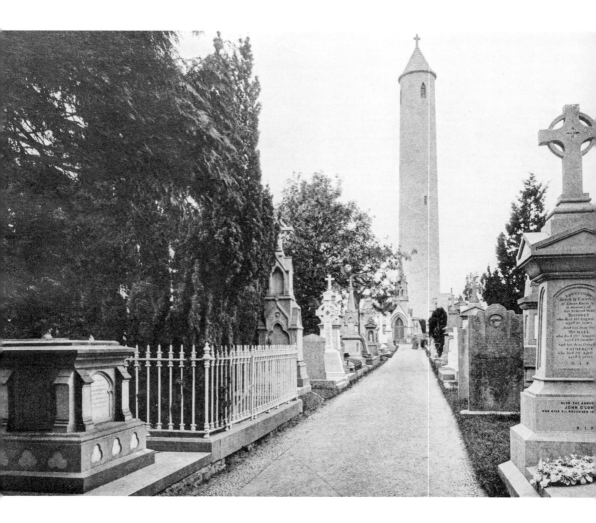

Glasnevin, Ireland's National Cemetery, Dublin, contains the graves of some of Ireland's key historical figures, including Daniel O'Connell and Éamon de Valera.

to continue using non-orthodox healing and health care. Doctors remained unable to cure any diseases until the following century. Controversies surrounding compulsory smallpox vaccinations and animal experimentation further tarnished the reputation of medical science. At worst, medicine was seen as a grotesque, morbid profession staffed by macabre doctors similar to those who populate novels such as *Dracula* and, further afield, *The Strange Case of Dr Jekyll and Mr Hyde*. Public health officials, the sorts who frowned upon traditional Irish customs such as wakes, were also viewed as intrusive and unnecessarily moralising.

Many aspects of nineteenth-century medicine looked suspiciously like a middle-class assault upon working-class bodies. Absconding with bodies was high on the list of complaints. The Dublin School of Medicine acquired its international ascendency largely due to its enthusiasm for dissecting dead bodies, but these were in short supply and hard to come by. Traditionally, the dissection of hanged criminals was seen as fair game, a way for sinners to finally contribute productively to society, despite now being dead. But prisons became more commonly used in the nineteenth century, and occasions for capital punishment declined. Doctors still needed to find bodies from somewhere.

Given the persistence of beliefs in the importance of caring for the recently deceased, the anger directed towards anatomists who cared little for these traditions, running roughshod over them for their own professional advancement, is understandable. As the supply of bodies dwindled, anatomists paid bodysnatchers to dig the bodies of newly deceased people up from their graves. Bully's Acre, a former cemetery near Kilmainham, Dublin, was a notably rich source of anatomical material that fuelled the work of the Dublin School of Medicine. A high wall was built around the largest cemetery in Ireland, at Glasnevin, complete with strategically placed watchtowers (and even bloodhounds) to deter grave robbers. However, such protection of bodies was normally an option only for those who could afford such luxuries. Legally speaking, a corpse was no one's property. It didn't really belong to anyone. Bodysnatchers often used the 'staggering home' technique, which involved dressing the corpse in clothes and having two people support it on either side. The corpse, so they pretended, was their drunken friend. Only if clothes or other items were removed from a grave would a bodysnatcher be liable for prosecution for theft.

In Dublin's medical schools, anatomy teachers expected medical students to dissect three bodies per year. In 1829, Dublin had around 500 dissecting

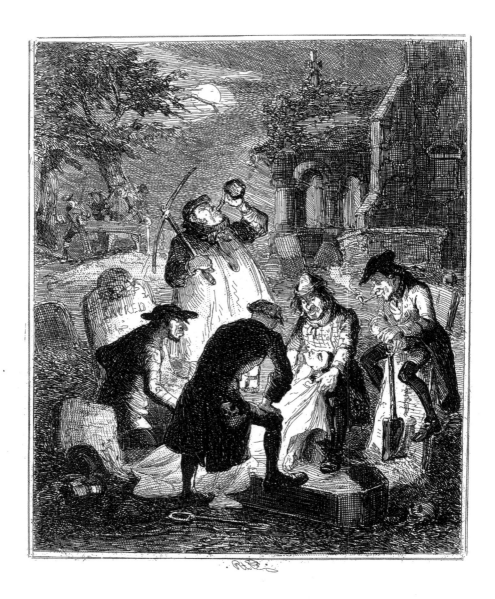

Resurrectionists

Bodysnatching was a serious
problem in early nineteenth-
century Ireland as anatomists
paid graverobbers handsomely
for securing fresh corpses.

pupils, meaning that 1,500 bodies had to be found from somewhere to keep up with demand. In the 1820s, the leading anatomist at Trinity College, James McCartney, called for the establishment of a body donation system. In the meantime, he continued to pay for fresh corpses, and it remains common on the campus to still discover buried bodies dating from that time. Public antipathy increased during the 1820s, the very same time that Dublin's global reputation for medical advancement ascended. Some newspaper accounts recorded bodies being stolen at wakes and mourners being held at gunpoint at graveyards while the dead body was taken. Major shootouts occurred at the old Merrion Cemetery in 1828 and at Glasnevin in 1830. An armed militia was called in temporarily to protect Bully's Acre, although the guards went rogue and became bodysnatchers themselves. McCartney remained largely oblivious to public feeling on the matter.[12]

The most notorious bodysnatchers were William Burke and William Hare, two men from the north of Ireland who operated in Edinburgh, which, like Dublin, was a major medical centre. Already in the 1820s, the residents of Edinburgh had taken to the streets in protest at increasing incidences of grave robbing. Grieving families hired guards to watch over graves, and watchtowers were built in some cemeteries. Wealthier families placed an impenetrable iron cage around their graves. Local anatomists started to entertain other options for securing dead bodies.

The fresher the corpse, the more money anatomists were willing to pay. Decayed, decomposed bodies were less useful anatomical specimens. Burke and Hare sped up the whole process by murdering 16 unfortunate victims and then selling their suspiciously fresh bodies to famed Edinburgh anatomist Robert Knox. They had first come up with the idea when a man died in their lodging house, and the pair decided to sell the corpse to pay off some debts. They were delighted to discover that Knox was willing to hand over £7 10s, a huge amount to two men who lived their poverty-stricken lives cobbling old shoes. When another lodger fell ill with fever, Burke and Hare smothered her. This time, they received £10. Fifteen more people, including 12 women, 2 disabled youths and

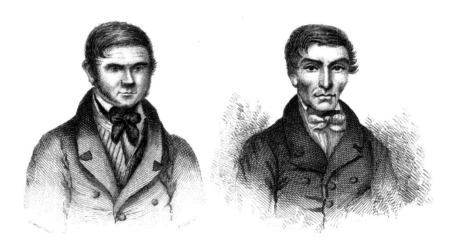

Above William Burke and William Hare, from the north of Ireland, were notorious for selling the corpses of their murder victims to anatomist Robert Knox at the Edinburgh Medical School.

Opposite William Burke's body was dissected after death and remains on display in Edinburgh.

an elderly man, were similarly murdered before the killers' source of income was discovered. All were poor vagrants or street folk, lured to their deaths by promises of drink and hospitality.

The story went public when an old lady's body was discovered in the straw of Burke's bed. Margaret Docherty had travelled to Edinburgh from Co. Donegal searching for her long-lost son. While she was begging in a gin shop, Burke noticed her and invited her home to eat. Margaret was murdered the same night, stripped and hidden in a straw bed until an opportune moment would arrive to package her body and deliver it to Knox. Other guests noticed her disappearance, and the pair's dastardly deeds were discovered.

Public outrage ensued. The police struggled to find decisive evidence that Burke and Hare had definitely committed the murder. To save his own neck, Hare provided evidence against Burke, confessing to 16 murders. Burke was hanged and dissected on 28 January 1829. As part of a punishment that has stretched on for two centuries, his skeleton remains grotesquely displayed at the Anatomical Museum, Edinburgh Medical School. Hare was escorted out of town and told to make his way to the English border. His fate remains uncertain. Knox's culpability was fiercely discussed in public and medical circles, but he was not asked to give evidence at Burke's trial. This caused public resentment and disbelief among working-class families, who had borne the brunt of the anatomists' work for decades.

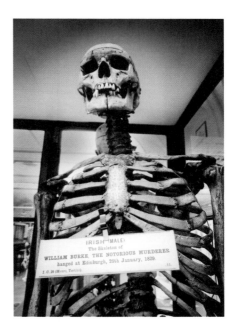

The murders raised public awareness of the need for bodies for medical research and encouraged discussion about the most appropriate sources. In 1832, the Anatomy Act was passed, which authorised workhouses to hand over unclaimed or abandoned corpses to the medical schools. A body was considered 'unclaimed' if relatives or friends did not arrive to identify it within 48 hours after death. For poorer communities, the association of workhouses with dissection, on top of the dreaded pauper's grave and the increasingly punitive ethos of these institutions, added further insult to injury and caused them to cast considerable suspicion on the doctors' morbid curiosity with their corpses.[13]

KEENERS

Until the mid-twentieth century, keeners attended Irish wakes. These were women paid (usually with money and whiskey) to wail and cry while mourners gathered around the deceased's body in the family home. Professional keeners travelled from funeral to funeral, with the ideal gig being a wealthy person's funeral. Traditionally, people in Ireland refrained from keening the dead until they were fairly certain that the soul had departed the body. No tears were to be shed until the body was laid out by a family member or neighbour. It was thought that the devil's dogs lay in wait for passing souls and might be roused from their sleep if keening took place too early. Once the body was laid out, danger had passed, and the keening might begin. Up to four keeners might be present, positioned around the corpse.

Keeners stood over the corpse and released a terrible wail. Their singing was deliberately off-note, producing an unsettling sound that mimicked the aching emotions of loss and grief. Their hands pounded frantically on their sides and hammered on the coffin. Keeners convulsed wildly, crying out in a spasm of all-consuming grief. These women might not have known the deceased, but this didn't matter much. Their role was to express personal loss when family members were still in shock or feeling unable, or unwilling, to articulate their confused feelings in public.

In Irish mythology, banshees sung keening laments. Keeners were essentially banshees in human form. The tradition features in Irish literature dating back to the eighth century. The Irish cultural revival became interested in keeners as they seemed to offer a tangible link between ancient and modern Ireland. Their mournful songs chimed through the millennia, providing another portal into long-gone times.

In the seventeenth century, the Church made keening punishable by excommunication. Priests were empowered to whip and beat keeners. Like so many other things that held deep meaning for the Irish, the Catholic Church made concerted efforts following independence to decisively stamp keening

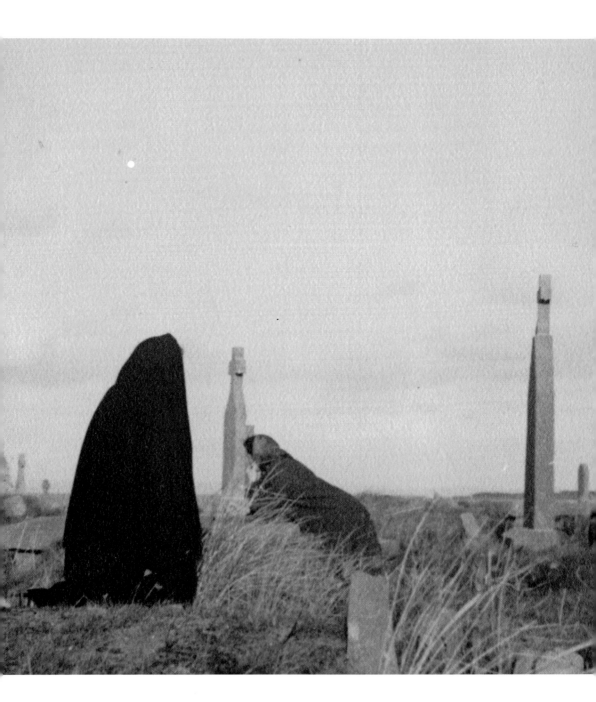

The keening tradition
remained popular
in Ireland until the
twentieth century.

out once and for all. To the Church, the practice seemed offensive and pagan, not the sort of thing wanted in the new Ireland. Much to the chagrin of priests, keeners drew attention away from the priests' role in praying over a body. Worse still for the Church, women threatened to overshadow their own sermons.

Twentieth-century priests still whipped and beat keeners while their singing was in full flow. Folklorist Seán Ó Súilleabháin recalls his father telling him about a funeral in the parish of Tuosist, south Co. Kerry:

> The parish priest, on horseback, met the funeral near Derreen, a few miles from the graveyard, and rode at its head along the road. As soon as he heard the three women howl loudly, he turned his horse about and trotted back until he reached them, where they sat on the coffin. He started to lash them with his whip as the cart passed by and ordered them to be silent.
>
> This they did, but on reaching the graveyard, they again took up their wailings, whereupon the priest forced them down from the coffin with his whip. They were afraid to enter the graveyard to howl at the graveside. That put an end to the hiring of keening women in that parish.[14]

Priests alleged that keeners were altogether tuneless, but people who actually understood music sprang to their defence by claiming that the music had structure provided by banging on the coffin, raw unearthly emotion, repeated motifs and elements of songs. Singing was carefully structured to allow feelings to flow. The vocals were a disciplined, powerful expression of the various stages of mourning, and also part of an oral culture too readily disregarded as non-modern.[15]

The lyrics, sung in Irish, were also beautiful and sophisticated, as evidenced in this translation made in the 1810s by antiquary T. Crofton Croker:

> Cold and silent is thy bed. Damp is the blessed dew of night, but the sun will bring warmth and heat in the morning and dry up

the dew. But thy heart cannot feel heat from the morning sun. No more will the print of your footsteps be seen in the morning dew, on the mountains of Ivera, where you have so often hunted the fox and the hare, ever foremost amongst young men. Cold and silent is now thy bed.

My sunshine you were. I loved you better than the sun itself, and when I see the sun going down in the west, I think of my boy and of my black night of sorrow, Like the rising sun, he had a red glow on his cheek. He was as bright as the sun at midday, but a dark storm came on, and my sunshine was lost to me for ever. My sunshine will never again come back. No! My boy cannot return. Cold and silent is his bed.[16]

However, the Church disliked the absence of a Christian sense of consolation or references to an afterlife. The keener's songs emitted grief, and grief alone. No hope. No God.

HUNGER STRIKES

In 1981, 10 men purposely starved themselves to death in a Northern Irish prison, attracting international attention. By then, the Troubles had been dragging on for 13 years. The 1981 hunger strikes marked the culmination of five years of prison protests by Irish republican prisoners which had started in 1976 when Kieran Nugent began his blanket protest. Denied political prisoner status, Nugent refused to wear a prison uniform and went naked (or wore only a blanket).

Two years later, the blanket protest was still underway, but few people outside the prison cared what Nugent and others wore (or not). The prisoners decided to escalate into a dirty protest. From 1978, prisoners refused to wash and smeared their excrement across the walls of their cells. They demanded the right not to wear a prison uniform or do prison work, free association with other prisoners, increased visiting rights and full restoration of remission lost through the protest. Initially, the protest received little attention. Even the IRA were not particularly interested. The protest attracted more support once Tomás Ó Fiaich, the Roman Catholic Archbishop of Armagh, visited the prison and condemned the conditions there and when MP Bernadette McAliskey led the National H-Block/Armagh Committee. Still, the prisoners thought a more effective means of protest had to be found.

Some people trace fasting as a form of protest back to ancient Ireland, and specifically the Brehon Laws. Aggrieved individuals protested against people who refused to pay their debts by publicly fasting outside their home. Those who owed an unpaid debt feared this tactic, though the process of death from hunger was rarely allowed to run its course as a protestor's death was feared to have magical consequences. In the early twentieth century, interest was renewed in the ancient Irish tactic of protesting by refusing to eat when literary figures including W.B. Yeats began writing about it. In some ways, the idea of hunger striking shared similarities with the blood sacrifice so revered by Patrick Pearse and others. Metaphorically, in modern Ireland, Britain was the aggressor against whom the Irish needed to fast to make their point clear.[17]

Through the decade of conflict that marked the 1910s–20s, numerous imprisoned Irish went on hunger strike. While acknowledging the pre-Christian roots of the practice, Irish republicans had a more immediate influence: suffragettes campaigning for women's right to vote. Between 1909 and 1914, hundreds of imprisoned suffragettes across Britain and Ireland went on hunger strike, much to the annoyance of the Home Office and the prison authorities, who decided to brutally feed them using stomach tubes forced down their throats. At Mountjoy Prison in Dublin, medical officer Raymond Granville Dowdall gleefully force-fed a number of suffragettes and labour leaders during the 1913 Dublin Lockout.

Dowdall is far better known for causing the death of Thomas Ashe in 1917. A stomach tube is difficult to insert. If it goes down the wrong way, the tube might snake through the windpipe into the lungs, without the doctors and nurses realising. When the liquid food is then poured in, a painful death from pneumonia results. The physical trauma of being force-fed can also aggravate heart conditions, and this seems to have been the case with Ashe. Ashe was a prominent IRA man, having played a leading role in events of the 1916 Rising outside of Dublin. His death caused a huge international controversy, being seen as further evidence of British brutality. A huge funeral procession took place which ran from City Hall to Glasnevin Cemetery.

After Ashe died, the government largely abandoned force-feeding, but this meant leaving hunger strikers alone to starve themselves to death. In 1920, this happened to the Lord Mayor of Cork, Terence MacSwiney. At the time, it was thought that prisoners could last only a week without food, two at best, before dying. MacSwiney proved them wrong. Unexpectedly, his fast in London's Brixton Prison lasted 74 days before he passed away. The world watched on, increasingly disgusted with Britain's behaviour in Ireland during the War of Independence. Meanwhile in Cork City Gaol, Michael Fitzgerald died after a 67-day fast. James Murphy died there after 76 days, on the very same day that MacSwiney died.

During much of the twentieth century, hunger strikes were actually far more common in British prisons than Irish ones. As well as the suffragettes, conscientious objectors staged hunger strikes during the First World War: Manchester silver engraver Emmanuel Ribeiro was force-fed for a staggering 17 months. During the Cold War, pacifists also regularly went on hunger strike. Over 800 convicted prisoners in Britain protested by fasting between 1913 and 1940, although the vast majority resumed eating after a brief bout of force-feeding.

Between 1973 and 1974, two Northern Irish republicans, sisters Dolours and Marian Price, attracted international sympathy when they were force-fed for six months in Brixton Prison. However, another force-feeding, that of Michael Gaughan, whose hunger strike in Parkhurst Prison on the Isle of Wight had gone virtually unnoticed, led to an excruciating death from pneumonia after milk and Complan were accidentally poured into his lungs.[18]

Force-feeding was abandoned in Britain and Ireland. Internationally, the World Medical Association formally condemned the practice, largely in response to controversies involving Northern Irish prisoners. The official policy became offering a hunger striker food but letting them starve if they refused to eat it.

In the Northern Irish prisons of 1980, hunger striking was called upon yet again as a progression from the ineffectual blanket and dirty protests. On 27 October, republican prisoners in the Maze/Long Kesh Prison, situated on the outskirts of Lisburn, went on hunger strike. Of the 148 Volunteers who signed up, only 7 were selected, the same number of men who had signed the 1916 Proclamation. In December, 3 prisoners in Armagh Women's Prison joined the strike. As Seán McKenna lapsed in and out of consciousness, fearsome British Prime Minister Margaret Thatcher started to feel edgy and presented the prisoners with a 30-page settlement document that appeared to concede to their demands. In reality, it didn't. McKenna's life was saved, and his hunger strike ended after 53 days, but the hunger strikers had been duped.

In 1981, the furious prisoners tried again. A second hunger strike commenced on 1 March when Bobby Sands refused food. Unlike the first strike, prisoners joined the protest at staggered intervals, meaning that the hunger strike might go on indefinitely. A seemingly endless supply of volunteers would join as other protestors passed away from the effects of hunger, placing overwhelming pressure on Thatcher. Even people opposed to IRA bombings and militancy were shocked by her adamant refusal to give in. In a curious, and unexpected, twist of events, Fermanagh and South Tyrone MP Frank Maguire died five days into Sands' hunger strike. Sands stood in the by-election, despite being in prison, and won a seat in the House of Commons. Thatcher was now threatening to condemn an elected official to death. Still, she would not budge. Famously, she said 'crime is crime is crime. It is not political'. The world was shocked by her intransigence.

On 5 May, Sands died after 66 days of hunger striking. The government dressed this up as deliberate suicide, but Thatcher could have intervened to save his life if she had wished. Instead, she commented that 'Mr Sands was a convicted criminal. He chose to take his own life. It was a choice that his organisation did not allow to many of its victims.' As the months passed, nine further hunger strikers died. Only in July did the protest begin to crumble when family members began to intervene, asking for medical treatment to save the lives of their sons. Perhaps they sensed that Thatcher was more than willing for the hunger strikes to go on forever. For close relatives, further deaths seemed pointless. The hunger strikes were finally called off on 3 October. The prisoners won some partial concessions. However, the deaths had not been altogether in vain. Sands' electoral victory encouraged Sinn Féin to move towards electoral politics. Eventually, in 2022, Sinn Féin received more votes than the Democratic Unionist Party, a historical turn of events.[19]

Bobby Sands died on hunger strike in 1981 at the Maze Prison/Long Kesh, causing international outrage at Margaret Thatcher's stubbornness.

POSTSCRIPT

As all these turbulent historical events took place, Clonycavan Man remained undisturbed, his preserved remains submerged deep below the surface of the waterlogged bogs of Co. Meath until 2003. If he miraculously materialised somehow today, what would he make of us? Would he see many similarities between us and him? And what would he think if he read this book and discovered all that had happened since his violent passing thousands of years ago? Once perhaps a prominent king or ruler himself, he might identify with the countless leaders and rulers who took his place, endlessly vying for control of parts of the land, sometimes even the whole island itself.

Our physical appearance wouldn't have changed too much, although Clonycavan Man might notice a greater preponderance of red hair than in his own time. He might be thankful that the Irish people's enthusiasm for sacrifice and beheading had waned, given his own gruesome end. If he had lived in the twenty-first century, he would probably have had a much longer life. Nonetheless, violence and bloodshed, usually to declare ownership of some territory, remained familiar across Irish history, as it still does today. Perhaps he might sympathise with noble beliefs such as blood sacrifice that permeated Irish history or have seen similarities in conflict between Catholics and Protestants and the intertribal rivalry of his own days. Clonycavan Man might resent hearing about the centuries of British influence in Ireland, but he was a man of the world with international connections, so he might not feel overly surprised.

Clonycavan Man would no doubt be fascinated by our hospitals, medical technologies and ability to cure many diseases. Particularly impressive to him would be the extensive reorganisation of global society that allowed us to survive through the COVID-19 pandemic. None of this would have been possible in his time. But what of all the fiddling around with human skulls and organs that has added such a grotesque element to modern medicine? Would he have been scared or fascinated by physical disabilities such as giantism or dwarfism? Would there be obvious similarities in how Irish society, ancient and modern, shunned those who appeared physically and mentally different? While hunger is still common across Ireland (nowadays known as 'food poverty'), mass starvation is not, and Clonycavan Man would no doubt be thankful for reawakening in a (western) world free from failed harvests and devastating famines.

Despite the obvious differences between our society and his own, Clonycavan Man would observe that we still fall in love, marry, have sex, give birth, speak, hear, dance and play sports in much the same way, even if different social customs and restrictions surround the various ways in which we use our bodies. We have faith and beliefs, just like he did, although the Catholic religion that dominates much of Ireland would have seemed very different, perhaps even fundamentally opposed, to the more liberal society of Celtic Ireland. Perhaps he would have been delighted that nineteenth and twentieth-century revivalists developed such a deep fascination for the Ireland that existed before the British came, just as we would be fascinated if we were able to listen to his stories of long ago.

ACKNOWLEDGEMENTS

I wish to thank Pauline Miller, Katie Powell, Sarah Miller and Miriam Trevor for their ongoing support. I am grateful for the ongoing enthusiasm within the School of History at Ulster University for my ideas, even the off-beat ones.

At the university, I wish to thank Ian Thatcher, Conor Heffernan, Gerard Leavey, Robert McNamara, Justin Magee, Kyle Hughes, Mark Benson, Rebecca Watterson, Michael Kinsella, Hannah Brown and Rebecca Brown. Further afield, I would like to thank Ida Milne, Bryce Evans, Máirtín Mac Con Iomaire and Rhianne Morgan.

While writing this book, I made extensive use of the Linen Hall Library, Belfast, whose staff were always helpful and supportive. I also wish to thank collaborators at National Museums Northern Ireland, the Northern Ireland War Memorial, the Healthcare Library of Northern Ireland, Northern Ireland Screen and EastSide Partnership.

I particularly wish to thank the team at Gill for helping to me develop my ideas for this book and bring the project into fruition.

Finally, I wish to thank Laura Garland for her ongoing support and love.

ENDNOTES

INTRODUCTION

1   'Clonycavan Man – a Bog Body.' *Meath History Hub with Noel French*, meathhistoryhub.ie/clonycavan-man-a-bog-body/. Accessed 22 Mar. 2024.
2   See, among others, Miranda Aldhouse-Green, *Bog Bodies Uncovered: Solving Europe's Ancient Mystery* (London: Thames and Hudson, 2015); Melanie Giles, *Bog Bodies: Face-to-Face with the Past* (Manchester: Manchester University Press, 2020).
3   Yair Field, Evan A. Boyle, Natalie Telis et al., 'Detection of Human Adaptation during the past 2000 Years', *Science*, 354 (2016), 760–4.
4   Francis Fukuyama, *Our Post-Human Future: Consequences of the Biotechnology Revolution* (London: Profile, 2006).
5   Roger Cooter and John V. Pickstone (eds), *Medicine in the Twentieth Century* (London: Routledge, 2000).
6   Richard Chambers, *A State of Emergency: The Story of Ireland's COVID Crisis* (London: Mudlark, 2022).

CHAPTER ONE

1   Daniel E. Lieberman, Brandeis M. McBratney and Gail Krovitz, 'The Evolution and Development of Cranial Form in *Homo Sapiens*', *Proceedings of the Natural Academy of Sciences*, 99 (2002), 1134–9.
2   Anthony C. Little, Benedict C. Jones and Lisa M. DeBruine, 'The Many Faces of Research on Face Perception', *Philosophical Transactions of the Royal Society B: Biological Sciences*, 366 (2011), 1634–7; Nicholas O. Rule, 'Introduction to the Special Issue on Face Perception', *Current Directions in Psychological Science*, 26 (2017), 211.
3   'Clonycavan Man – a Bog Body.' *Meath History Hub with Noel French*, meathhistoryhub.ie/clonycavan-man-a-bog-body/. Accessed 22 Mar. 2024.
4   Lady Moira, 'Particulars Relative to a Human Skeleton and the Garments that were Found thereon when Dug Out of a Bog at the Foot of Drumkeragh, a Mountain in the County Down', *Archaeologia*, 7 (1785), 90–110.
5   William R. Wilde, 'On the Antiquities and Human Remains Found in the County of Down in 1870 and Described by the Countess of Moira in the *Archaeologia* Volume Seven', *Proceedings of the Royal Irish Academy*, 9 (1864–6), 101–4.
6   Jon C. Henderson, *Settlement and Identity in the First Millennium BC* (London: Routledge, 2007); Francis Pryor, *Britain BC: Life in Britain and Ireland before the Romans* (London: Harper Perennial, 2003).
7   'Clonycavan Man – a Bog Body.' *Meath History Hub with Noel French*, meathhistoryhub.ie/clonycavan-man-a-bog-body/. Accessed 22 Mar. 2024.
8   James Owen. 'Murdered "Bog Men" Found with Hair Gel, Manicured Nails.' *Science*, 17 Jan. 2006, www.nationalgeographic.com/science/article/ireland-ancient-bog-men-science. Accessed 22 Mar. 2024.
9   'Clonycavan Man – a Bog Body.' *Meath History Hub with Noel French*, meathhistoryhub.ie/clonycavan-man-a-bog-body/. Accessed 22 Mar. 2024.
10   'Kingship & Sacrifice – a New Theory of Sacrifice.' *National Museum of Ireland*, www.museum.ie/en-IE/Collections-Research/Irish-Antiquities-Division-Collections/Collections-List-(1)/Iron-Age/Kingship-Sacrifice-A-New-Theory-of-Sacrifice. Accessed 22 Mar. 2024.
11   Charles A. Coulombe, *The Pope's Legion: The Multinational Fighting Force That Defended the Vatican* (Basingstoke: St Martin's, 2008).
12   'Are the Irish a Red-Haired Race?', *Donahoe's Monthly Magazine*, 28 (June 1892), 563–4.
13   A.G. Richey, *A Short History of the Irish People* (Dublin: Hodges, Figgis and Co., 1887), 26.
14   Jacky Colliss Harvey, *Red: A Natural History of the Redhead* (London: Allen and Unwin, 2015), 1–2.
15   Jonathan Swift, *Gulliver's Travels* (Oxford: Oxford University Press, 2005 [1726]). See also Donald T. Torchiana, 'Jonathan Swift, the Irish and the Yahoos: The Case Reconsidered', *Philological Quarterly*, 54 (1975), 195–212.
16   Brenda Ayres and Sarah E. Maier, *A Vindication of the Redhead: The Typology of Red Hair through the Literary and Visual Arts* (Basingstoke: Palgrave Macmillan, 2021), 6–8.
17   Charles de Kay, 'Fairies and Druids of Ireland', *Century Illustrated Monthly Magazine*, 37 (1889), 591–9.
18   Francecsa Speranza Wilde, *Ancient Legends, Mystic Charms and Superstitions of Ireland* (Boston: Ticknor & Co., 1887), 21, 158, 161.
19   Plympton Southwick, Albert. *Wisps of Wit and Wisdom.* (New York: A. Lovell, 1892), 127.
20   'Irish Fairy Lore', *New Monthly Magazine*, 122 (1861), 329–36 on 333.
21   See, among others, Micheál Ó Siochrú, *God's Executioner: Oliver Cromwell and the Conquest of Ireland* (London: Faber and Faber, 2009); Martyn Bennett, Raymond Gillespie and Scott Spurlock (eds), *Cromwell and Ireland: New Perspectives* (Liverpool: Liverpool University Press, 2020).
22   Sarah Covington, *The Devil from Over the Sea: Remembering and Forgetting Oliver Cromwell in Ireland* (Oxford: Oxford University Press, 2022), 233–4.

23   C. Parish, 'The Posthumous History of Oliver
     Cromwell's Head', in Derek Edward Dawson
     Beales and Hugh Barr Nisbet (eds) *Historical Essays
     in Commemoration of the Quatercentenary* Suffolk:
     Boydell Press, 1996, 105–10; Jonathan Fitzgibbons,
     Cromwell's Head (London: Bloomsbury, 2008);
     Frances Larson, *Severed: A History of Heads Found and
     Lost* (London: Granta, 2014), xiii–xiv.

24   Larson, *Severed*, 89.

25   'Beheaded Chicken Calmly Lives On', *Salt Lake
     Tribune* (19 September 1945), 17.

26   Frances Larson. 'What a Beheading Feels Like:
     The Science, the Gruesome Spectacle -- and Why
     We Can't Look Away.' *Salon*, Salon.com, 3 Feb. 2015,
     www.salon.com/2015/02/03/what_a_beheading_
     feels_like_the_science_the_gruesome_spectacle_
     and_why_we_cant_look_away/. Accessed 22 Mar.
     2024.

27   Matthew D. Turner, '"The Most Gentle of
     Lethal Methods": The Question of Retained
     Consciousness Following Decapitation', *Cureus*, 15
     (2023).

28   See Tobias Cheung, 'Limits of Life and Death:
     Legallois's Decapitation Experiments', *Journal of the
     History of Biology*, 46 (2013), 283–313.

29   K. Kongara, A.E. McIlhone, N.J. Kells and C.B.
     Johnson, 'Electroencephalographic Evolution of
     Decapitation of the Anaesthetised Rat', *Laboratory
     Animals*, 48 (2014), 15–19.

30   Aine Foley. *Who Was Murcod Ballagh?* irishplearolls.
     blogspot.com/2015/06/who-was-murcod-ballagh.
     html. Accessed 22 Mar. 2024.

31   Elizabeth Brewer, *From Cuchulainn to Gawain: Sources
     and Analogues of Sir Gawain and the Green Knight*
     (Totowa: Rowman and Littlefield, 1973), 8; B.K.
     Martin, 'The Medieval Irish Stories about Bricriu's
     Feast and Mac Dathó's Pig', *Parergon*, 10 (1992), 71–93

32   Niamh Carty, '"The Halved Heads": Osteological
     Evidence for Decapitation in Medieval Ireland',
     Papers from the Institute of Archaeology, 25 (2015), 1–20.

33   Thomas Charles-Edwards, *Early Christian Ireland*
     (Cambridge: Cambridge University Press, 2008).

34   Barra Ó Donnabháin, 'The Social Lives of Severed
     Heads: Skull Collection and Display in Medieval
     and Early Modern Ireland', in Michelle Bonogofsky
     (ed.), *The Bioarchaeology of the Human Head* (Miami:
     University Press of Florida, 2011), 122–38.

35   See, among others, Clare Downham, *Medieval
     Ireland* (Cambridge: Cambridge University Press,
     2018).

36   Carty, '"The Halved Heads"'.

37   Quoted in Barra Ó Donnabháin, 'Monuments
     of Shame: Some Probable Trophy Heads from
     Medieval Dublin', *Archaeology Ireland*, 9 (1995), 12–15
     on 13.

38   David Edwards, 'The Escalation of Violence in

39   Steven Ellis, *Ireland in the Age of Tudors, 1447–1603:
     English Expansion and the End of Gaelic Rule* (London:
     Routledge, 1995).

40   Barra Ó Donnabháin, 'Monuments of Shame: Some
     Probable Trophy Heads from Medieval Dublin',
     Archaeology Ireland, 9 (Winter 1995), 12–15 on 14.

41   Patricia Palmer, '"An Headless Ladie" and "A
     Horseloade of Heades": Writing the Beheading',
     Renaissance Quarterly, 60 (2007), 25–57.

42   David Edwards, '"Some Days Two Heads, and Some
     Days Four"', *History Ireland*, 17 (2009), 18–21.

43   Diodorus Siculus, *History*, 5.29.

44   Strabo, *Geographica*, IV.4.5.

45   Barry Cunliffe, *Druids: A Very Short Introduction*
     (Oxford: Oxford University Press, 2010), 71–2.

46   Palmer, '"An Headless Ladie"'.

47   Victor Gatrell, *The Hanging Tree: Execution and the
     English People, 1770–1868* (Oxford: Oxford University
     Press, 1994).

48   James Kelly, 'Punishing the Dead: Execution and
     the Executed Body in Eighteenth-Century Ireland',
     in Richard Ward, *A Global History of Execution and the
     Criminal Corpse* (Basingstoke: Palgrave Macmillan,
     2015), 37–70.

49   Ó Donnabháin, 'Monuments of Shame', 15.

50   For a recent biography see Micháél Ó Siochrú, *God's
     Executioner: Oliver Cromwell and the Conquest of Ireland*
     (London: Faber and Faber, 2008).

51   Sean O'Callaghan, *To Hell or Barbados: The Ethnic
     Cleansing of Ireland* (Dublin: Brandon, 2001); Liam
     Hogan, Laura McAtackney and Matthew C. Reilly,
     'The Irish in the Anglo-Caribbean: Servants or
     Slaves?', *History Ireland*, 24 (2016); Finola O'Kane and
     Ciaran O'Neill (eds), *Ireland, Slavery and the Caribbean*
     (Manchester: Manchester University Press, 2022).

52   Catrien Santing and Barbara Baert, 'Introduction',
     in Catrien Santing, Barbara Baert and Anita
     Traninger (eds), *Disembodied Heads in Medieval and
     Early Modern Culture* (Leiden: Brill, 2013), 2–3.

53   Larson, *Severed*, 137–42.

54   Alfred C. Haddon, *Head-Hunters: Black, White and
     Brown* (London: Methuen & Co., 1901).

55   Haddon, *Head-Hunters*, 394–5.

56   For an influential critique of this, see Stephen Jay
     Gould, *The Mismeasure of Man* (New York: W.W.
     Norton & Co., 1981).

57   Franz Joseph Gall, *On the Functions of the Brain and
     Each of Its Parts* (Boston: Marsh, Capen and Lyon,
     1835).

58   Larson, *Severed*, 172–3.

59   Larson, *Severed*, 176–7.

60   Alfred Cort Haddon, 'Studies in Irish Craniology:

The Aran Islands, Co. Galway', *Proceedings of the Royal Irish Academy*, 2 (1891–3), 759–67 on 759.

61 John Grattan, 'Notes on the Human Remains Discovered within the Round Towers of Ulster', *Ulster Journal of Archaeology*, 6 (1858), 27–39 and 221–46; Johnson Symington, 'John Grattan's Craniometer and Craniometric Methods', *Journal of Anatomy and Physiology*, 38 (1904), 259–74. For a thorough biography, see Alun Evans, 'John Grattan: Pharmacist, Phrenologist and Physical Anthropologist', *Ulster Journal of Archaeology*, 76 (2021), 109–44.

62 John Grattan, 'On the Importance to the Archaeologist and Ethnologist of an Accurate Mode of Measuring Human Crania', *Ulster Journal of Archaeology*, 1 (1853), 198–208.

63 'Descriptive Catalogue of Skulls and Caste of Skulls from Various Irish Sources, Collected by the late John Grattan, Esq., now the Property of the Belfast Natural History and Philosophical Society', *Proceedings of the Belfast Natural History and Philosophical Society for the Session 1873–74* (1873–4), 121–6.

64 John Beddoe, *The Races of Britain: A Contribution to the Anthropology of Western Europe* (Bristol: J.W. Arrowsmith, 1885), 1–3.

65 John Beddoe, 'The Kelts of Ireland', *Journal of Anthropology*, 1 (October 1870), 117–31.

66 A.C. Haddon, 'Peasant Life and Industries in Ireland', *Journal of the Society of Arts*, 44 (1896), 387–91 on 388–9.

67 Haddon, 'Studies in Irish Craniology', 759.

68 William Frazer, 'A Contribution to Irish Anthropology', *Journal of the Royal Society of Antiquarians of Ireland*, 1 (1891), 391–404.

69 Alfred C. Haddon, 'Studies in Irish Craniology: II. Inishbofin, Co. Galway', *Proceedings of the Royal Irish Academy (1889–1901)*, 3 (1893–1896), 311–16 on 311.

70 Alfred Cort Haddon, *The Races of Man* (Cambridge: Cambridge University Press, 1924), esp. 88.

71 Haddon, 'Studies in Irish Craniology', 760.

72 Scott Ashley, 'The Poetics of Race in 1890s Ireland: An Ethnography of the Aran Islands', *Patterns of Prejudice*, 35 (2001), 5–18 on 12.

73 Larson, *Severed*, 196.

74 Ashley, 'The Poetics of Race in 1890s Ireland', 16–17.

75 See also Sinéad Garrigan Matter, *Primitivism, Science and the Irish Revival* (Oxford: Oxford University Press, 2004); Maria McGarrity and Claire A. Culleton (eds), *Irish Modernism and the Irish Primitive* (Basingstoke: Palgrave, 2009).

76 Douglas Hyde, 'The Necessity for De-Anglicising Ireland', in Charles Gavan Duffy, George Sigerson and Douglas Hyde (eds), *The Revival of Irish Literature* (London: T. Fisher Unwin, 1894), 117–61.

77 See, among others, Timothy J. McMahon, *Grand Opportunity: The Gaelic Revival and Irish Society, 1893–1910* (New York: Syracuse University Press, 2008); Declan Kiberd and P.J. Mathews (eds), *Handbook of the Irish Revival: An Anthology of Irish Cultural and Political Writings, 1891–1922* (Dublin: Abbey Theatre Press, 2015); Caoimhín De Barra, *The Coming of the Celts, AD 1860* (Notre Dame: University of Notre Dame Press, 2018).

78 John Wilson Foster, 'The Western Island in the Irish Renaissance', *Studies: An Irish Quarterly Review*, 66 (1977), 261–74.

79 Greta Jones, 'Contested Territories: Alfred Cort Haddon, Progressive Evolutionism and Ireland', *History of European Ideas*, 24 (1998), 195–211.

80 John Millington Synge, *The Aran Islands* (Belfast: Blackstaff Press, 1988 [1906]), 32–3.

81 John Millington Synge, *The Playboy of the Western World: A Comedy in Three Acts* (Dublin: Maunsel, 1907), Act III.

82 Gregory Castle, *Modernism and the Celtic Revival* (Cambridge: Cambridge University Press, 2001), 112–13.

83 Charles R. Browne, 'The Ethnology of Inishbofin and Inishshark, County Galway', *Proceedings of the Royal Irish Academy*, 3 (1893–6), 317–70 on 321–2.

CHAPTER TWO

1 *Finn McCool: Irish Heroes* (History Nerds, 2022).

2 Dáithí Ó hÓgáin, *Fionn Mac Cumhail: Images of the Gaelic Hero* (Dublin: Gill & Macmillan, 1988).

3 Terri M. Roberts, *Fionn MacCool and the Salmon of Knowledge* (Dartmouth, Nova Scotia: Bradan Press, 2017).

4 Jacqueline Borsje and Fergus Kelly, *The Celtic Evil Eye and Related Mythological Motifs in Medieval Ireland* (Leuven: Peeters, 2012).

5 Agnes McMahon, *Celtic Way of Life* (Dublin: O'Brien Press, 1998), 72–9.

6 Jeffrey Gantz (ed.), *Early Irish Myths and Sagas* (London: Penguin, 1981), introduction.

7 Mark Williams, *Ireland's Immortals: A History of the Gods of Irish Myth* (Princeton: Princeton University Press, 2018).

8 Ronan McGreevy. 'Study Suggests Tall Tales of Irish Giants Had a Grain of Truth' *The Irish Times*, The Irish Times, 7 Jan. 2011, www.irishtimes.com/news/study-suggests-tall-tales-of-irish-giants-had-a-grain-of-truth-1.1276552. Accessed 22 Mar. 2024.

9 Niall O Ciosáin, *Print and Popular Culture in Ireland, 1750–1850* (Basingstoke: Palgrave Macmillan, 2016).

10 Glenn Hooper, *Travel Writing and Ireland, 1760–1860* (Basingstoke: Palgrave Macmillan, 2005).

11 Later books include G.N. Wright, *A Guide to the Giant's Causeway* (London: Baldwin Cradock and Joy, 1823).

12 Thomas Muinzer, 'The Giant', *Freckle Magazine*, 1 (2015).

13 Hilary Mantel, *The Giant, O'Brien* (New York: Fourth Estate, 1998).

14 This was originally recorded in Harvey Cushing, 'The Hypophysis Cerebri: Clinical Aspects of Hyperpituitarism and of Hypopituitarism', *Journal of the American Medical Association*, 53 (1909), 249–55.

15 Robert Chambers, *The Book of Days: A Miscellany of Popular Antiquities Volume Two* (London: W.R. Chambers, 1864), 325–7 on 326.

16 *London Magazine* (August 1752), 381; *Faulkner's Journal* (16 May 1760); Chambers, *The Book of Days*, 325–7; D.J. Cunningham, 'The Skeleton of the Irish Giant, Cornelius Magrath', *Transactions of the Royal Irish Academy*, 29 (1887–92), 553–612; H.R. Swanzy, 'Note of Defective Vision and other Ocular Derangements in Cornelius Magrath, the Irish Giant', *Proceedings of the Royal Irish Academy*, 3 (1893–96), 524–8; Breda Moloney *Cornelius McGrath, the Silvermines Giant*, www.ouririshheritage.org/wp-content/uploads/2021/06/1622915070953_Breda-Moloney-Cornelius-Mcgrath-Silvermines-Giant.pdf. Accessed 22 Mar. 2024.

17 Cunningham, 'The Skeleton of the Irish Giant', 553–612.

18 Chambers, *Book of Days*, 325–7; Edward J. Wood, *Giants and Dwarfs* (London: R. Bentley, 1868), 166–97; G. Frankcom and J.H. Musgrave, *The Irish Giant* (London: Duckworth, 1976).

19 *The Living Age*, 57 (1858), 89; 'O'Brien, The Irish Giant', *Cork Historical and Archaeological Society*, 2 (1896), 231–2 on 231.

20 'There Were Giants in Those Days', *Harper's Young People* (1 March 1892), 314–5.

21 Nadja Durbach, *Spectacle of Deformity: Freak Shows and Modern British Culture* (Berkeley: University of California Press, 2010).

22 '"He Did Not Want This": No Rest in Quest to End Display of Irish Giant.' *The Guardian*, Guardian News and Media, 14 Jan. 2023, www.theguardian.com/culture/2023/jan/14/he-did-not-want-this-one-mans-two-decade-quest-to-let-the-irish-giant-rest-in-peace. Accessed 22 Mar. 2024.

23 David Wolfe, 'TCDSU Council Passes Motion Calling for Burial of Remains of Eighteenth Century "Giant".' *Trinity News*, 6 Nov. 2022, trinitynews.ie/2022/11/tcdsu-council-passes-motion-calling-for-burial-of-remains-of-eighteenth-century-giant/. Accessed 22 Mar. 2024.

24 Roger Chatterton Newman, *Brian Boru: King of Ireland* (Cork: Mercier Press, 2011); Morgan Llywelyn, *1014: Brian Boru and the Battle for Ireland* (Dublin: O'Brien Press, 2014).

25 Nancy Hurrell, 'The "Brian Boru" Harp', *History Ireland*, 22 (2014).

26 Patrick Joyce, *The Origin and History of Irish Names of Places* (Dublin: McGlashan and Gill, 1875), 319.

27 John Carey, 'Tuath Dé', in John T. Koch (ed.), *Celtic Culture: A Historical Encyclopedia* (Santa Barbara: ABC Clio, 2006), 1693–7.

28 Carolyn White, *A History of Irish Fairies* (Dublin: Mercier Press, 1976).

29 White, *History of Irish Fairies*.

30 Diarmuid Arthur Mac Manus, *The Middle Kingdom: The Faerie World of Ireland* (London: Max Parrish, 1959).

31 Timothy Corrigan Correll, 'Believers, Sceptics and Charlatans: Evidential Rhetoric, the Irish Oral Narrative and Belief', *Folklore*, 116 (2005), 1–18.

32 Thomas Crofton Croker, *Fairy Legends and Traditions of the South of Ireland*, 2nd ed. (London: John Murray, 1825), 117–25.

33 Mac Manus, *The Middle Kingdom*, 23.

34 Elizabeth Andrews, *Ulster Folklore* (London: Elliot Stock, 1913), 1–2.

35 William Butler Yeats, *Fairies and Folk Tales of the Irish Peasantry* (London: Walter Scott, 1888), xii.

36 Mary Helen Thuente, *W.B. Yeats and Irish Folklore* (Dublin: Gill & Macmillan, 1980).

37 Jeremiah Curtin, *Irish Tales of the Fairies and the Ghost World* (Boston: Little, Brown and Company, 1895).

38 Ríonach Uí Ógáin, 'Music Learned from the Fairies', *Béaloideas*, 60/61 (1992–3), 197–214.

39 White, *History of Irish Fairies*, 57.

40 Daniel A. Binchy, 'The Saga of Fergus Mac Léti', *Ériu*, 16 (1955), 33–48.

CHAPTER THREE

1 Recent books include Peter Heather, *The Fall of the Roman Empire: A New History of Rome and the Barbarians* (Oxford: Oxford University Press, 2007).

2 Thomas Cahill, *How the Irish Saved Civilisation* (London: Hodder and Staughton, 1995), 164.

3 Vittorio di Martino, *Roman Ireland* (Cork: Collins Press, 2003).

4 Cahill, *How the Irish Saved Civilisation*, 151.

5 Liz Fitzpatrick, 'Raiding and Warrin in Monastic Ireland', *History Ireland*, 3 (1993).

6 Roy Flechner and Sven Meeder (eds), *The Irish in Early Medieval Europe: Identity, Culture and Religion* (London: Palgrave, 2017).

7 J.J. O'Meara (trans.), *The Voyage of St Brendan: Journey to the Promised Land* (Gerrards Cross: Colin Smythe, 1991); Tim Severin, *The Brendan Voyage: Across the Atlantic in a Leather Boat* (Dublin: Gill & Macmillan, 2005).

8 Timothy O'Neill, *The Irish Hand: Scribes and Their Manuscripts from the Earliest Times* (Cork: Cork University Press, 2014).

9 Cahill, *How the Irish Saved Civilisation*, 170.

10 William Reeves St Adamnan, *Prophecies, Miracles and Visions of St Columba (Columcille): First Abbot of Iona, AD 563–597* (Oxford: Clarendon Press, 1894).

11 Cahill, *How the Irish Saved Civilisation*, 181–2.

12 Cahill, *How the Irish Saved Civilisation*, 168.

13 Bernard Meehan, *The Book of Durrow: A Medieval Masterpiece at Trinity College Dublin* (Dublin: Town House, 1996); Rachel Moss, *The Book of Durrow* (Dublin: Trinity College Library, 2018).

14 Peter Brown, *The Book of Kells: Forty-Eight Pages and Details in Color from the Manuscript in Trinity College Dublin* (New York: Alfred A. Knopf, 1980); George Henderson, *From Durrow to Kells: The Insular Gospel Books, 650–800* (New York: Thames and Hudson, 1987); Heather Pulliam, *Word and Image in the Book of Kells* (Dublin: Four Courts Press, 2006).

15 For a recent biography, see Roy Flechner, *St Patrick Retold: The Legend and History of Ireland's Patron St* (Princeton: Princeton University Press, 2019). See also E.A. Thompson, *Who Was St Patrick?* (Woodbridge: Boydell Press, 1985); Liam de Paor, *St Patrick's World: The Christian Culture of Ireland's Apostolic Age* (Dublin: Four Courts Press, 1993); David Howlett (ed.), *The Book of Letters of St Patrick the Bishop* (Dublin: Four Courts Press, 1994); Cahill, *How the Irish Saved Civilisation*, 101–19; Thomas O'Laughlin, *St Patrick: The Man and his Works* (London: S.P.C.K., 1999); Thomas O'Laughlin, *Discovering St Patrick* (New York: Orbis, 2005).

16 Edna Barth, *Shamrocks, Harps, and Shillelaghs: The Story of the St Patrick's Day Symbols* (Dublin: Houghton Mifflin Harcourt, 2001 [1977]); Mike Cronin and Daryl Adair, *The Wearing of the Green: A History of St Patrick's Day* (London: Routledge, 2002).

17 Thomas Frances O'Rahilly, *The Two Patricks: A Lecture on the History of Christianity in Fifth-Century Ireland* (Dublin: Dublin Institute for Advanced Studies, 1942).

18 Cormac Bourke, 'The Shrine of St Patrick's Hand', *Irish Arts Review*, 4 (1987), 25–7.

19 Royal Society of Antiquarians of Ireland, *The Western Islands and the Antiquities of Galway, Athenry, Roscommon &c.* (Dublin: Hodges, Figgis and Co., 1897), 295–6; Sean McMahon, *The Story of the Claddagh Ring* (Boulder: Irish American Book Co., 1997), 27–42; Malachy McCourt, *The Claddagh Ring: Ireland's Cherished Symbol of Friendship, Loyalty and Love* (Philadelphia: Running Press, 2003), 50–61.

20 McCourt, *Claddagh Ring*, 40–4.

21 George Quinn, 'The Claddagh Ring', *The Mantle*, 13 (1970), 9–13; Ida Delamer, 'The Claddagh Ring', *Irish Arts Review*, 12 (1996), 181–7; Adrian James Martyn, *The Tribes of Galway, 1124–1642* (Self-published: Adrian Martyn, 2016); 'Claddagh Ring', in Judy Pearsall (ed.), *The Concise Oxford Dictionary* (Oxford: Oxford University Press, 2004); Seán McMahon, *Story of the Claddagh Ring* (Cork: Mercier Press, 2001).

22 Edward J. Wood, *The Wedding Day in All Ages and Countries Volume Two* (London: Richard Bentley, 1869), 55.

23 Linda May Ballard, *Forgetting Frolic: Marriage Traditions in Ireland* (Belfast: Institute of Irish Studies, 1998), 74.

24 Gillian Kenny, 'Anglo-Irish and Gaelic Marriage Laws and Traditions in Late Medieval Ireland', *Journal of Medieval History*, 32 (2006), 27–42.

25 Oliver P. Rafferty, 'Mixed Marriages in Pre-Independence Ireland', in Salvador Ryan (ed.), *Marriage and the Irish: A Miscellany* (Dublin: Wordwell, 2019), 172.

26 Fiona Fitzsimons, 'Bedding Ceremonies', *History Ireland*, 27 (January/February 2019).

27 Ballard, *Forgetting Frolic*.

28 Maria Luddy and Mary O'Dowd, *Marriage in Ireland, 1600–1925* (Cambridge: Cambridge University Press, 2020), chapter 6.

29 Maria Luddy, 'Abductions in Eighteenth- and Nineteenth-Century Ireland', in Ryan (ed.), *Marriage and the Irish*, 143–4.

30 Kenny, 'Anglo-Irish and Gaelic Marriage Laws'.

31 Janet Nolan, *Ourselves Alone: Women's Emigration from Ireland, 1885–1925* (Kentucky: University of Kentucky Press, 1989); Patrick O'Sullivan (ed.), *Irish Women and Irish Migration* (Leicester: Leicester University Press, 1995); Bernadette Whelan, 'Women on the Move: A Review of the Historiography of Irish Emigration to the USA, 1750–1900', *Women's History Review*, 24 (2015), 900–16.

32 'Result of Consanguineous Marriages', *Dublin Journal of Medical Science*, 75 (1883), 514–16.

33 Discussed in 'First-Cousin Marriages', *Knowledge: An Illustrated Magazine of Science* (15 June 1883), 357–8.

34 S.J. Kilpatrick, J.D. Mathers and A.C. Stevenson, 'The Importance of Population Fertility and Consanguinity Data being Available in Medico-Social Studies: Some Data on Consanguineous Marriages in Northern Ireland', *Ulster Medical Journal*, 24 (1955), 113–22.

35 Pollak, Sorcha. 'Every Irish Person Has More than 14,000 Living Relatives, Research Finds.' *The Irish Times*, 24 Apr. 2018, www.irishtimes.com/news/ireland/irish-news/every-irish-person-has-more-than-14-000-living-relatives-research-finds-1.3473134. Accessed 22 Mar. 2024.

36 Gráinne Healy, Brian Sheehan and Noel Whelan, *Ireland Says Yes: The Inside Story of How the Vote for Marriage Equality Was Won* (Dublin: Merrion Press, 2015); Sonja Tiernan, *The History of Marriage Equality in Ireland: A Social Revolution Begins* (Manchester: Manchester University Press, 2021).

37 'Flags used in Northern Ireland', Conflict Archive on the Internet (CAIN).

38 Francis John Byrne, *The Rise of the Uí Néill and the High-Kingship of Ireland* (Dublin: National University of Ireland, 1969).

39 Patricia Moir, 'The Red Hand of Ulster', *Worldview Magazine* (1975).

40 'Hand over Fist: The Red Hand of Ulster Still Has the Power to Divide'. *The Independent*, Independent Digital News and Media, 24 Apr. 2010, www.independent.co.uk/news/uk/politics/hand-over-fist-the-red-hand-of-ulster-still-has-the-power-to-divide-northern-ireland-1950412.html. Accessed 22 Mar. 2024.

41 Gareth Mulvenna, *Tartan Gangs and Paramilitaries* (Oxford: Oxford University Press, 2016).

CHAPTER FOUR

1 William H.E. Harcourt-Smith, 'The First Hominins and the Origins of Bipedalism', *Evolution: Education and Outreach*, 3 (2010), 333–40; Jeremy Desilva, *First Steps: How Upright Walking Made Us Human* (New York: HarperCollins, 2021).

2 Michael Cusack, 'A Word about Irish Athletics', *The Irishman* (11 October 1884).

3 T.H. Nally, *The Aonac Tailteann and the Tailteann Games: Their History and Ancient Associations* (Jesson Press, 2008).

4 Art Ó Maolfabhail, *Camán: Two Thousand Years of Hurling in Ireland* (Dundalk: Dundalgan Press, 1973); Ian Prior, *The History of Gaelic Games* (Belfast: Appletree Press, 1997); Seamus J. King, *A History of Hurling*, 2nd ed. (Dublin: Gill & Macmillan, 2005); Seamus J. King, *The Little Book of Hurling* (Cheltenham: History Press, 2020); Loren Berlin 'Irish Hurling: The Ball Moves 100 Miles per Hour. so Why Don't Goalkeepers Want to Wear Facemasks?' *Slate Magazine*, Slate, 13 Apr. 2011, slate.com/culture/2011/04/irish-hurling-the-ball-moves-100-miles-per-hour-so-why-don-t-goalkeepers-want-to-wear-facemasks.html. Accessed 22 Mar. 2024.

5 Anne Dolan, 'Killing and Bloody Sunday', *Historical Journal*, 49 (2006), 789–810; Michael Foley, *The Bloodied Field: Croke Park, Sunday 21 November 1920* (Dublin: O'Brien Press, 2014).

6 For broader context, see Michael T. Foy, *Michael Collins's Intelligence War: The Struggle between the British and the IRA, 1919-1921* (Stroud: History Press, 2006).

7 Neil Richardson, *A Coward If I Return, A Hero If I Fall: Stories of Irishmen in World War One* (Dublin: O'Brien Press, 2010).

8 Paul Taylor, *Heroes or Traitors? Experiences of Southern Irish Soldiers Returning from the Great War, 1919–1939* (Liverpool: Liverpool University Press, 2015); Michael Robinson, '"Nobody's Children?": The Ministry of Pensions and the Treatment of Disabled Great War Veterans in the Irish Free State, 1921–1939', *Irish Studies Review*, 25 (2017), 316–35; Anthony Farrell, '"A Forgotten Generation": Medical Care for Disabled Veterans of the First World War in Independent Ireland', *Irish Studies Review*, 29 (2021), 142–55.

9 Jane Leonard, 'Getting Them at Last: The IRA and Ex-Servicemen', in David Fitzpatrick (ed.), *Revolution? Ireland, 1917–23* (Dublin: Trinity History Workshop, 1990), 118–29.

10 John Horne, *Our War: Ireland and the Great War* (Dublin: RTÉ, 2008); Steven O'Connor, *Irish Officers in the British Forces, 1922–45* (Basingstoke: Palgrave Macmillan, 2014).

11 Marie Coleman, 'Military Service Pensions for Veterans of the Irish Revolution, 1916–1923', *War in History*, 20 (2013), 201–21.

12 Bureau of Military History, WS Ref 1283, Patrick Ormond, OC Republican Police, West Waterford, 1921, 23.

13 Bureau of Military History, WS Ref 1194, Bernard Sweeney, Member IV, Leitrim, 1917–19, Officer, IRA Leitrim, 1921, 6.

14 Bureau of Military History, WS Ref 1504, Seumas O'Meara, OC Athlone Brigade, IRA, 1921, 51.

15 Bureau of Military History, WS Ref 1336, Patrick Lennon, Member IV and IRA, Westmeath, 1917–21, 12–13.

16 Liam Kennedy, *They Shoot Children, Don't They? An Analysis of the Age and Gender of Victims of Paramilitary 'Punishments' in Northern Ireland*. Report to the Northern Ireland Committee against Terror and the House of Commons, 2001.

17 For medical perspectives on the Troubles, see James McKenna, Farhat Manzoor and Greta Jones, *Candles in the Dark: Medical Ethical Issues in Northern Ireland during the Troubles* (London: Nuffield Trust, 2009).

18 Michael Flatley, *Lord of the Dance: My Story* (London: Sidgwick and Jackson, 2006).

19 Helen Brennan, *The Story of Irish Dance* (Lanham: Rowman and Littlefield, 2022 [1999]), 16.

20 Breandán Breathnach, *Folk Music and Dances of Ireland* (Dublin: Educational Company of Ireland, 1971).

21 Nigel Boulliler, *Handed Down: Country Fiddling and Dancing in East and Central Down* (Newtownards: Ulster Historical Foundation, 2012).

22 Breathnach, *Folk Music and Dances*.

23 Catherine E. Foley, *Step Dancing in Ireland: Culture and History* (London: Routledge, 2013).

24 Arthur Young, *Arthur Young's Tour in Ireland (1776–1779)* (London: George Bell, 1892 [1780]), 147.

25 Brennan, *Story of Irish Dance*, 31–9.

26 John P. Cullinane, *Aspects of the History of Irish Céilí Dancing, 1897-1997* (Cork: John Cullinane, 1998).

27 Frank Whelan, *The Complete Guide to Irish Dance* (Belfast: Appletree, 2000).

28 Jim Smyth, 'Dancing, Depravity and all the Jazz: The Public Dance Halls Act of 1935', *History Ireland*, 2 (Summer 1993); Gearóid Ó hAllmhuráin, 'Dancing on the Hobs of Hell: Rural Communities in Clare

and the Dance Halls Act of 1935', *New Hibernia Review*, 9 (2005), 9–18; Barbara O'Connor, 'Sexing the Nation: Discourses of the Dancing Body in Ireland in the 1930s', *Journal of Gender Studies*, 14 (2005), 89–105.

CHAPTER FIVE

1   'Ancient Irish Sex Thirst Crushed by Church, Claims Australian TV Show'. *Irish Independent*, Irish Independent, 7 Aug. 2004, www.independent.ie/life/ancient-irish-sex-thirst-crushed-by-church-claims-australian-tv-show/26223324.html. See also Peter Cherici, *Celtic Sexuality: Power, Paradigms and Passions* (London: Duckworth, 1984). Accessed 22 Mar. 2024.

2   Patrick Power, *Sex and Marriage in Ancient Ireland* (Dublin and Cork: Mercier Press, 1976).

3   Salvador Ryan (ed.), *Marriage and the Irish: A Miscellany* (Dublin: Wordwell, 2019), 22.

4   Leanne Calvert, 'Your Marage Will Make a Change with Them All … When You Get Another Famely': Illegitimate Children, Parenthood and Siblinghood in Ireland, c.1759–1832', *English Historical Review*, 137 (2022), 1144–73.

5   *Calendar of the Justiciary Rolls* (London: HMSO, 1914), 1307.

6   Jörgen Hartogs and Findwyer. 'Sex and Scandal in Medieval Ireland.' *Irish History, Folklore and All That*, 16 Dec. 2014, irishhistoryfiles.wordpress.com/2014/12/16/sex-and-scandal-in-medieval-ireland/. Accessed 22 Mar. 2024.

7   Eamon Darcy, *The World of Thomas Ward: Sex and Scandal in Late Seventeenth-Century Co. Antrim* (Dublin: Four Courts Press, 2016).

8   Julie Peakman, *Peg Plunkett: Memoirs of a Whore* (London: Quercus, 2015).

9   Rónán Gearóid Ó Domhnaill, *Fadó: Tales of Lesser Known Irish History* (Kibworth: Matador, 2013), 207.

10 Maurice Curtis, *To Hell or Monto: The Story of Dublin's Most Notorious Districts* (Cheltenham: History Press, 2015).

11 Maria Luddy, *Prostitution and Irish Society, 1800–1940* (Cambridge: Cambridge University Press, 2007).

12 Glenn Chandler, *The Sins of Jack Saul: The True Story of Dublin Jack and the Cleveland Street Scandal* (Tolworth: Grosvenor House Publishing, 2016).

13 For an extensive list, see Edith M. Guest, 'Irish Sheela-na-Gigs in 1935', *Journal of the Royal Society of Antiquaries of Ireland*, 6 (1936), 107–29; 'Ireland's Síle Na Gig.' Ireland's Síle Na Gig, www.irelands-sheelanagigs.org/. Accessed 22 Mar. 2024. See also Maureen Concannon, *The Sacred Whore: Sheela Goddess of the Celts* (Cork: Collins Press, 2004).

14 John O'Donovan, *Ordnance Survey of Ireland: Letters: Tipperary Volume 1* (1839–40), 541–9.

15 Discussed in Barbara Freitag, *Sheela-na-Gigs:*

Unravelling an Enigma (London: Routledge, 2004), 17–18.

16 Freitag, *Sheela-na-Gigs*, 1.

17 Jørgen Andersen, *The Witch on the Wall: Medieval Erotic Sculpture in the British Isles* (Copenhagen: Rosenkilde and Bagger, 1977); James Jerman and Anthony Weir, *Images of Lust: Sexual Carvings on Medieval Churches* (London: T. Batsford, 1986).

18 Patricia Monaghan, *The Red-Haired Girl from the Bog: The Landscape of Celtic Myth and Spirit* (Novato: New World Library, 2010), chapter 2.

19 Andersen, *Witch on the Wall*.

20 Joanne McMahon and Jack Roberts, *The Sheela-na-Gigs of Ireland and Britain: The Divine Hag of the Catholic Celts – An Illustrated Guide* (Cork: Mercier Press, 2000); Jack Roberts, *Sheela-na-Gig: Sacred Celtic Images of Feminine Divinity* (Process, 2020).

21 Miriam Dexter and Starr Goode, 'The Sheela-na-Gigs, Sexuality and the Goddess in Ancient Ireland', *Irish Journal of Feminist Studies*, 4 (2002), 50–75.

22 Senan Molony, *The Phoenix Park Murders: Conspiracy, Betrayal and Retribution* (Dublin: Mercier Press, 2006).

23 Margery Brady, *The Love Story of Parnell and Katharine O'Shea* (Cork: Mercier Press, 1991), 12.

24 Quoted in Jane Jordan, *Kitty O'Shea: An Irish Affair* (Stroud: Sutton, 2005), 22–3.

25 Katharine Parnell [nee O'Shea], *Charles Stewart Parnell: His Love Story and Political Life* (London: Cassell and Co., 1914). Recent biographies include Myles Dungan, *The Captain and the King: William O'Shea, Parnell and Late Victorian Ireland* (Dublin: New Island, 2009); Paul Bew, *Enigma: A New Life of Charles Stewart Parnell* (Dublin: Gill, 2011).

26 Margaret Brady, *The Love Story of Yeats and Maud Gonne* (Cork: Mercier Press, 1998); Anthony J. Jordan, *The Yeats, Gonne, MacBride Triangle* (Dublin: Westport, 2000).

27 John Wilson Foster, 'Yeats and the Easter Rising', *Canadian Journal of Irish Studies*, 11 (1985), 21–34.

28 See, among others, Trevor Fisher, *Oscar and Bosie: A Fatal Passion* (Stroud: Sutton, 2002); Douglas Murray, *Bosie: A Biography of Lord Alfred Douglas* (London: Hodder and Stoughton, 2020).

29 For a broad overview across time, see Salvador Ryan (ed.), *Birth and the Irish: A Miscellany* (Dublin: Wordwell, 2021).

30 Eileen M. Murphy, '"The Child that is Born of One's Fair Body": Maternal and Infant Death in Medieval Ireland', *Childhood in the Past: An International Journal*, 14 (2021), 13–37.

31 Clodagh Tait, 'Safely Delivered: Childbirth, Wet Nursing, Gossip Feasts and Churching in Ireland, 1530–1690', *Irish Economic and Social History*, 30 (2003), 1–23.

32 Tait, 'Safely Delivered'.

33 T. Percy C. Kirkpatrick, *The Book of the Rotunda Hospital* (London: Adlard and Son, 1913); Julia Anne Bergin, 'Birth and Death in Nineteenth-Century Dublin's Lying-In Hospitals', in Elaine Farrell (ed.), *'She Said She Was in the Family Way': Pregnancy and Infancy in Modern Ireland* (London: Institute of Historical Research, 2012), 91–111.

34 Tait, 'Safely Delivered'; Clodagh Tait, '"Kindred Without End": Wet-Nursing, Fosterage and Emotion in Ireland, c.1550–1720', *Irish Economic and Social History*, 47 (2020), 10–35.

35 Gerard M. Fealy (ed.), *Care to Remember: Nursing and Midwifery in Ireland* (Cork: Mercier Press, 2001).

36 Ian Miller, *Reforming Food in Post-Famine Ireland: Medicine, Science and Improvement, 1845–1922* (Manchester: Manchester University Press, 2014), chapter 7.

37 Cara Delay, 'Women, Childbirth Customs and Authority in Ireland, 1850–1930', *Lilith: A Feminist History Journal*, 21 (2015), 6–18; Maryann Valiulis, 'Neither Feminist nor Flapper: The Ecclesiastical Construction of the Ideal Irish Woman', in Mary O'Dowd and Sabine Wichert (eds), *Chattel, Servant or Citizen? Women's Status in Church, State and Society* (Belfast: Institute of Irish Studies, 1995), 168–78.

38 Delay, 'Women, Childbirth Customs and Authority'.

39 Diarmaid Ferriter, *Judging Dev: A Reassessment of the Life and Legacy of Éamon De Valera* (Dublin: Royal Irish Academy, 2007).

40 Maryann Gialanella Valiulis, *The Making of Inequality: Women, Power and Gender Ideology in the Irish Free State, 1922–1937* (Dublin: Four Courts Press, 2019), 118, 120.

41 Éamon de Valera, 'On Language and the Irish Nation', in Maurice Moynihan (ed.), *Speeches and Statements by Eamon De Valera: 1917–73* (Dublin: Gill and Macmillan, 1980), 466.

42 I borrow extensively here from Caitriona Beaumont, 'Women, Citizenship and Catholicism in the Irish Free State, 1922–1948', *Women's History Review*, 6 (1997), 563–85.

43 https://teletronic.co.uk/television-history/the-history-television-in-ireland.

44 Elaine Farrell, *'A Most Diabolical Deed': Infanticide and Irish Society, 1850–1900* (Manchester: Manchester University Press, 2013).

45 Maeve B. Callan, 'Of Vanishing Fetuses and Maidens Made-Again: Abortion, Restored Virginity, and Similar Scenarios in Medieval Irish Hagiography and Penitentials', *Journal of the History of Sexuality*, 21 (2012), 282–96.

46 *The Irish Journey: Women's Stories of Abortion* (Dublin: Irish Family Planning Association, 2000), 6.

47 Lindsey Earner-Byrne and Diane Urquhart, *The Irish Abortion Journey, 1920–2018* (London: Palgrave Macmillan, 2019); Therese Caherty, Pauline Conroy and Derek Speirs (eds), *Road to Repeal: Fifty Years of Struggle in Ireland for Contraception and Abortion* (Dublin: Lilliput Press, 2022).

48 Earner-Byrne and Urquhart, *Irish Abortion Journey*, 121.

49 Women's Committee of National Union of Public Employers, *Women's Voices: An Oral History of Women's Health in Northern Ireland (1900–1990)* (Dublin: Attic Press, 1992), 96–7.

50 Greta Jones, 'Eugenics in Ireland: The Belfast Eugenics Society, 1911–15', *Irish Historical Studies*, 28 (1992), 81–95.

51 Women's Committee of National Union of Public Employers, *Women's Voices*; Sandra McAvoy, '"Its Effect on Public Morality is Vicious in the Extreme": Defining Birth Control as Obscene and Unethical, 1926–32' in Farrell (ed.), *'She Said She Was In the Family Way'*, 35–52; Máiréad Enright and Emilie Cloatre, 'Transformative Illegality: How Condoms "Became Legal" in Ireland, 1991–1993', *Feminist Legal Studies*, 26 (2018), 261–84; Therese Caherty, Pauline Conroy and Derek Speirs (eds), *Road to Repeal: Fifty Years of Struggle in Ireland for Contraception and Abortion* (Dublin: Lilliput Press, 2022).

52 Women's Committee of National Union of Public Employers, *Women's Voices*, 100–1.

53 Katherine O'Donnell and Maeve O'Rourke, *Ireland and the Magdalene Laundries: A Campaign for Justice* (London: I.B. Tauris, 2021).

54 James M. Smith, *Ireland's Magdalen Laundries and the Nation's Architecture of Confinement* (Notre Dame: University of Notre Dame Press, 2007).

55 Moira J. Maguire, *Precarious Childhood in Post-Independence Ireland* (Manchester: Manchester University Press, 2009), 49.

56 Martin Sixsmith, *The Lost Child of Philomena Lee: A Mother, Her Son and a Fifty-Year Search* (London: Macmillan, 2010); Paul Jude Redmond, *The Adoption Machine: The Dark History of Ireland's Mother and Baby Homes and the Inside Story of How Tuam 800 Became a Global Scandal* (Newbridge: Merrion Press, 2018).

57 Mike Milotte, *Banished Babies: The Secret History of Ireland's Baby Export Business* (Dublin: New Island, 1997).

CHAPTER SIX

1 Olivier Garraud and Jean-Jacques Lefrère, 'Blood and Blood-Associated Symbols Beyond Medicine and Transfusion', *Blood Transfusion*, 12 (2014), 14–21.

2 Lara M. Cassidy, Ros Ó Maoldúin, Thomas Kador et al., 'A Dynastic Elite in Monumental Neolithic Society', *Nature*, 582 (2020), 384–88.

3 New Scientist and Afp, "Medieval Irish Warlord Boasts Three Million Descendants", *New Scientist*, New Scientist, 18 Jan. 2006, www.newscientiStcom/article/dn8600-medieval-irish-warlord-boasts-

three-million-descendants/. Accessed 22 Mar. 2024.
4   Edmund Gilbert, Seamus O'Reilly, Michael Merrigan et al., 'The Irish DNA Atlas: Revealing Fine-Scale Population Structure and History within Ireland', *Scientific Reports*, 7 (2017).
5   Claire Downham, 'The Viking Slave Trade: Entrepreneurs or Heathen Slavers?', *History Ireland*, 17 (2009).
6   Edmund Gilbert, Shai Carmi, Sean Ennis et al., 'Genomic Insights into the Population Structure and History of the Irish Travellers', *Scientific Reports*, 7 (2017).
7   'Homepage', *Irish Haemochromatosis Association*, 8 Feb. 2024, haemochromatosis.ie/. Accessed 22 Mar. 2024.
8   Keith Haines, *Fred Crawford: Carson's Gunrunner* (Donaghadee: Ballyhay Books, 2009).
9   Frederick H. Crawford, *Guns for Ulster* (Belfast: Graham and Heslip, 1947).
10 Biographies include Joost Augusteijn, *Patrick Pearse: The Making of a Revolutionary* (Basingstoke: Palgrave Macmillan, 2010); Ruán O'Donnell, *Patrick Pearse: 16 Lives* (Dublin: O'Brien Press, 2016).
11 Francis Shaw, 'The Canon of Irish History: A Challenge', *Studies*, 56 (1972), 113–53; James Heaney, 'Chesterton, Pearse and the Blood Sacrifice Theory of the 1916 Rising', *Studies: An Irish Quarterly Review*, 103 (2014), 307–17.
12 Owen McGee, *The IRB: The Irish Republican Brotherhood from the Land League to Sinn Féin* (Dublin: Four Courts Press, 2007).
13 For differing perspectives on war, faith and bloodshed, see Philip Jenkins, *The Great and Holy War: How World War One Changed Religion Forever* (Kidderminster: Lion Books, 2014).

CHAPTER SEVEN

1   Ian Miller, 'The Gut-Brain Axis: Historical Reflections', *Microbial Ecology in Health and Disease*, 20 (2020); Matthew Cobb, *The Idea of the Brain* (London: Profile, 2021).
2   Barra Ó Donnabhain, 'Trepanations and Pseudotrepanations: Evidence of Cranial Surgery from Prehistoric and Early Historic Ireland' in Robert Arnott, Stanley Finger, Chris Smith et al. (eds), *Trepanation* (London: CRC Press, 2003).
3   Patrick W. Joyce, *A Smaller Social History of Ancient Ireland* (London: Longmans, Green and Co., 1906), chapter 14.
4   Geoffrey Keating, *The General History of Ireland* (J. Bettenham, 1723 [1634], 182–7.
5   Sylvester O'Halloran, *A New Treatise on the Different Disorders Arising from External Injuries of the Head* (Dublin, 1793), 4.
6   Charles Bell, *The Anatomy of the Brain* (London: Longman, Rees, Cadell and Davies, 1802).
7   David Ferrier, *The Functions of the Brain* (London:

Smith, Elder & Co., 1876); David Ferrier, *The Localisation of Cerebral Disease* (London: Smith, Elder and Co., 1878).
8   Anne Stiles, 'Bram Stoker's Brother, the Brain Surgeon', in Anne Stiles, Stanley Finger and François Boiler (eds), *Literature, Neurology and Neuroscience: Historical and Literary Connections* (Amsterdam: Elsevier, 2013), 197–218.
9   Brendan Kelly, *Hearing Voices: The History of Psychiatry in Ireland* (Dublin: Irish Academic Press, 2019); 'Lobotomies in 20th-Century Belfast Asylums.' *Epidemic Belfast*, epidemic-belfaStcom/podcast/lobotomies-in-belfast-asylums-during-the-20th-century. Accessed 22 Mar. 2024.
10 Lisa Feldman Barrett, *How Emotions are Made: The Secret Life of the Brain* (London: Picador, 2017).
11 Alfred Crowquill (music by Edward Loder), 'The Tears on the Shamrock', *Illustrated London News* (29 May 1847).
12 Lady Wilde, *Ancient Legends, Mystic Charms and Superstitions of Ireland, Volume One* (Boston: Tickner and Co., 1887), 259–60.
13 Croker, *Fairy Legends and Traditions*, 233.
14 Wilde, *Ancient Legends*, 260–1.
15 For more on families and banshees, see Patricia Lysaght, *The Banshee: A Study in Beliefs and Legends about the Irish Supernatural Death Messenger* (Dublin: O'Brien Press, 1986), chapter 3.
16 'The Banshee', *Weekly Irish Times* (27 May 1893).
17 'The Coolock Banshee', *Irish Times* (9 January 1931).
18 Eoin O'Sullivan and Ian O'Donnell (eds), *Coercive Confinement in Ireland: Patients, Prisoners and Penitents* (Manchester: Manchester University Press, 2012).
19 For good overviews of the nineteenth and twentieth centuries, see Pauline Prior (ed.), *Asylums, Mental Health Care and the Irish, 1800–2010* (Dublin: Irish Academic Press, 2012); Kelly, *Hearing Voices*.
20 Siobhan O'Neill and Nichola Rooney, 'Mental Health in Northern Ireland: An Urgent Situation', *The Lancet (Psychiatry)*, 5 (2018), 965–66.

CHAPTER EIGHT

1   William Grattan, *Adventures with the Connaught Rangers from 1809 to 1814, Volume One* (London: Henry Colburn, 1847), 118.
2   John Pope-Hennessy, *Sir Walter Raleigh in Ireland* (London: Kegan Paul, Trench and Co., 1883).
3   Leitch Ritchie, *Ireland: Picturesque and Romantic* (London: Longman, Rees, Orme, Brown, Green and Longman, 1837), 179.
4   Regina Sexton, 'Food and Culinary Cultures in Pre-Famine Ireland', *Proceedings of the Royal Irish Academy; Archaeology, Culture, History, Literature*, 115C (2015), 257–306.
5   Leslie A. Clarkson and Elizabeth Margaret Crawford, *Feast and Famine: A History of Food and*

Nutrition in Ireland, 1500–1920 (Oxford: Oxford University Press, 2001), 88–111.

6 William and Robert Chambers, *Chambers's Information for the People, Volume One* (Edinburgh: William and Robert Chambers, 1848 [1842]), 708.

7 Clarkson and Crawford, *Feast and Famine*, 88–111.

8 Robert Allan, *The Sportsman in Ireland* (London: Henry Colburn, 1840), 237.

9 Juliana Adelman, 'Food in Ireland since 1740', in Eugenio F. Biagini and Mary E. Daly (eds), *Cambridge Social History of Modern Ireland* (Cambridge: Cambridge University Press, 2017), 233–43 on 234.

10 William Cobbett, *Cottage Economy* (London: William Cobbett, 1821), 44.

11 David Gentilcore, *Italy and the Potato: A History, 1550-2000* (London: Bloomsbury, 2012).

12 Thomas Campbell Foster, *Letters on the Condition of the People of Ireland* (London: Chapman and Hall, 1846), 558.

13 Robert Bentley Todd, 'Clinical Lecture on Dilatation of the Stomach and Sarcinae Ventriculi', *London Medical Gazette*, 47 (1851), 749–55 on 750.

14 James Johnson, *A Tour in Ireland with Meditations and Reflections* (London: S. Highley, 1844), 313–14.

15 William Wilde, 'The Food of the Irish', *Dublin University Magazine*, 43 (1854), 127–46 on 131.

16 Leith Ritchie, *Ireland: Picturesque and Romantic, Volume Two* (London: Longman, Rees, Orme, Brown, Green and Longman 1837), p. 133.

17 Ritchie, *Ireland*, 133–4.

18 'Review of Reports of the Commission on Irish Railways', *Edinburgh Review*, 69 (1839), 156–88.

19 Recorded in *Western Journal of the Medical and Physical Sciences*, 7 (1834), 596–7.

20 Sandham Elly, *Potatoes, Pigs and Politics: The Curse of Ireland and the Cause of England's Embarrassments* (London: Kent and Richards, 1848), 7, 16, 34.

21 Edward B. McGuire, *Irish Whiskey: A History of Distilling, the Spirit Trade and Excise Controls in Ireland* (Dublin: Gill & Macmillan, 1973), 91; Brian Townsend, *The Lost Distilleries of Ireland* (Glasgow: Neil Wilson, 1997), 11.

22 *The Annals of Clonmacnoise from the Creation to AD 1408*, trans. Conell Mageoghagan, ed. Denis Murphy (Dublin: University Press, 1896), 325.

23 Frederic Richard Lees, *The Condensed Argument for the Legislative Prohibition of the Liquor Traffic* (London: J. Caudwell, 1864). 54.

24 John McGuffin, *In Praise of Poteen* (Belfast: Appletree Press, 1978), 10–11.

25 Brian Townsend, *The Lost Distilleries of Ireland* (Glasgow: Neil Wilson, 1997), 16.

26 Elizabeth Malcolm, *Ireland Sober, Ireland Free* (Syracuse: Syracuse University Press, 1986), 23.

27 McGuffin, *In Praise of Poteen*, 10–11.

28 Townsend, *The Lost Distilleries of Ireland*, 3.

29 Clarkson and Crawford, *Feast and Famine*, 56.

30 Ken H. Connell, *Irish Peasant Society: Four Historical Essays* (Dublin: Irish Academic Press, 1996 [1968]), 25.

31 Clarkson and Crawford, *Feast and Famine*, 85.

32 Matthew Woods, *Rambles of a Physician, or A Midsummer Dream* (Philadelphia: Dunlap and Clarke, 1889), 93.

33 Clarkson and Crawford, *Feast and Famine*, 84.

34 *The Bould Sojer Boy's Irish Comic Song Book* (Glasgow: Cameron and Ferguson, 1871), 6.

35 *Irish National Magazine* (23 May 1846), 32.

36 Connell, *Irish Peasant Society*, 3–6.

37 William Richard Le Fanu, *Seventy Years of Irish Life, being Anecdotes and Reminiscences*, 2nd ed. (London and New York: Edward Arnold, 1896 [1893]), 290.

38 'The Poteen Still', *Dublin Penny Journal* (13 September 1834), 85–8 on 85.

39 David Russell McAnally, *Irish Wonders: The Ghosts, Giants, Pookas, Demons, Leprechawns, Banshees, Fairies, Witches, Widows, Old Maids and other Marvels of the Emerald Isle* (Boston and New York: Houghton, Mifflin and Co., 1888), 134–5.

40 Connell, *Irish Peasant Society*, 10–11.

41 Larry Conlon, 'A Poteen Affray at Ardee in 1808', *Journal of the County Louth Archaeological and Historical Society*, 25 (2003), 336–50.

42 'Illicit Distillation in County Fermanagh', *Freeman's Journal* (29 August 1899).

43 'Disarming Police in Donegal', *Belfast Newsletter* (13 February 1885).

44 'Tobacco and Poteen for Somebody', *Belfast Newsletter* (11 December 1872).

45 *An Irish Heart*, 7th ed. (Boston: Whipple and Damrell, 1837), xv.

46 George Nicholls, *Poor Law, Ireland: Three Reports* (London: HMSO, 1838), 7.

47 *Christian Examiner and Church of Ireland Magazine*, 5 (May 1832), 351.

48 'The Irish Woman', *Lady's Home Magazine of Literature, Art and Fashion*, 11 (February 1858), 93–5.

49 McGuffin, *In Praise of Poteen*, 7.

50 Johnson, *A Tour in Ireland*, 315.

51 Johnson, *A Tour in Ireland*, 316.

52 Ian Miller, *A Modern History of the Stomach: Gastric Illness, Medicine and British Society, 1800-1950* (London: Pickering and Chatto, 2011), 1–38.

53 James Johnson, *An Essay on Morbid Sensibility of the Stomach and Bowels*, 4th ed. (London: Thomas and George Underwood, 1827), 2.

54 Johnson, *Essay on Morbid Sensibility*, 3–4.

55 Johnson, *Essay on Morbid Sensibility*, 6.

56 Johnson, *Essay on Morbid Sensibility*, 20.

57 Johnson, *Essay on Morbid Sensibility*, 20.

58 David Dickson, *Artic Ireland: The Extraordinary Story*

of the Great Frost and Forgotten Famine of 1740–41
(Belfast: White Row Press, 1997).

59 Many books have been written on the famine. For
    a thorough overview, see John Crowley, William J.
    Smyth, Mike Murphy and William J. Smyth (eds),
    Atlas of the Great Irish Famine (Cork: Cork University
    Press, 2012).

60 I draw here from Miller, *Reforming Food*, 33–7.

61 James Simpson, *On the More Effective Application
    of the System of Relief by Means of Soup Kitchens*
    (London: Whittaker and Co., 1847).

62 *Lancet*, 49 (27 February 1847), 232.

63 Henry Marsh, *On the Preparation of Food for the
    Labourer* (Dublin: James McGlashan, 1847).

64 Miller, *Reforming Food*, chapter 4.

65 'A Cup of Tea', *Freeman's Journal* (4 June 1872).

66 Miller, *Reforming Food*, 100.

67 *Alleged Increasing Prevalence of Insanity in Ireland:
    Special Report from the Inspectors of Lunatics to the
    Chief Secretary*, House of Commons Papers, 1894
    [C.7331], xliii.647.

68 Thomas Drapes, 'On the Alleged Increase of
    Insanity in Ireland', *Journal of Mental Science*, 40
    (October 1894), 519–48 on 535–6.

69 Tricia Cusack, '"This Pernicious Tea Drinking
    Habit": Women, Tea and Respectability in
    Nineteenth-Century Ireland', *Canadian Journal of
    Irish Studies*, 41 (2018), 178–209.

70 'The Abuse of Tea', *Belfast Newsletter* (27 September
    1887).

71 'Ether Drinking in Ireland', *The Times* (27 March
    1891), 6.

72 Mike Jay, *Emperors of Dreams: Drugs in the Nineteenth
    Century* (Sawtry: Dedalus, 2000), 124–6, 137.

73 'House of Commons: Ether Drinking', *Belfast News-
    letter* (12 August 1890), 6.

74 C. Kerrigan, *Father Mathew and the Irish Temperance
    Movement 1838–1849* (Cork: Cork University Press,
    1992); John F. Quinn, *Father Mathew's Crusade:
    Temperance in Nineteenth-Century Ireland and Irish
    America* (Dublin: Irish Academic Press, 2002); Paul
    A. Townend, *Father Mathew, Temperance and Irish
    Identity* (Dublin: Irish Academic Press, 2002).

75 Elizabeth Malcolm, 'The Catholic Church and the
    Irish Temperance Movement, 1838–1901', *Irish
    Historical Studies*, 23 (1982), 1–16.

76 McGuffin, *In Praise of Poteen*, 29, 36.

77 Diarmaid Ferriter, 'Drink and Society in Twentieth-
    Century Ireland', *Proceedings of the Royal Irish
    Academy: Archaeology, Culture, History, Literature*, 115C
    (2015), 349–69 on 350.

78 Bradley Kabel, *Drink and Culture in Nineteenth-
    Century Ireland: The Alcohol Trade and the Politics of the
    Irish Public House* (London: Bloomsbury, 2020).

79 William Calwell, 'Ether Drinking in Ulster', *British
    Medical Journal*, ii (13 August 1910), 388.

80 McGuffin, *In Praise of Poteen*, 90.

81 'Ether Drinkers in Ireland', *Irish Times* (14 October
    1890), 7.

82 'Ether Drinkers in Ireland'.

83 H.N. Draper, 'Ether Drinking in the North of
    Ireland', *Medical Press and Circular*, 73 (30 May 1877),
    425.

84 'Ether as an Intoxicant', *Medical Press and Circular*, 65
    (9 May 1888), 493; 'Ether as an Intoxicant', *Medical
    Press and Circular*, 66 (3 April 1889), 367–8.

85 Ernest Hart, 'An Address on Ether Drinking: Its
    Prevalence and Results', *British Medical Journal*, ii (18
    October 1890), 885–90.

86 'Ether Drinkers in Ireland', 7.

87 'House of Commons Yesterday', *Belfast News-letter*
    (22 August 1889), 4.

88 'Ether Drinking in Ireland', *Belfast News-letter* (30
    January 1891), 5.

89 'House of Commons Yesterday'.

90 'Ether Drinking in Ireland: Evidence from Ireland',
    Belfast News-letter (11 March 1891), 5.

91 *Freeman's Journal* (4 September 1890), 4.

92 *Alleged Increasing Prevalence of Insanity in Ireland*, 16.

93 *Report from Dr T.J. Stafford, Medical Inspector on Ether
    Drinking in the North of Ireland*, Local Government
    Board for Ireland, Nineteenth Report, 1890–1
    [C.6439], 136.

94 Draper, 'Ether Drinking'.

95 'Ether Drinkers in Ireland,' *Belfast News-letter* (15
    October 1890), 3; Calwell, 'Ether Drinking in Ulster',
    389.

96 'Ether Drinking in Ireland: Evidence from Ireland'.

97 'Ether Drinkers in Ireland', *Irish Times*, 7; *Freeman's
    Journal and Daily Commercial Advertiser* (4 September
    1890), 4.

98 McGuffin, *In Praise of Poteen*, 91.

CHAPTER NINE

1   David Stitfer, 'Early Irish', in Martin J. Ball and
    Nicole Müller (eds), *The Celtic Languages* (London:
    Routledge, 2009).

2   David Stifter, *Sengoidelc: Old Irish for Beginners*
    (Syracuse: Syracuse University Press, 2006).

3   Diarmuid Ó Breasláin and Padaí Dwyer, *A Short
    History of the Irish Language* (Belfast: Nova, 1995), 8–12.

4   Liam Mac Mathúna, 'From Early Modern Ireland
    to the Great Famine', in Raymond Hickey (ed.),
    Sociolinguistics in Ireland (Basingstoke: Palgrave
    Macmillan, 2016), 154–75.

5   Patricia Palmer, *Language and Conquest in Early
    Modern Ireland: English Renaissance Literature
    and Elizabethan Imperial Expansion* (Cambridge:
    Cambridge University Press, 2001).

6   Willy Maley, *Salvaging Spenser: Colonialism, Culture
    and Identity* (Basingstoke: Palgrave Macmillan,
    1997), chapter 2.

7   Nicholas M. Wolf, *An Irish-Speaking Island: State, Religion, Community and the Linguistic Landscape in Ireland, 1770–1870* (Madison: University of Wisconsin Press, 2014), 1–2.

8   Ó Breasláin and Dwyer, *Short History of the Irish Language*, 17–25.

9   Aidan Doyle, *A History of the Irish Language: From the Norman Invasion to Independence* (Oxford: Oxford University Press, 2015); Olga Balaeva, *Ireland as Gaeilge: A User-Friendly Guide to the Irish Language* (Dublin: Orpen Press, 2017).

10 Fionntán de Brún (ed.), *Belfast and the Irish Language* (Dublin: Four Courts Press, 2006).

11 Camille C. O'Reilly, *The Irish Language in Northern Ireland: The Politics of Culture and Identity* (Basingstoke: Macmillan, 1999); Lisa Goldenberg, *The Symbolic Significance of the Irish Language in the Northern Irish Conflict* (Dublin: Columba Press, 2002).

12 William Kelly, William P. Kelly and John R. Young, *Ulster and Scotland, 1600–2000: History, Language and Identity* (Dublin: Four Courts Press, 2004).

13 Michael Sheane, *King William's Victory: The Battle of the Boyne* (Ilfracombe: Arthur H. Stockwell, 2006).

14 Nelson McCausland, 'Scotch Town': Ulster-Scots Language and Literature in Belfast* (Belfast: Ulster-Scots Agency, 2015).

15 Henry Parnell, *A History of the Penal Laws against the Irish Catholics from the Year 1869 to the Union*, 4th ed. (London: Longman, Hurst, Rees, Orme, Brown and Greene. 1825).

16 Ian McBride, *Eighteenth-Century Ireland: The Isle of Slaves – The Protestant Ascendancy in Ireland* (Dublin: Gill, 2009).

17 Helen Litton, *Irish Rebellions 1798–1921* (Dublin: O'Brien Press, 2018).

18 John Mitchel, *The Crusade of the Period and Last Conquest of Ireland (Perhaps)* (New York: Lynch, Cole and Meehan, 1878), 119.

19 Quoted in J.A.L.F., 'The Oratory of Daniel O'Connell', *Irish Review*, 3 (1913), 175–8.

20 Frederick Douglass, *Life and Times of Frederick Douglass: His Early Life as a Slave, His Escape from Bondage and His Complete History* (Boston: De Wolfe, Fiske and Co., 1881), 295.

21 Daniel O'Connell and Arthur Houston, *Daniel O'Connell: His Early Life and Journal, 1795–1802* (London: Isaac Pitman and Sons, 1906), 57.

22 Biographies include Patrick M. Geoghegan, *King Dan: The Rise of Daniel O'Connell, 1775–1829* (Dublin: Gill & Macmillan, 2010); Patrick M. Geoghegan, *Liberator: The Life and Death of Daniel O'Connell, 1830–1847* (Dublin: Gill & Macmillan, 2012).

23 William J. O'Daunt, *Personal Recollections of the Late Daniel O'Connell Volume One* (London: Chapman and Hall, 1848), 14–15.

24 Rachel Pollard, *The Avenue: A History of the Claremont Institution* (Dublin: Denzille Press, 2006).

25 'Deaf Records', *History Ireland*, 25 (2017); Cormac Leonard, 'Deaf People in Ireland: Education, Poverty and the Law'. Unpublished PhD thesis. Trinity College Dublin, 2023.

26 Noel O'Connell, '"Deaf Liberator": The Life and Times of Francis Maginn, 1861–1918', *History Ireland*, 29 (2021).

27 Cormac Leonard, 'Deaf Activists and the Irish Sign Language Movement, 1980–2017', *Sign Language Studies*, 21 (2021), 263–89.

28 Edward J. Crean, *Breaking the Silence: The Education of the Deaf in Ireland, 1816–1996* (Dublin: Irish Deaf Society, 1997), xv–xvii.

29 Patrick A. Matthews, *The Irish Deaf Community, Volume One* (Dublin: Linguistics Institute of Ireland, 1996), 74–103.

CHAPTER TEN

1   Julie-Marie Strange, *Death, Grief and Poverty in Britain, 1870–1914* (Manchester: Manchester University Press, 2005); Patricia Lysaght, 'Old Age, Death and Mourning', in Eugenio F. Biagini and Mary E. Daly (eds), *Cambridge Social History of Modern Ireland* (Cambridge: Cambridge University Press, 2017), 282–96.

2   James Mooney, 'The Funeral Customs of Ireland', *Proceedings of the American Philosophical Society*, 22 (19 October 1888), 243–96 on 266.

3   Mooney, 'The Funeral Customs of Ireland', 267.

4   Mooney, 'The Funeral Customs of Ireland', 270.

5   *Report on the Sanitary Condition of the Labouring Population of Great Britain: A Supplementary Report on the Results of a Special Inquiry into Practice of Internment in Towns* (London: W. Clowes, 1843), 46.

6   For an extensive discussion of the games, see Seán Ó Súilleabháin, *Irish Wake Amusements* (Cork: Mercier Press, 1967).

7   Croker, *Researches in the South of Ireland* (London: John Murray, 1824), 166–7.

8   Linda G. Lynch, 'Death and Burial in the Poor Law Union Workhouses in Ireland', *Journal of Irish Archaeology*, 23 (2014), 189–203; Aoife Breathnach, 'Without a Friend? Burial of the Destitute Poor in Cork, 1830–1900', *Irish Economic and Social History* (forthcoming).

9   Mooney, 'The Funeral Customs of Ireland', 265.

10 Greta Jones, *'Doctors for Export': Medical Migration from Ireland, c.1860–1960* (Amsterdam: Clio Medica, 2021).

11 James McGeachie, '"Normal" Development in an "Abnormal" Place: Sir William Wilde and the Irish School of Medicine', in Greta Jones and Elizabeth Malcolm (eds), *Medicine, Disease and the State in Ireland, 1650–1940* (Cork: Cork University Press, 1999); Greta Jones, *'Captain of All These Men of*

Death': The History of Tuberculosis in Nineteenth- and Twentieth-Century Ireland (Amsterdam: Clio Medica, 2001), 1–29.

12   John F. Fleetwood, *The Irish Body Snatchers: A History of Body Snatching in Ireland* (Dublin: Tomar, 1988).

13   For a nineteenth-century account, see George MacGregor, *The History of Burke and Hare and of the Resurrectionist Times* (Glasgow: Thomas Morison, 1884).

14   Seán Ó Súilleabháin, *Irish Wake Amusements* (Cork: Mercier Press, 1967), 143.

15   Ó Súilleabháin, *Irish Wake Amusements*, 130–45; Angela Bourke, 'The Irish Traditional Lament and the Grieving Process', *Women's Studies International Forum*, 11 (1988), 287–91; Patrick Lysaght, 'Caoineadh os Cionn Coirp: The Lament for the Dead in Ireland', *Folklore*, 108 (1997), 65–82; Henry N. Gifford, 'No Keening Carried on Nowadays', *Lapham's Quarterly* (2021); 'The Keening Wake', *Keening Tradition : The Keening Wake*, www.keeningwake.com/keening-tradition. Accessed 22 Mar. 2024.

16   T. Crofton Croker, *The Keen of South of Ireland* (London: Percy Society, 1844), xxi–xxii.

17   George Sweeney, 'Irish Hunger Strikes and the Cult of Self-Sacrifice', *Journal of Contemporary History*, 28 (1993), 421–37.

18   Ian Miller, *A History of Force Feeding: Hunger Strikes, Prisons and Medical Ethics, 1909–74* (Basingstoke: Palgrave Macmillan, 2016).

19   David Beresford, *Ten Men Dead: The Story of the 1981 Hunger Strike* (London: HarperCollins, 1987); Padraig O'Malley, *Biting at the Grave: The Irish Hunger Strikes and the Politics of Despair* (Belfast: Blackstaff Press, 1990); Richard O'Rawe, *Blanketmen: An Untold Story of the H-Block Hunger Strike* (Dublin: New Island, 2005); Thomas Hennessey, *Hunger Strike: Margaret Thatcher's Battle with the IRA, 1980–1981* (Dublin: Irish Academic Press, 2013).

INDEX